International Standard Library of Chi

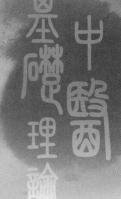

Fundamentals
of Chinese Medicine

Project Editors: Huang Lei, Zhou Ling & Liu Shui
Copy Editors: Harry Lardner, Zhou Ling
Book Designer: Li Xi
Cover Designer: Li Xi
Typesetter: Zhao Lu

International Standard Library of Chinese Medicine

Fundamentals
of Chinese Medicine

Sun Guang-ren (孙广仁), M. S. TCM
Professor of TCM Fundamentals,
Shandong University of TCM,
Jinan, China

Douglas Darwin Eisenstark, L. Ac.
Professor of Chinese Medicine,
Emperor's College,
Los Angeles, USA

Zhang Qing-rong (张庆荣)
Professor of TCM Fundamentals,
Liaoning University of TCM,
Shenyang, China

Associate editor
Zhang Zhe (张喆), Ph. D. TCM
Associate Professor of TCM Fundamentals,
Shandong University of TCM,
Jinan, China

人民卫生出版社
PMPH PEOPLE'S MEDICAL PUBLISHING HOUSE

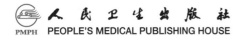

PMPH PEOPLE'S MEDICAL PUBLISHING HOUSE

Website: http://www.pmph.com/en

Book Title: Fundamentals of Chinese Medicine (International Standard Library of Chinese Medicine)
中医基础理论（国际标准化英文版中医教材）

Contact address: No. 19, Pan Jia Yuan Nan Li, Chaoyang District, Beijing 100021, P.R. China, phone/fax: 8610 5978 7352, E-mail: pmph@pmph.com

For text and trade sales, as well as review copy enquiries, please contact PMPH at pmphsales@gmail.com

First published: 2014
ISBN: 978-7-117-18726-8/R·18727

Cataloguing in Publication Data:
A catalogue record for this book is available from the
CIP-Database China.

ISBN 978-7-117-18726-8

Printed in The People's Republic of China

Contributors

Sun Guang-ren (孙广仁), M.S. TCM
Professor, School of Basic Medical Science, Shandong University of TCM, Jinan, China

Zhang Zhe (张喆), Ph.D. TCM
Associate Professor, School of Foreign Languages, Shandong University of TCM, Jinan, China

Liu Xiao-yan (刘晓艳), M.S. TCM
Professor, School of Basic Medical Science, Changchun University of CM, Changchun, China

Li Yi-qi (李奕祺), Ph.D. TCM
Associate Professor, School of Traditional Chinese Medicine, Fujian University of TCM, Fuzhou, China

Xu Ning (徐宁), Ph.D. TCM
Associate Professor, School of Acupuncture, Moxibustion and Tuina, Shandong University of TCM, Jinan, China

Wang Hong-wu (王洪武), Ph.D. TCM
Associate Professor, School of Traditional Chinese Medicine, Tianjin University of TCM, Tianjin, China

Wang Yong (王勇), Ph.D. TCM
Associate Professor, Department of Traditional Chinese Medicine, Jinan Military General Hospital, Jinan, China

Yu Shao-hong (于少泓), M.S. TCM
Associate Professor, School of International Education, Shandong University of TCM, Jinan, China

Zhang Jin-bo (张金波), M.S. TCM
Associate Professor and Associate Chief Physician, Prevention Center, Yantai Hospital of Traditional Chinese Medicine, Yantai, China

Li Lei (李磊), Ph.D. TCM
Attending Physician, Guangcai Clinic of Traditional Chinese Medicine, Taian, China

Translators

Zhang Qing-rong (张庆荣)
Professor and Chief Physician of Chinese Medicine, Liaoning University of TCM, Shenyang, China

Song Hai-ying (宋海英), Ph.D.TCM
Instructor and Attending Physician of Chinese Medicine, Shengjing Hospital Affiliated to China Medical University, Shenyang, China

Yi Jie (易杰), Ph.D.TCM
Professor of Chinese Medicine, Liaoning University of TCM, Shenyang, China

Liu Jing-feng (刘景峰), Ph.D.TCM
Associate Professor of Chinese Medicine, Liaoning University of TCM, Shenyang, China

Cui Jia-peng (崔家鵬), Ph.D.TCM
Associate Professor of Chinese Medicine,
Liaoning University of TCM, Shenyang,
China

Li Xi-ming (李曦明), Ph.D.TCM
Associate Professor of Chinese Medicine,
Liaoning University of TCM, Shenyang, China

Shang De-yang (尚德阳), Ph.D.TCM
Associate Professor of Chinese Medicine,
Liaoning University of TCM, Shenyang,
China

Liu Ning (刘宁), Ph.D.TCM
Attending Physician of Chinese Medicine,
Liaoning Provincial Cancer Hospital,
Shenyang, China

English copy editors

Holly Goguen, DAOM
Professor of Chinese Medicine, Emperor's
College, Los Angeles, USA

Lucy Lau, DAOM
Emperor's College, Los Angeles, USA

Amanda Millie Raynor, MTOM
Emperor's College, Los Angeles, USA

About the Authors

Prof. Sun Guang-ren has served for many years at the Shandong University of TCM where he was awarded as Distinguished Teacher of Higher Education by the Shandong Provincial Government, and also honored as a Leading National Faculty Member by the National Health and Family Planning Commission of the People's Republic of China.

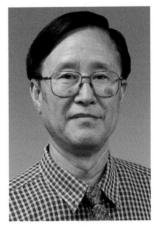

Prof. Sun's main research interests include visceral state theory, TCM thinking methodology, and physical constitution and health cultivation. He is also Director of the Yi-Jing Science Branch of the China Natural Dialectics Research Association, and director of the TCM Philosophy and History Association.

Sun Guang-ren

He has acted as Chief Editor for the textbooks, *Basic Theory of TCM*, the *National Standard Textbook for TCM Higher Education, Chinese Philosophy and TCM*, the *National Standard Textbook for Graduate Students*, and the *Basic TCM Theory* for the International TCM Acupuncture Training Course. Prof. Sun has compiled 10 textbooks, and published more than 100 peer-reviewed papers.

Douglas Eisenstark graduated from Emperor's College in Santa Monica, California in 1996 and currently is a professor at Emperor's. He has taught a wide range of subjects including Fundamentals of Chinese Medicine, Advanced Herbal Formulas and Clinical Point Selection. He currently supervises students in the clinics of Emperor's College and Yo-san University. In addition to his private practice, he has worked for the Turnabout ASAP Acupuncture Detox Center, Venice Family Clinic and the L.A. Free Clinic. He served previously as editor for several PMPH publications including *The Clinical Practice of Chinese Medicine: Eczema* and *The Treatment of Depressive*

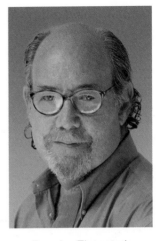

Douglas Eisenstark

Disorder with Chinese Medicine- An Integrative Approach. He has written for several journals including the *Journal of Chinese Medicine.* Douglas has made three trips to China for specialized studies in liver diseases, dermatology and oncology.

Prof. Zhang Qing-rong is Chief Physician and Doctoral Supervisor at Liaoning University of TCM, where he has been engaged in clinical practice, teaching and scientific research on TCM since 1976. He practices at the First Affiliated Chinese Medical University Hospital and Basic Medical College. Prof. Zhang has remained devoted to the research and practice of TCM translation for more than 20 years, with too many great achievements to list here.

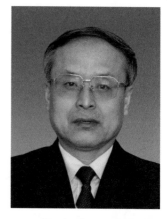

Zhang Qing-rong

After passing the "English Proficiency Test" of the State Education Ministry of P.R. China, Prof. Zhang was appointed as visiting scholar working with Northwest University Medical School in Chicago for one year. He is Vice Director of the Translation Society of the China Association of Traditional Chinese Medicine, and Vice President of the Translation Association of the World Federation of Chinese Medicine Societies. He is now a member of the Expert Communication Committee of the Life Science Departments of both Liaoning Provincial and National Foundations of Natural Science. Prof. Zhang also serves as a part-time English editor of *Chinese General Practice.*

Hu Jun (胡俊), B.A. Medical English
Currently Pursuing Master's of Science in Social History of Medicine, Peking University, Beijing, China

Hu Ke-xin (胡克信), Ph.D. TCM
Professor of Otorhinolaryngology, Keelung City Municipal Hospital, Taiwan, China

Hu Zhen (胡臻)
Professor and Head of Department of Traditional Chinese Medicine, Wenzhou Medical College, Wenzhou, China

Huang Fei-li (黄霏莉)
Professor of Cosmetology, Hong Kong Baptist University, Hong Kong, China

Russell William James, M.S. TCM
IELTS Examiner & Marker, Beijing, China

Jia De-xian (贾德贤), Ph.D. TCM
Professor of Chinese Materia Medica, Beijing University of CM, Beijing, China

Jin Hong-zhu (金宏柱)
Professor of Acupuncture & Tui Na, Nanjing University of TCM, Nanjing, China

Lao Li-xing (劳力行), Ph.D.
Professor of Family and Community Medicine, University of Maryland School of Medicine, Baltimore, USA
Professor and Director, School of Chinese Medicine, The University of Hong Kong, Hong Kong, China
Past Co-President of the Society for Acupuncture Research

Hon K. Lee (李汉光), Dipl. OM, L.Ac.
Director of the Jow Ga Shaolin Institute, Herndon, Virginia, USA

Li Dao-fang (李道坊), Ph.D. TCM
President of Florida Acupuncture Association; Executive Board Director, National Federation of Chinese TCM Organizations, Kissimmee, USA

Mei Li (李梅), M.S. TOM, L.Ac.
Translator and Editor, People's Medical Publishing House, Beijing, China

Li Ming-dong (李名栋), Ph.D. OMD, L.Ac.
Professor of Chinese Internal Medicine, Yo San University of Traditional Chinese Medicine, Los Angeles, USA

Li Wan-ling (李云宁)
Qi Gong and TCM Translator, Beijing, China

Liang Li-na (梁丽娜), Ph.D. TCM
Associate Professor of Ophthalmology, Eye Hospital of China Academy of Chinese Medical Sciences, Beijing, China

Liu Zhan-wen (刘占文)
Professor of Chinese Medicine, Beijing University of CM, Beijing, China

Lü Ming (吕明)
Professor of Tui Na, Changchun University of CM, Changchun, China

Mark L. Mondot, B.A. Chinese Language, L.Ac.

Translator and Editor, People's Medical Publishing House, Beijing, China

Julie Mulin Qiao-Wong (乔木林)

Professor of Chinese Medicine, Victoria University, Melbourne, Australia

Paul F. Ryan, M.S., Dipl. OM, L.Ac.

Acupuncture Preceptor, Lutheran Medical Center, Department of Neurotogy, Brooklyn, New York, USA

Secondo Scarsella, MD, DDS

Visiting Professor of Tui Na, Nanjing University of TCM, China Department of Maxillofacial Surgery, San Salvatore Hospital, L'Aquila, Italy

Tsai Chun-hui, Ph.D.

Associate Professor of Pediatrics, School of Medicine, University of Colorado, Denver, USA

Wang Shou-chuan (汪受传)

Professor of TCM Pediatrics, Nanjing University of TCM, Nanjing, China

Douglas Wile, Ph.D.

Former Professor of History & Philosophy of Chinese Medicine and of Chinese Language at Pacific College of Oriental Medicine, New York,USA Professor of Chinese Language at Alverno College, Milwaukee, USA

Xiao Ping (肖平)

Associate Professor, Hunan University of TCM, Changsha, China

Yan Dao-nan (严道南)

Professor of Otorhinolaryngology, Nanjing University of TCM, Nanjing, China

Jane Lyttleton, Hons, M Phil, Dip TCM, Cert Ac.

Lecturer, University of Western Sydney, Sydney, Australia

Andy Rosenfarb, M.S. TOM, L.Ac.

Acupuncture Health Associates, New Jersey, USA

Martin Schweizer, Ph.D. Molecular Biology, L.Ac.

Emeritus Professor of Medicinal Chemistry, University of Utah, USA

Sun Guang-ren (孙广仁), M.S. TCM

Professor of TCM Fundamentals, Shandong University of TCM, Jinan, China

Tu Ya (图娅)

Professor of Acupuncture and Moxibustion, Beijing University of CM, Beijing, China

Wei Qi-ping (韦企平)

Professor of Ophthalmology, Beijing University of CM, Beijing

Jane Frances Wilson, M.S., L.Ac.

Senior Lecturer of School of Life Sciences, University of Westminster, London, UK

Xu Shi-zu (徐士祖), M.A. Chinese Martial Arts

Chinese Traditional Sports and Health Cultivation Instructor, School of Physical Education in Wenzhou Medical College, Wenzhou, China

Ye Qiao-bo (叶俏波), Ph.D. TCM

Lecturer of Chinese Medicinal Formulae, Chengdu University of TCM, Chengdu, China

Zhang Ji (张吉)
Professor of Acupuncture and Moxibustion, Beijing University of CM, Beijing, China

Zhang Ji (张季), Ph.D. TCM
Professor of Chinese Materia Medica, Emperor's College of Oriental Medicine, Alhambra University, Dongguk University, Los Angeles, USA

Helen Q. Zhang (张齐), Ph.D. TCM, L.Ac.
Director of Qi TCM Clinic, New York, USA

Zhang Qing-rong (张庆荣)
Professor of TCM Fundamentals, Liaoning University of TCM, Shenyang, China

Zhao Bai-xiao (赵百孝), Ph.D. TCM
Professor of Acupuncture and Moxibustion, Dean, School of Acupuncture and Moxibustion, Beijing University of CM, China

Zhao Xia (赵霞), Ph.D. TCM
Professor of TCM Pediatrics, Nanjing University of TCM, Nanjing, China

Zhou Gang (周刚), Ph.D. TCM
Lecturer of Shāng Hán Lùn, Beijing University of CM, Beijing, China

Gregory Zimmerman, M.S., L.Ac.
Lecturer, Southern California University of Health Sciences (Formerly LACC), California, USA

Sponsored by

World Federation of Chinese Medical Societies

Preface

Fundamentals of Chinese Medicine introduces and explains in-depth the basic theory, knowledge, and thinking methods of traditional Chinese medicine (TCM).

The material in this text comprises course material for a professional course of training in TCM, also being the basic material for studying and comprehension of other more advanced courses in TCM. The main contents include the physiological basis of essence-qi, yin-yang and the five phases, followed by the theories of essence, qi and blood, fluids, and spirit. Organ manifestation, channel and collateral theory, constitutional theory, etiology and pathomechanism, and also principles of prevention and treatment are expounded upon. The knowledge in this textbook is approximately equal to that for students of TCM colleges in China, and coincides with the requirements in the *Examination Syllabus for TCM Professional Practitioners Worldwide*.

The compilation carries forward the achievements and clinical experiences of ancient experts throughout the ages so as to maintain the authenticity of TCM knowledge. At the same time, we have adopted current findings in TCM research so that the further developments in TCM theory can be embodied.

Application is emphasized here along with theory and practice; the guiding principles of ancient Chinese philosophy influenced both the establishment of the theoretical system of TCM and its practice. Application of basic theory and knowledge in clinical practice is also emphasized here. Furthermore, the relationships between philosophical and medical concepts are clarified; similar concepts in ancient Chinese philosophy and TCM such as essence, qi, spirit, and original qi are clearly distinguished.

The theories of TCM are explained in as much as possible in a simple way so as to cater to the thinking and study habits of native English speakers. By consulting teaching textbooks from the West, a teaching mode of "introduction-extension-summary" has been adapted. Many of the more abstract concepts are expressed with auxiliary illustrations which help students to understand the concepts and theories of TCM.

Relevant literatures from recent decades on research are also referred to in this textbook; we also wish to express our gratitude to the authors of this original material. Finally, we earnestly ask our readers to point out any errors or shortcomings that may appear here to help us improve future editions of this text.

Sun Guang-ren   Zhang Qing-rong
January 2014

Note

Modern Chinese medicine texts are the interpretation and synthesis of texts over the millennia written in "classical Chinese". For the modern native Chinese speaker these texts are opaque and students in a traditional medical program in China may have several semesters of training in how to read these classical books. The core texts of Chinese medicine are often themselves compilations of books from several authors and are not without their own contradictions and ambiguities. Subsequent writings over the thousands of years, including this book, are attempts to clarify, interpret and supplement the original intent of these ancient texts.

This book is an outgrowth of the consolidation, in China's mainland in the 1950's, of many Chinese traditions and is now referred to in the West as Traditional Chinese Medicine (TCM). Throughout the centuries, many concepts in the original texts of *The Yellow Emperor's Inner Classic (Huáng Dì Nèi Jīng, 黄帝内经)* and *The Classic of Difficult Issues (Nàn Jīng, 难经)* have been filtered out. Likewise, although permeating the roots of the medicine, modern texts are largely (but not always) quiet on the *Book of Changes (Yì Jīng, 易经)*, astronomy and astrology, numerology, branches and stems. The result is a science and medicine that endures into the modern age yet debate continues as to the "true medicine". This mixture of ancient "esoteric" practices with the modern and scientific is what appeals and makes accessible the medicine to a wide range of practitioners and patients.

Chinese medicine always pays homage to the original texts even as the discussion of the appropriateness of innovation versus tradition is one that has touched every generation of writings since the original texts were first written. The modern Chinese medical student is then reading their own versions of translations of the classics. Western students additionally face language issues as they learn non-romance language terminology but understanding traditional classical medicine is not simply a matter of cultural understanding. Whether the word is known in Chinese or English, the concepts of Chinese medicine must be explained accurately.

The beginning student will probably be blissfully unaware of the often heated debates among Chinese medical practitioners and publishers concerning language and translation. Since the first books to be published in English, the "right" English words for Chinese terms have been debated. As a result, few English language texts will agree totally with one another. Linguists in China and West have created dictionaries of terms that if not universally accepted by all interested parties, have furthered the discussion. The publisher of this book, (PMPH) has its own term list that is largely but not exclusively followed in this book. Where appropriate these deviations are noted and clarified. For example, the word *zheng* can be termed "upright" and/or "healthy" qi or anti-pathogenic qi. However, in current discourse, *zheng*[1] is the common verbal term that is used. Beginning students are best served by learning the one or more terms rather than learning one and then be confronted with another in a different text. Therefore, in this book, there are terms such as "*zheng*/upright", "*zheng*", "healthy" or "upright" that may be used in combination or interchangeably. It's correlative, "*xie*" qi, may be translated as pathogenic or evil qi. Learning a nominal amount of the Chinese words will also serve the student when conversing with Chinese native speakers. It is only these Chinese words that create commonality among all practitioners. Although use of these "technical" words may displease those looking for an perfectly rendered translation, this is the best way that a student can best understand not only this text but others that they will soon or concurrently be studying.

The French scholar and writer of Chinese medicine, Elizabeth de la Valle, makes this important point: that one shouldn't try to analyze a term of Chinese medicine from the meaning in English (or French)[2]. If we use the above as an example, it is neither useful nor accurate to dissect the meaning of "upright". Only looking at *zheng* or more importantly, the character "正", will we get a better sense of its meaning.[3] With study and good teachers, there is no reason that anyone needs to read the Chinese language in order to practice Chinese medicine. However, those with scholarly aspirations would be best served by knowing as much of the language as possible.

Introductory books on Chinese medicine can either fall into consumer level texts explaining the medicine or textbooks to prepare students for a strenuous and challenging course of study that will last at least for several years. This text puts itself in the latter category. We hope that anyone who reads this text will fall in love with Chinese medicine and continue to study it in the future. We must also acknowledge that many beginning students have come to this book with little background in neither Chinese medicine nor Asian culture and may actually be still undecided whether to pursue the path of Chinese medicine. For that reason, we attempt to provide context and background that can be expanded upon by a student's teacher as well as other texts.

Chinese medicine is the culmination of thousands of years of Chinese history

---

[1] Pronounced with a hard j as in "just" added to the front of "jung". This is an approximation of the sound, as the true tones or accents of Chinese are best discussed in a Chinese class.

[2] Lecture Emperor's College 2010.

[3] There are many internet resources and the computer program called Wenlin which can greatly facilitate understanding the meaning of Chinese characters.

and culture. It has developed into a unique theoretical and clinical science involving the natural sciences, spiritual exploration, the humanities and the social sciences. Chinese medicine has now spread throughout all countries and regions of the world and where its theories and concepts have become increasingly relevant for the reassessment of contemporary Western medicine.

Chinese medicine is best known in the West through acupuncture but the medicine encompasses much more than that. Acupuncturists in China are known as *zhenjiu* (针灸) doctors or acupuncture and moxibustion doctors. Moxibustion is the burning of special herbs near the acupuncture points and many practitioners only do moxibustion. The field also has specialties of tui na (推拿) or manual massage therapy, as well as qi gong (气功), tai ji quan (太极拳) and other adjunct therapies. Whether a person is practicing herbs, acupuncture or tui na, the fundamentals of medicine remain the same and vital to clinical success.

Douglas Eisenstark
January 2014

Table of Contents

Chapter 2   Essence, Qi, Blood, Fluids and Spirit ·· 51

Chapter 3   Organ Manifestation (*Zàng Xiàng*, 藏象) ·············· 94

Chapter 4   Etiology and Pathogenic Factors ······· 181

Chapter 5   The Onset and Transmission of Disease

Chapter 6   Pathomechanisms

Chapter 7   Constitutional Theory ·············· 263

Chapter 8   Prevention, Principles and Methods of Treatment ·············· 277

Chapter 9   Diagnosis·············· 304

Chapter 10   Channel and Collateral Theory ······· 318

Chapter 11   The History of Chinese Medical Theory ······· 427

Introduction

FUNDAMENTALS OF CHINESE MEDICINE

The Fundamentals of Chinese Medicine serves as the foundation for the basic theories, facts and methodology for Chinese medicine. It lays out the theoretical framework for the further study of diagnostics, acupuncture techniques, Chinese herbs and formulas, clinical disciplines and the study of the classic texts of Chinese medicine. This is the core of the theoretical system of Chinese medicine and is crucial to understanding and practicing Chinese medicine.

Unlike the constant innovations of Western medicine (biomedicine), Chinese medicine, no matter how advanced or sophisticated, always circles back to ancient and fundamental paradigms. For this reason, Chinese medical fundamentals can be viewed as a discipline of basic facts that one is always contemplating and refining through clinical experience.

This chapter is an introduction to some of the major points that distinguish Chinese medicine.

Holism

Holism[①] is a philosophy that says that any one phenomenon is larger than just itself and that in medicine any one part of the body has a relationship with not only the other parts of the body but with the whole of the outside world. Human beings are part of a universe of objects that are common in their origins with all other living things.

Ancient Chinese philosophers held that the universe is produced from *"dao"*, "tai ji" or by "qi". The interaction of yin and yang created the qi that generated the universe or what is called "heaven and earth". Humans are said to exist between heaven and earth. The interaction of the qi which is yin and the qi which is yang gives shape and form to everything in the universe. The process of life is inevitably molded and impacted by nature and changes in the natural environment and will, either directly or indirectly yet inevitably, influence human health and disease.

---

① (*zhěng tǐ guān niàn*, 整体观念) holism

Direct and Indirect Observation

Chinese people in ancient times, in order to explore the secrets of the relationship between human life and the natural environment, applied two different observational methods. In the *Spiritual Pivot* (*Líng Shū*, 灵枢) section of *The Yellow Emperor's Inner Classic* (*Huáng Dì Nèi Jīng*, 黄帝内经), it is written that "the body can be examined by anatomical methods after a person has died". Driven by the need to understand how to treat disease, the dissection of cadavers allowed early doctors to see both the shape and form of the internal organs and to begin to recognize some of their functions. This is called the direct method of observation.

Performing autopsies is not the only way to understand the human body, however. Although anatomical knowledge at that time in China was advanced in comparison to many cultures, it could not explain concretely matters such as the cause of disease nor abstract concepts such as thinking nor emotions nor produce theories that are necessary for treatment. Consequently, these early doctors and scientists also attempted to understand human life by conceptualizing it at its broadest and most organic whole. Lacking the microscopic tools of lab tests, X-rays and ultrasounds, these early doctors turned to the largest view possible, that of the entire universe. In combination with their anatomical knowledge, they came to understand life's activity by reasoning from analogy. This second, holistic way of observing the human body is called the indirect method and is applied through the theories of qi, yin and yang, and the five phases.

Holistic observation is based on the analysis of reactions in the body to environmental and internal conditions. The state of the internal organs is often reflected on the surface of the body and external signs and symptoms can be correlated to changes in the internal organs. Through clinical observation, Chinese medicine recognized that one kind of disease creates a group of approximately similar symptoms and this group of symptoms correlates with dysfunctions of particular organs and systems.

The human body functions so that if an internal organ gets ill it will be inevitably reflected elsewhere on the exterior. For example, according to Chinese medicine, an eye disease may be caused by the liver system or a dysfunction originating from one of the other internal organs. Therefore, an eye disease cannot be simply analyzed based on the eye itself but also on the connections between the organs. For example, liver issues may not only result in a disorder of the eyes and liver, but also may affect the spleen as well as create stomach symptoms, blood deficiency or disorders of the heart. In addition, the summer environment, anger or political turmoil can create conditions which will disturb the liver and create the above cascade of symptoms. This is a concept that runs through every aspect of the theories and clinical practices of Chinese medicine.

Patterns and Metaphors

With their observations of the phenomena of human life, the early creators of Chinese philosophy and medicine developed the concepts of essence, qi, blood and fluids and the relationships between them. This developed into the ideas of the *zang-fu* organs and the channels and collaterals. Eventually "patterns" developed and treatments according to "pattern differentiation" (*biàn zhèng*, 辨证) became the major focus of diagnosis and treatment. Pattern differentiation remains a unique contribution of Chinese medicine.

In order to explain the systems involved, certain metaphors are applied to fundamental principles. The metaphors and analogies that appear over and over again are those of waterways and of military and bureaucratic functions.[1] Acupuncture channels and collaterals are seen as rivers, seas, and streams of energy. Even the name for an acupuncture point (*jǐng*, 井) evokes the water well which the qi of the needle descends into and influences.

Coming later as the more theoretical and sophisticated aspects of the medicine were developed, there are overlapping metaphors of military, commercial and bureaucratic systems. Herbal formulas are organized into herbs that are designated "king", "ministers", "assistants" and "envoys". Describing the organs, we see phrases such as "the lung governs the skin", the heart is the "emperor/sovereign" and the spleen is the "ministry of grains".

Body and Spirit

In Chinese medicine, the organs are all considered to be under the guidance of the heart. The heart stores and governs the "spirit". Therefore, the heart spirit can control and regulate all the functions of the body so that a person's emotional state influences the functions of the entire body.

The body's form and its spirit depend on each other for their existence even as they appear at times to constrain one another. The body is the structure that houses the spirit, and the spirit gives expression to the body's life force. In Chinese language and culture, the human body refers to a "self" which includes body and the spirit.[2] From this viewpoint, the human is an inseparable body-spirit. Disorders of the body cause disorders of the spirit, and vice versa. Treatment of the attitudes and emotions of the patient necessarily involves treating the body because the body is also a reflection of

---

[1] Tangentially, one sees hints in these two metaphors, two major strands of Chinese medicine and culture: that of the Taoist emphasis on nature and the Confucian preoccupation with society and its structures.

[2] Yanhua Zhang. *Transforming Emotions with Chinese Medicine: An Ethnographic Account from Contemporary China*. Albany: State University of New York Press; 2007. p. 35.

the interiority of the patient. In this sense, Chinese medicine makes concurrent use of both the body and spirit for issues that might be seen as separate in Western culture and medicine. The body itself is simply a more condensed version of the spirit, and movements of particular energies (qi) create the conditions for emotional life. Although we may talk about the "unity of body and mind", in Chinese medicine and philosophy, the two have never been separated.

ORGANS, QI, YIN AND YANG, FIVE PHASES AND CHANNELS AND COLLATERALS

The most relevant theories and concepts of human physiology in Chinese medicine include the theories of visceral/organ manifestations, essence-qi-blood-fluids-spirit, channels and collaterals, and the constitution.

Organ Manifestation

"Organ manifestation" theory states that both the healthy and diseased states of the internal organs appears ("manifests") to the careful observer. In Chinese medicine, the organ system includes the five yin organs, six yang organs and the six "extraordinary" organs. Most of the organs have both a structure and a functional aspect which when viewed in its totality creates the physiology of Chinese medicine. Therefore, we don't attempt to only understand the actual organ itself but also its "manifestations" of specific and broad influences.

Vital Substances

Essence-qi-blood-fluids are collectively called the "vital substances" or "essential qi". In Chinese medicine, essence, qi, blood and fluids are the most important components of the body and the essential materials to maintain various functions of the body. They circulate among all the organs to support their functions and in turn, the organs produce, circulate, distribute, store and metabolize essence, qi, blood and fluids.

Ancient philosophers thought that essence-qi (*jīng qì*, 精气) is the common origin of the universe. The movement of qi promotes and regulates the creation, development and change of everything in the universe. Qi is a very fine yet powerfully energetic material which is constantly moving and transforming throughout the universe as well as in the body. It is the fundamental power to promote and regulate the activities of life. Qi is also the essential material for the production of the spirit.

The *Chinese Medicine Study Guide: Fundamentals* says, "The scientific theories of the natural sciences cannot evolve or develop without a strong philosophical grounding and are guided and bounded by philosophical thought. During the course of the evolution and development of the theoretical system of Chinese medicine, it is inevitable that ancient philosophical thought would exert a strong influence. Amidst this influence, the doctrines of essence and qi, yin-yang and the five phases have exerted the most profound influence on Chinese medicine. "[①]

An individual's constitutional physiological background is created from what Chinese medicine calls "prenatal (pre-birth) qi and essence". This can be seen in modern terms as genetics and is influenced throughout a lifetime by diet, life-style, thoughts, moods and social and environmental conditions. Chinese medicine says that essence (*jīng,*精) is the most essential material of the body and is able to transform into qi and produce spirit. In turn, the essence stored in the organs depends upon the regulation of the spirit and qi.

The essence, qi and spirit are the "three treasures" of the body. The body is composed of essence as its basis, qi as its power, and spirit as its regulator. Together these bring about a "coexistence of the body and the spirit". Because the circulation of qi is dependent on the control and regulation of the spirit, there is the saying that "the spirit masters the qi".

Yin and Yang

Yin and yang theory is seemingly simple and serves as the central paradigm of all the materiality and functions of the world. The material substance of the world can be broadly associated with yin. Movement, function, process and communication can be broadly associated with yang. The theory of yin and yang is an infinitely expansive methodology that recognizes the origin of the universe and how it progresses. Chinese medicine, by applying yin and yang to all phenomenon, understands that the body is an organic whole consisting of both various body structures and physiological functions.

Five Phases

The theory of the five phases is both a world view and methodology that holds that objects and phenomena in the universe may be divided into five different categories of wood, fire, earth, metal and water. The motion of these five different categories of objects and phenomena create a constantly evolving and changing world. Applying the five-phase theory of Chinese medicine to the human body, creates both real and metaphorical relationships with the natural environment. The term "five phases" is translated in many ways including the five elements, five agents or five movements.

---

① Zhou Xue-sheng. *Chinese Medicine Study Guide: Fundamentals*. Beijing: People's Medical Publishing House; 2007. p. 17.

Channels and Collaterals

The channels and collaterals are referred to in Chinese as the "*jīng luò* (经络)". These are best known as the lines or "meridians" on an acupuncture chart. Usually these charts depict just the 12 major channels but channel and collateral theory also incorporates the functions of other channels and smaller networks called "collaterals". It is the communication of the channel and collateral system that forms a healthy and well functioning person. The channel and collateral system is what allows an acupuncture needle in the foot to help heal a headache or a needle in the hand to heal a chronic stomach problem. The channel and collateral system is like a never-ending loop for the passage of qi throughout the body.

SIGNS AND SYMPTOMS, DISEASES AND PATTERN DIFFERENTIATION

The concepts of holism and treatment according to pattern differentiation are two of the major features of Chinese medicine which differentiate it from many other forms of medicine. A practitioner must apply these two concepts in order to step over the threshold into Chinese medicine. To create effective treatments, the practitioner must consider and understand symptoms, diseases, pattern differentiation and diagnosis.

Signs and Symptoms[1]

Signs and symptoms are the beginnings of any diagnostic encounter between the patient and doctor. Symptoms are verbal descriptions (usually complaints) from the patient while signs are observations by the doctor. A description of symptoms often quickly (but not always) reveals a disease category such as sore throat, palpitations, insomnia or stomach pains. Chinese medicine practitioners may ask questions about symptoms and view the signs in order to determine the correct disease category and then the correct pattern. A rash on the skin, whether red or pale, can change a diagnosis from a "heat" to a "cold" pattern that can inform the diagnosis and treatment of a disease.

Diseases

In Chinese medicine, diseases are a disharmony of yin and yang which causes damage to the organs and creates physiological and psychological disturbances. Jiao Shu-de writes, "The Chinese character for 'disease' actually has a double meaning: the first meaning is disease or illness, and the second meaning is a shortcoming, insufficiency, flaw or error."[2] Disease is the result of upright qi being in conflict with

---

① (*zhèng zhuàng*, 症状) signs and symptoms
② Jiao Shu-de. *Case Studies on Patterns Identification*. Taos: Paradigm Press; 2006. p. 247.

unhealthy qi (pathogens)[1]. During the process of disease, there always exists to some degree a fight between a pathogen and upright qi.

Because of the modernization and incorporation of biomedicine into mainland Chinese medicine, there has been a much debated tendency to relate conditions of biomedicine diseases to those of the traditional Chinese medical system. The issue of diseases becomes compounded when translated into English and thus taken as one-to-one correspondence with biomedicine disease names. For example, anemia usually has "blood deficiency", yet "blood deficiency" in Chinese medicine has a multitude of other signs and symptoms that may not show up as anemia with biomedical tests. The current trend in English texts is to carefully distinguish between biomedical and Chinese terms.

There are many diseases in Chinese medicine that are exactly the same as biomedical counterparts, others that roughly correspond and still others that are unique to Chinese medicine. Indeed, within this and other books, sometimes there are attempts to explain traditional concepts through analogies to biomedicine. But these must be taken as correlations and correspondences and not as interchangeable. We make these associations because many of us often understand mechanisms of biomedicine better than we understand the nuances of traditional Chinese medical concepts. For example, a fuller understanding of the functions of the kidney (as conceived of in Chinese medicine) can be had by looking at the adrenal cortex. Yet it would be inaccurate to limit the Chinese kidney function to the adrenals or to its hormones. In fact, a careful analysis of the TCM conception of the kidney gives a deeper understanding of its biomedical function. Increasingly modern knowledge is proving the accuracy of traditional Chinese medicine in its emphasis on specific and systemic functions.

As biomedicine research improves and validates original Chinese medicine theories, the cross categorization of diseases will undoubtedly lead to advancements in both fields. Yet we must be careful that biomedical terms do not become substitutes for Chinese medical diagnosis and treatment. This last point cannot be emphasized enough as the Chinese system must exist fully on its own to be employed to its potential.

Another important point is that different patterns present in the same disease and that the same pattern presents in different diseases.[2] "Disease categories" generally consist of an agreed upon fixed group of signs and symptoms. A "pattern" is a unique

---

[1] Pathogentic (*xie*) and upright (*zheng*) qi oppose each other in the disease process. Pathogenic, *xie*/evil qi is that which disrupts the healthy processes while *zheng*/ upright qi is the sum all of the forces that fights the pathogenic qi.

[2] Chinese textbooks often are organized in chapters of disease categories with multiple possible pattern differentiations following.

system that uses the terminology of Chinese medicine and philosophy. A disease can be caused by any one of a dozen possible patterns and a pattern might be the cause of a dozen diseases. Therefore, treating blood deficiency can potentially treat everything from infertility to acne. Depending on the pattern, a headache might be treated by "supplementing the spleen" or "subduing liver yang" or any number of other treatment methods. The strength of the use of patterns arises from a conception of a holistic model of a well functioning, healthy body. Whether it is Chinese medicine or biomedicine, diagnosis is the key to all treatments.

Diagnosis

Chinese diagnosis has historically used what are called the "four pillars of diagnosis" of 1) inspection; 2) listening and smelling; 3) questioning and 4) palpation (from pressing the body and taking the pulse). Practitioners become adept at discovering signs and symptoms in the tone of voice, the way a person walks in the room as well as the content of their words. A patient with a persistent cough may be asked questions about the quality of sleep, their bowel and urinary patterns and their emotional life. In addition, the sound and quality of the cough itself can be quite revealing. Small details can be vital for a skilled practitioner to develop the proper pattern diagnosis.

Diagnosis primarily consists of talking with and observing the patient, taking the pulse and looking at the tongue. Many practitioners will touch (palpate) the body for specific aches and pains as well as signs of hard and softness on the channels. An experienced doctor can look at the patient's face to sense the underlying problems. Pulse taking is a secondary modality for some doctors while others are known as masters of discovering internal problems by the pulse. Pulse taking is considered by many to be a refined art and throughout the history of Chinese medicine has been much debated and discussed. The tongue is observed for the color and shape of the tongue body as well as the coating or "fur" which may be on it. The underside of the tongue can also show signs of the state of the blood. Sometimes a diagnosis can be made from the way the patient coughs, talks or sighs. From any of these signs and symptoms, the doctor will arrive at a pattern differentiation or a syndrome.

Treatment

Chinese medicine is a part of Asian culture and thus permeates all levels of the society. Parents may perform "cupping" on their children with colds; martial art teachers may give their students herbs for their bruises or be adept at setting bones; mothers may cook special foods and herbs at certain times of the years; an herbalist may have two chairs and a small desk in the back of a grocery and herb store and some doctors may spend decades of study on the classics of Chinese philosophy. All of these are facets of Chinese medicine.

Treatment in Chinese medicine is as varied as there are practitioners. In general, treatment can classified as preventative, internal medicine using herbs ("medicinals"), acupuncture, acupressure, moxibustion, massage (tui na) and dietary. Practitioners can specialize and make exclusive use of any of the therapies or be adept at many of them. In general, modern practitioners learn acupuncture, some adjunct modalities and possibly herbs. There has been, and will continue to be, much discussion as to the degree to which each of the above can and should overlap and as to what modalities are best suited for particular issues.

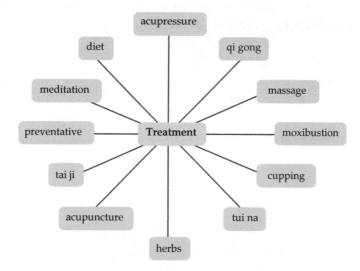

Preventative medicine can include any of the above modalities. Certainly doing supervised qi gong or tai ji exercise, as well as practicing good dietary practices and meditation is a good start to preventing disease. Each of these has a rich history and the focus of medical studies.

Herbs (medicinals) are thought to be the domain of "internal medicine" and primarily involve the organs, essence, qi and blood. Herbal "formulas" are the mainstay of herbal treatment and are made up of one to more than a dozen herbs. Herbal prescription writing is considered a highly skilled discipline and much of the medical literature concerns itself with its intricacies. Herbs are drunk as raw tea, made into pills or used externally as compresses and less often, internally as suppositories. In the last twenty years, the use of powdered extracts has grown in popularity among both patients and practitioners. Herbs are often plants and foods but also include minerals, insect and animal products. For this reason, many English language books will refer to "medicinals" when discussing herbs.

Acupuncture is best known for the treatment of aches and pains but an experienced acupuncturist can also treat internal organs and systems with the same efficacy as herbal medicine. A single acupuncture treatment may use one to several dozen acupuncture needles at a time. Cupping and *gua sha* (scraping the skin) is also very commonly used in conjunction with an acupuncture treatment.

Moxibustion is considered an art within itself and goes back to the most distant path of the medicine. Moxibustion involves the burning of herbs, particularly *ài yè* (Artemisiae Argyi Folium), on or near the surface of the skin. Often times the herbs are placed on top of a slice a ginger or in a ball on top of an acupuncture needle. Treatment is at the end of a long line of decisions from the practitioner and is certainly not limited to just acupuncture and herbs.

This extremely brief outline is to anticipate some of the basic questions that beginning students often have.

Chapter 1

The Fundamental Philosophy of Chinese Medicine

Section 1   Theory of Essence-Qi
(Jīng Qì Xué Shuō, 精气学说)

Essence-qi is one of the most important concepts within Chinese philosophy. It is the origin of that which constitutes all things in the universe and the medium that links all things together. The motion of essence-qi regulates the creation, progression and change of all things. Therefore, essence-qi can be seen as both the creator and the medium for the inter-connections among all things.

Chinese medicine is derived from and deeply with intertwined Chinese philosophy. During the Warring States Period and the Qin and Han Dynasties (ending in 220 AD), advanced philosophies were assimilated into a medical system to explain human life, health, and disease. From that time on, there has been a progression from these concepts and methods to a complete and unique theoretical system of Chinese medicine. This ancient time was the founding period of the theoretical system of Chinese medicine that is in use to this day.

Modern Chinese medicine has evolved to incorporate (and in some cases underplay) traditions of the *Book of Changes* (*Yì Jīng*, 易经), numerology, stems and branches, among others. While many of these philosophical paradigms are intrinsic to modern Chinese medicine, they are not usually elucidated in (fundamental) Chinese texts. In this book, we explore some basic philosophical concepts that inform modern mainland Chinese medicine, or what is called in the West, traditional Chinese medicine (TCM).

We begin this chapter with the broadest concept of essence-qi, which involves the creation of the universe. In this text we refer to this as "essence-qi" but we could also refer to it as "universal qi". In the narrower medical sense, essence-qi is produced within and circulates throughout the body.

Essence and qi almost mean the same within Chinese philosophy, while they are different in Chinese medicine.

ESSENCE-QI OF PHILOSOPHY

The Concept of Qi within Chinese Philosophy

Qi in ancient Chinese philosophy refers to an invisible and extremely fine substance that is in constant motion. The initial connotation for qi was that of a cloud floating in the sky. By observing the motions of the clouds (ascending, descending, accumulating and dispersing), Chinese philosophers formulated a concept that all substances in nature that have form are generated by a formless substance that is in continual and endless motion. This substance is qi. These early philosophers also perceived the existence and influence of qi in the body by observing the phenomena of human life such as the qi of breathing, hot qi over the body during exercise, and so on. After further considering cloud-qi and water-qi, as well as breathing qi and the hot qi of the body, additional general concepts of qi and its nature were formed. They postulated that qi begins as an extremely fine substance with no form and is in perpetual motion. As qi accumulates, it acquires form, and is thus responsible for creating all the physical manifestations we perceive in the universe.

The Concept of Essence within Chinese Philosophy

Essence within Chinese philosophy is also called as *jīng qì* (精气), an invisible and extremely fine substance (invisible) that is in constant motion, the basic unit to form the universe.

One early concept of essence derived from the essence of the human body (reproduction) and "water". Ancient Chinese held that water or earth is the origin of the source for life forms to generate and develop while water being the essence of earth. Based on such understanding, a primitive concept of "essence" formed. However, both have form, and as such contradicts the idea that "the formed is from the formless". Because of this, essence as the source of the universe was not accepted and this theory was not further developed.

Since then, the concept of essence was combined with the concept of qi and celled essence-qi, which is formless, and considered the origin of universe. Therefore in ancient philosophy, the concept of essence combined with the concept of qi, and gradually evolved into one concept. Therefore, essence-qi is often simplified as qi in Chinese philosophy.

Ancient philosophy holds that essence-qi is the origin of the universe, its movement regulates the development of the universe, and it is the media to link things within the universe.

Though physical objects and the extremely fine invisible substance moving around them are both forms of essence-qi, the invisible form is considered the basic state of existence for essence-qi. This version of essence-qi is what is usually referred to as "qi", while the qi that accumulates and is in a relatively stable and tangible state is named "form" (*xíng*, 形). Formless essence-qi is extremely fine, and is in a constant state of dispersion and motion; it is considered "intangible" or "formless" because it cannot (usually) be seen with the naked eye. When this invisible and intangible essence-qi accumulates, it becomes a stable form, which then can be seen and identified as a tangible "thing" or object.

These two states of essence-qi are perpetually in a state of transition. As part of the process of life, the formless and intangible (qi) and the tangible (form) transform into each other. Formless qi accumulates and becomes a tangible substance just as tangible substances disperse and revert to formless qi. All things in the universe change from the formless to the tangible and then in turn from the tangible to the formless. Therefore, essence-qi is both the starting point and the ending point of a thing or phenomenon within an endless cycle.

Essence-qi produces various phenomena and forms because of its different properties or ways in which it accumulates. Qi can transform not only into form, but also can change back into formless yin qi and formless yang qi. Yang essence-qi is characterized by clarity and lightness with an ascending motion; yang qi that has ascended fully then accumulates and transforms into what is referred to as heaven. Yin qi is characterized by condensation and descending, and thus yin qi has fully descended forms what is referred to as earth. Because yin and yang change into each other, after the formation of heaven and earth, the yang qi from heaven descends, and the yin qi of the earth ascends. Yang qi and yin qi interact with each other between heaven and earth, where the innumerable things of the universe are generated. Human beings, also generated by the accumulation of essence-qi, are therefore seen as existing "between heaven and earth".

In the Han Dynasties, essence-qi theory evolved into the "monism of original qi", which holds that qi is the most original and basic unit to form the universe, and therefore, qi in the universe is also called "original qi".

Ancient philosophy holds that the universe consists of essence-qi, and the human body also consists of qi. The life process of the human body is the process in which essence-qi accumulates and disperses.

THE MOTION AND CHANGES OF ESSENCE-QI

Qi Transformation

The various changes that result from the movements of qi are called "qi transformation". The process of qi transformation exists only through the motion of qi, and this is divided into two types. The first type refers to changes induced by a small movement of qi resulting in a small quantitative change. The second change implies significant changes caused by dramatic movements of qi which result in a qualitative change. In the first case, the object or phenomenon changes only by being more or less of it. In the second case, the object or phenomenon changes into something else altogether. Indeed with a dramatic change, an object may transit from form to formlessness, thus ceasing to exist as an independent "thing" and becoming formless, or vice versa.

Qi Movement

Qi is in constant motion, and it is because of this motion that the universe exists. We can also say that the changes of all things in the universe result from the motion of qi. The movements of qi are described as ascending, descending, accumulating, dispersing, exiting and entering. "Heaven-qi" from above moves downward, while "earth-qi" moves upward from below. When they interact, all the things in the universe are produced as a result. Accumulation and dispersion refer to the motion of qi as it condenses and scatters. New formed things come into existence when qi accumulates, and formed things revert to the formless qi when qi disperses. Life and death is also a result of this accumulation and dispersion of qi. The movements of qi are what make the universe full of life, and the movement of qi exists within every physical object. While the movement of qi promotes and generates all new things, it also causes their decline and demise into the formless.

Qi movement and qi transformation are eternal and uninterrupted, being the inner mechanism of the creation, development, and change of all things in the universe. Different kinds of qi convert into other forms of qi through a process of transformation between qi and the physical form. As an observable tangible object dies and disperses, it will transform back into formless intangible qi through the process of qi transformation.

Transformation can also happen between different physical forms under the action of qi. In nature, ice transforms into water, and water into fog, frost, rain or snow. A seed also matures into a tree, which eventually produces its own seeds. All living things experience the changes of birth, growth, development, aging and death. These phases of life exhibit the process of qi transformation that is unceasing and ever changing. In this way, the balance of nature is maintained.

Qi Links the Universe As the Intermediary

Essence-qi connects everything as a coordinated and unified whole, which is in constant motion; it exists both within and without, filling the entire world of things. Essence-qi penetrates into all forms, and activates the qi that has formed into an object. So, qi is not only a material or element that constitutes all things in the universe, but is also an intermediary through which all things in the world communicate, interconnect and interact with each other. As one of the universal things that exists within this integrated whole, the human being also responds to changes in the order of things, however slight or subtle the change may be.

All things are composed of qi, and all the gaps between are also filled with qi. The resonance of musical instruments, the attraction of iron by a magnet, the formation of the tides caused by the moon, and the physiological processes of the human body are all natural and interactive phenomena made possible by qi. Essence-qi is therefore the basis of all that constitutes the myriad of things in the universe. The motions and transitions of essence-qi cause all things in the universe evolve and develop in a more or less orderly manner, and because of this, the dynamic balance of the material world is maintained.

ESSENCE-QI OF MEDICINE

Essence-qi of Chinese medicine is different from that of ancient philosophy. TCM combined the essence-qi of the universe with medical theory and practice to form its own essence-qi concept and theory. TCM holds that essence is the origin of the human body, and qi is the force to promote life activities, and the medium to link the human body.

Ancient Chinese philosophy posits that essence-qi is the basis for the unity of nature, society and human beings. Essence-qi, moving in the universe, fills up the tangible and intangible to serve as the medium for transmission of information that allows things to interact. Chinese medicine understands that human beings live in natural and social environments. Qi inside the body exchanges and transmits information from the natural and social environments through the lung, nose, skin and other sensory organs. Due to changes within the natural and social environment, the physiology and pathology of the human body are necessarily influenced as the body attempts to adapt.

In Chinese medicine, qi transformation between tangible things and the intangible processes of the body allow the qi of the body to invigorate and regulate itself. For example, the digestion of food creates an intangible process of qi that eventually produces the function and growth of tangible substances such as blood, fluids and the internal organs. The internal organs, when well functioning, then create the conditions necessary for the production of qi within the body. The qi of the body converts the intangible into the tangible, and the tangible produces qi, which is intangible. From this, we derive the Chinese medical view of physiology.

Ancient Chinese philosophy holds that essence-qi is the origin of the universe. TCM, influenced by this thought, also holds that the essence of the human body is the origin of human body. Essence in TCM is a fluid, essential substance that forms and sustains the human body.

Ancient Chinese philosophy holds that qi is always in movement, and is the promoting force for the generation and development of the things in the universe. Influenced by this thought, TCM holds that qi is the promoting force for life activities. Based on the monism of original qi, TCM holds that qi in the human body is generated from the same origin, the essence of the human body. Essence-qi of the philosophy consists of yin qi and yang qi, so does the qi of the medicine. In ancient Chinese philosophy, essence-qi is the intermediary, so is the qi of the human body. The concept of essence-qi in TCM is greatly influenced by the concept of essence-qi in ancient Chinese philosophy.

ESSENCE IN MEDICINE

In Chinese medicine, essence refers specifically to the fundamental formation of qi that is responsible for the creation of the human body. Essence, therefore, has two equally important and impressive connotations. One, which we call in this book "essence-qi", is aligned with the largest philosophical and cosmological concerns, while the other, which we call "essence", is the basis of life that is passed on from generation to generation. In this view, "essence-qi" is a universal philosophical concept, while medically speaking, "essence" begins and ends with the creation and the death of the body. As stated above, essence in medical terms is differentiated from that of qi in the broadest sense. In yet another context, the term "essence-qi" refers to a form of qi comprised of qi, essence, body fluids and blood.

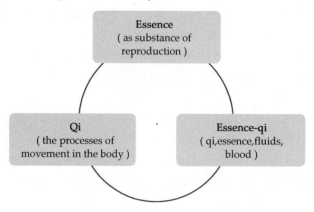

3 Inter-related Terms of Chinese Medicine

The modern person can understand essence most basically as the combination of genetic material in men and women. As the primary substance that constitutes the embryo, this essence acts to generate a new life. Chinese medicine believes that human life is composed of essence, and maintained by qi. In a developed human, qi is first transformed from essence, after which it combines with the qi that the lungs inhale and the qi that the digestive system obtains from food and water. The qi acquired from the essence of the parents (congenital essence) and qi derived from the daily processes of the body (acquired essence) combine to maintain the physical and mental processes of human beings. Essence, therefore, has two interrelated forms; that which develops in the womb and that which develops and is created throughout a lifetime.

"Essence-qi" in Chinese medicine refers to the essential substances stored in the organs; this includes qi, essence, fluids and blood. Essence-qi is regarded as the source material used for generating both body and spirit.

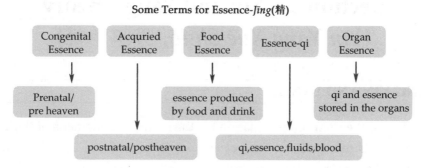

Some Terms for Essence-*Jīng*(精)

Chinese medicine holds that essence generates the internal organs, the sense organs, and also the spirit, thus all are closely connected. Ancient philosophy tells us that essence-qi first divides into yin and yang, and that their balanced coordination is required to maintain the orderly motion of all things. The essence of the body is also divided into yin-essence and yang-essence, where accordingly, their balanced coordination is also required to maintain the health of the body.

Because everything is made up of essence-qi, the human being is also a coagulation and accumulation of essence-qi. After death, the qi of the individual will disperse and return to its original and more primordial form of essence-qi.

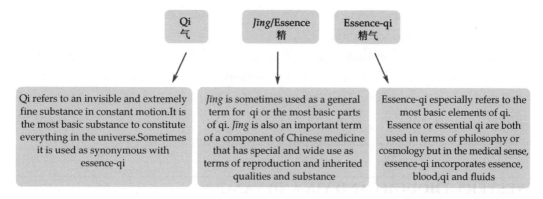

SUMMARY

Qi is both a philosophical and vernacular term that is incorporated within

Chinese culture. Students of Chinese medicine will study the more narrow medical applications of qi that are inseparable from these broader concepts. Understanding that qi is not necessarily only a "material" but also a "phenomenon" is important as one becomes immersed in the details of Chinese medical diagnosis and treatment. Return to this chapter section in a few weeks, months or years to see if your appreciation of its content has deepened after further study.

Section 2   Yin and Yang Theory
(*Yīn Yáng Xué Shuō*, 阴阳学说)

DEFINING YIN AND YANG

Yin and yang theory is an explanation for the natural phenomena of the universe. According to this theory, the whole of the universe is made up of two forces in opposition, and yet each contains aspects of the other. These opposites can be called yin qi and yang qi, which function as abstract concepts for describing the nature of both material objects and their relationships within the world. Because of the interactions of yin qi and yang qi, the world is made up of objects and phenomenon that are all subject to transformation.

In general, things that are bright, hot, active, ascending, external or related to functional activity pertain to yang, while those that are dull, cold, unmoving, descending, internal or related to material form pertain to yin. Therefore, all processes and objects can be said to pertain to these abstract concepts in varying intensities depending upon their natures and the context of their surroundings. Although seemingly simple at first, these are complex relationships that can take a lifetime of study to appreciate and understand.

As a uniquely Chinese philosophy, the implications of yin and yang resonate from philosophy and culture to the depth of the needle put into the body in an acupuncture treatment. After it was introduced into the medical field, yin and yang theory became the most important theoretical and practical component in the Chinese medical system for guiding the diagnosis, prevention and treatment of disease.

WESTERN THOUGHT AND YIN AND YANG

Western thought and Western medicine emphasize finding the particulars and unique qualities of objects, even down to their microscopic components. This microscopic and molecular viewpoint becomes the essence of what is examined, also being the main evidence used to diagnose and cure disease. Chinese philosophical and medical thought is less concerned with a microscopic perspective, but rather emphasizes more observable qualities and behaviors. Yin and yang (and the five phases) do not assign static "realities" to objects and phenomena, but only describe properties within the context of other objects and phenomena. Consequently, yin and yang medical philosophy holds that all medical conditions and "realities" are not definitive, but rather that they remain in a relative state of continual process.

> "Under the rubric of yin and yang, it is not a matter of establishing classifications, but of describing the dynamic responsible for the relationship of all the elements within the defined whole."[1]

A chair in Western thought is a chair, and with further categorization, an armchair or dining room chair. It may be made of maple wood or cedar, but is still primarily identified as being a chair. From the viewpoint of Western science, to understand the chair better one may run tests to determine its molecular makeup. Further study and measurement will reveal more and more about what the chair "really is".[2] In yin and yang terms, because it is solid and "substance", a chair is first considered to have predominantly yin qualities. However, in relation to the floor, it has yang properties because yang is above yin when considering direction. A chair resting on the floor of a room is yin because it is still and immobile and is relatively low within the space of the room. Yet, this same yin-related chair develops yang properties when thrown up into the air and across the room, because it now is in action and has the moving properties of yang.

The chair therefore has both yin and yang potentials within it and we see that indeed (with few exceptions) all objects and phenomena have the potential to manifest properties of both yin and yang. If one were to consider the ceiling above your head, it would be considered yang, because yang is above yin. Yet, to a person standing on the roof of your building, that same ceiling would have yin properties. Furthermore, the yin-related chair has the potential to transform and be set a fire, burn, and thus have more properties of yang. Because every object and phenomenon has yin and yang qualities, the description of any object's "reality" is dependent upon the placement of the viewer and their circumstances as well as the qualities of the object or phenomenon themselves.

---

① Laure, Schatz, Rochat de la Vallee. *Survey of Traditional Chinese Medicine*. Paris: Institut Ricci; 1986. p. 44.

② David Bohm writes "… to Western society, as it derives from the Greeks, measure, with all that this word implies, is the very essence of reality, or at least the key to this essence…" *Wholeness and the Implicate Order*. London: Routeledge and Paul; 1980. p. 23.

Many Chinese books and their translations will refer to yin "belonging to", "pertaining to", "refers to" or is "associated with" substance, immobility or a quality of cold, etc. As another example, wood is "associated with" wind. For the student (perhaps especially for those used to the relative precision of the English language) this may seem frustratingly vague. Such language is used because of Chinese grammar and syntax. Yet more broadly in Chinese philosophy, things of the world are not objects of certainty, but rather things with qualities; these are things known only through their appearance at particular times and places. (Astute readers may note the similarity of this thought to some concepts described by modern quantum physics.) Yin and yang, the five phases, and indeed all the medical processes of the body thoroughly discussed in this and countless other books are only reflections and "manifestations".

There is a saying in Chinese medicine that "Yang transforms qi, yin constitutes form" (*yáng huà qì, yīn chéng xíng* - 阳化气, 阴成形). Some texts will refer to yin as "substance" and yang as "function" or "movement". However, this idea requires further context because yin and yang are abstractions of the tendencies present in all objects and phenomena. "Substances" or "objects" refer to those material objects that constitute "things". Function or phenomena reflect the forces which bring into motion the potential of things. Objects and phenomena can transform from one to another, from object to phenomenon and from phenomenon to object, or to put it simply, from yin to yang and yang to yin.

All objects or things have physical shapes and patterns that are formed by the qualities of the yang from which they were created. Referring back to the chair mentioned above, the qualities of that chair were determined by the location of the tree that grew the wood. A tree grown in a rainforest at the equator has a different quality from one grown in a northern climate. This shows how the yang processes of growth and nourishment at different locations would affect the yin-object of wood that results.

Similarly, yang actions are dependent upon the shape of yin from which they were transformed. The sound of a guitar made from wood grown at the equator is different from that made of wood grown in a northern forest. In another example, the fire and smoke produced from coal and those from wet grass are very different. So within substance and function are evidences of both yin and yang properties. Looked at in this way, yin and yang are not simply synonymous with matter-substance.

Although this way of thinking has any number of complexities, none of this should imply that it is in any way imprecise. The laws of yin and yang as expanded upon below are descriptions of both material properties and change. Because yin and yang are opposites, yet always changing, what may be obvious at first often becomes fluid; this changing quality makes yin and yang philosophy a discipline of properties, time and space. The overall impression of these laws may appear simple (that things change from one to another) but in order to understand health and illness in our patients, it is vitally important to understand how these particular laws of yin and yang are revealed. The understanding of yin and yang comes through study and deep reflection along with clinical practice and personal experience.

"Yin-yang is an abstract concept without form." - *The Spiritual Pivot*

ATTRIBUTES OF YIN AND YANG

Opposite

Yin and yang are the attributes of two opposite aspects of related things or phenomena in the universe. Yin and yang can be applied to two different things or phenomenon, or to one object or phenomenon with the aspects of yin and yang within it. The original meaning of yin and yang was very simple, referring to places and their position relative to the sun. A place exposed to the sunlight is warm and bright, while a place in the shadows is relatively cold and dim. That is also to say, the side of an object facing the sun pertains to yang, while the side facing away from the sun pertains to yin. So, millennia ago, Chinese philosophers attributed the things or phenomena which are bright and warm to yang, and the things or phenomena which are dark and cold to yin. In looking at the seasons, it is warm in spring and summer and cold in the autumn and winter. Spring and summer are then attributed to yang, and autumn and winter to yin. Taking a day as another example, it is warm and bright in the daytime while cold and dark at night. So, daytime is attributed to yang and night to yin.

By further observation, it was found that the body of an animal or human being can be warmed to withstand cold through exercise and activity. In contrast, when the body is exposed to cold and remains inactive, it will feel cold. So, activity is attributed to yang, and inactivity to yin. Plants grow rapidly under the sunlight, and slower without the sunlight. Therefore,

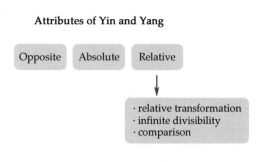

Attributes of Yin and Yang

Opposite   Absolute   Relative

· relative transformation
· infinite divisibility
· comparison

things or phenomena in an active or excited state are attributed to yang, while those that are in an inhibitory or inactive state are attributed to yin. The theory of yin and yang has evolved into a philosophical and abstract concept used to generalize those things or phenomena with opposite aspects. We can say that yin and yang refer to a pair of standards with opposite properties.

The categorization of things or phenomena into yin and yang refers to the particular properties by which the yin or yang attributes of things or phenomena can be determined. Cold and heat are one of the primary pairs of opposites where things with signs of relative cold are attributed to yin, while those with relative warmth are attributed to yang. Motion and stillness form another primary pair of characteristics of which one can determine yin or yang attributes. Something in nature that is relatively active and excited is attributed to yang, while things that are relatively still, inactive or inhibited are attributed to yin. Considering the natures of cold/heat and motion/stillness, many other yin and yang attributes have evolved over time. For example, yang features include activity, outward movement, ascending, warmth, brightness, dispersing, outside and hyperactivity. Yin features include stasis, inward movement, descending, accumulating, contraction, and inhibition.

Attribute	Yang	Yin
Space (Direction)	upside, outside, left, south	downside, inside, right, north
Space (Location)	heaven	earth
Time	day	night
Season	spring and summer	autumn and winter
Temperature	warm and hot	cool and cold
Humidity	dry	moist
Weight	light	heavy
Fluid Character	clear	turbid
Light	bright	dim
Motion	dispersion, ascent, activity	accumulation, descent, inactivity
Action	exiting, activity, transformation	inhibition, decline, formation

Again, it must be noted that the theory of yin and yang does not refer to concrete things or objects, but that yin and yang are abstracted concepts concerned only with properties. Many phenomena or objects are not related nor have opposite qualities, and for practical reasons there is no need to divide or compare them as yin or yang. For example, the couch in a living room has no relationship with the house across the street and so there is little reason to call one more yin or yang than the other.[1]

---

[1] To analyze the yin and yang attributes of two things or phenomena, two conditions must be met. The first condition is that these things or phenomena have some correlation or defined relationship with each other. Second, these two things or phenomena must in some way be in opposition to each other. Therefore, only two related yet opposite things or phenomena or two opposite aspects within one thing or phenomena can be generalized and analyzed with attributes of yin and yang. For example, cold and heat, both of which are used to describe temperature and are opposite in nature, can be symbolized with yin and yang. If two things or phenomena do not correlate to each other, or they are correlated but their features are not opposite, they cannot be explained with yin and yang. For example, ice and snow, both of which are the crystal transformed from water, do not have opposite features, so their relationship cannot be as easily described with yin and yang.

Lao Zi said, "All things embrace yang and carry yin."

Absolute

Yin and yang have both relative and absolute aspects. For example, regarding water and fire, water pertains to yin and fire to yang. Water, no matter how hot, is always yin when compared with fire. Fire, no matter how weak, always belongs to yang when compared with water. The yin and yang attributes are fixed, and thus absolute.

Relative

Because the qualities of things naturally change, things with yin and yang attributes also change over time. Therefore, the yin and yang attributes of things can be absolute, but also relative. The relative attributes of yin and yang manifest in three ways:

Mutual transformation

The first of the relative attributes is the mutual transformation of yin and yang. Under certain conditions, the yin and yang attributes of things may change into their polar opposites. A bright flame will eventually burn out and become cold. A night will always turn back into day. In the clinic, we see that when the cold or heat nature of a disease changes, the yin or yang attribute of the condition will also change. For example, a common cold caused by what Chinese medicine calls "wind-cold" has manifestations that include physical coldness and a whitish coating on the tongue. Both of these are signs of cold, which is yin. If treatment is delayed, then the cold pattern may turn into a heat pattern with manifestations that include fever with a yellow coating on the tongue. In this case we can observe that a yin-type condition has transformed into a yang-type condition. Conversely, it is also possible for a heat/yang condition to transform into a cold/yin condition.

Infinite divisibility

The second relative attribute is that yin and yang are said to have infinite divisibility. Two things that are related yet contrary can be further divided into yin and yang; in other words, the yin or the yang aspects themselves can also be divided into another pair of yin and yang, and this kind of subdivision can be continued infinitely. However, each yin and yang aspect always includes the other aspect, so they will never be complete yin or complete yang. Within any yang object there is a yin aspect, called the "yin within yang". A yin object also contains a yang aspect within it, called the "yang within yin".

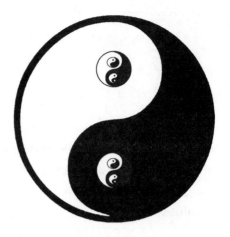

The yin and yang attributes of things or phenomena are determined according to the proportions of the yin or yang components. For example, if one thing or phenomenon pertaining to yang contains a small yin component, its general attribute still belongs to yang. Our basic example of day and night is informative. The daytime is yang because it is active and bright and warm. Yet, as it declines into night we have aspects of yin. The late afternoon is called "yin within yang". Night time is yin and falls deeper and deeper into yin. This period of dark is called "yin within yin." Yet as the night reaches its darkest, it can go no farther into yin and thus its movement changes in the direction of yang (the morning). The latter half of the night is therefore called "yang within yin". The morning signifies the full beginning of the new day as the sun rises to its zenith, so the morning is therefore called "yang within yang".[1]

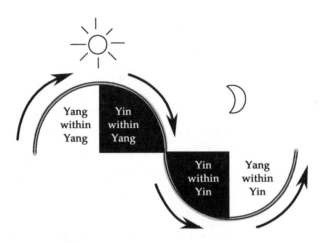

Relative comparison

The third relative attribute involves the comparison of different objects. An object can only be known as "yin" or "yang" in comparison with other things. If the objects being compared change, the yin and yang attributes of these things will also change. For example, when a flat piece of land is compared with a mountain, the mountain

---

[1] This description is more than a simple naming of the times of day. Remember it as a natural progression of yang and yin within body processes.

pertains to yang, and the flatland to yin. But when a flatland is compared with a deep valley or canyon, the flatland pertains to yang and the valley to yin. Therefore, we come back to this idea that an object is known by the position of the person who is viewing it, and then only in contrast to the surroundings or other objects of comparison which gives it context.

Yin and yang are always interacting. Yang qi ascends to generate the heaven, and yin qi descends to form the earth. Yang qi of heaven contains a small amount of yin qi. The yin qi within the yang qi of heaven brings the heaven qi downward to seek the yin qi of the earth, and in turn, the yin qi of earth goes upward to heaven through the quality of the yang qi included within it. This interaction of yin and yang where heaven-qi descends and the earth-qi ascends also causes the two to mingle and interact with each other. As a result, wind, clouds, rain, fog, thunder, lightning, and animals and plants all come into being. These things grow and develop because of both sunshine and rain showers. As for many animals, the interaction of the genetic essence of a female and a male (yin and yang) reproduces new life, and thus beings multiply. We see how important, at all levels, the interaction of yin and yang is to the fundamental conditions for the generation, development and change in all things.

The balance between yin and yang is dynamic, with the ratio of yin and yang constantly changing within normal limits (if a person or situation is relatively healthy). Even though the change between yin and yang can be relatively abrupt or slow, the two aspects most often exist together and transform into each other in order to create a harmonized state of being; it can even be said that this spontaneous harmonization of yin and yang is what enables the universe to continue its existence. So this idea refers to the inherent ability of yin and yang to maintain and restore a state of coordination and equilibrium along with spontaneous development through the motion of yin and yang. Harmonization restores the balance of yin and yang, and is reflected in the ability of the body to restore health after becoming ill or otherwise imbalanced. However, when the dynamic balance of yin and yang within the body is impaired, the resulting disharmony manifests as disease.

LAWS OF YIN AND YANG

Every object or phenomenon which can be classified as yin or yang has rules by which it exists. These are called the laws and doctrines of yin and yang. [1]

---

[1] Note that not all fundamentals texts conform to these exact classifications. *Chinese Acupuncture and Moxibustion* (Beijing: Foreign Language Press; 2010), for example, puts the "infinite divisibility" of yin and yang as a 5th doctrine instead of an attribute as discussed in this text.

- Opposition and Restraint
- Interdependence
- Growth and Decline
- Transformation

Opposition and Restraint between Yin and Yang

There are two opposite aspects of yin and yang present in all things and phenomena in nature. One aspect inhibits and restrains the other. Opposition and restraint between yin and yang means that the two opposite aspects of yin and yang within a single object or phenomena struggle to restrain and repel each other. This contention maintains a dynamic balance between yin and yang and also, most importantly promotes creation, development and change in all things.

Heaven, earth and people are the "3 realms" of the universe. Discussions of heaven (*tiān*, 天) date back to the original Chinese religions, but from the Zhou Dynasty (1046–256 BC) onward, philosophers have proposed many different theories regarding the idea of heaven, including the concepts that *tiān* was a material that covered the earth, that the planets were attached to *tiān* and that they rotated around the earth, or that *tiān* was an infinite space where the planets moved due to the actions of qi. Chinese medicine, except those traditions explicitly tied to Taoism, has long disregarded many of these cosmological and theological concerns.

Opposition and restraint of yin and yang are the basic factors for the decline and growth of yin and yang. When yin grows, yang then declines, and restraint ensures that neither yin nor yang will grow excessively. In a healthy body, opposition and restraint means that the movement of yang will be restrained by inward-moving yin. Conversely, active yang will prevent yin from becoming more and more static.

As an example, cold is associated with yin, and heat is associated with yang. These two properties are opposite and contrary to each other. Heat can disperse and dispel cold, and cold can reduce heat. We also see this natural opposition in the phenomena of the seasons (spring, summer, autumn and winter), in the daytime and nighttime cycle of a day, and in the cycle of exhalation and inhalation which maintains the metabolism of life within the body.

When the relationship of opposition and restraint between yin and yang becomes disordered, the dynamic equilibrium will be destroyed; such imbalances symbolize the onset of disease. Therefore, the most basic therapeutic principle of Chinese medicine is to adjust yin and yang within the body to achieve balance. Note that being "in balance" does not mean a static pairing of yin and yang, but rather a dynamic and ever-changing "dance" between the actions of yang and the form of yin.

Interdependence of Yin and Yang

The interdependence of yin and yang means that yin and yang are "rooted in" and dependent on each other. Yin and yang take the existence of the other as the prerequisite for their own existence, and neither of them can exist by themselves. Without a context, they are devoid of meaning. Without heaven, there would be no earth. The upper is yang, and the lower is yin. Without the upper, there would be no lower. This is called the interdependence of yin and yang, and it is the basis for the "grounding" and "supplementation" of yin and yang. Because yang contains yin, yin is the source of the generation of yang. Because yin contains yang, yin's existence is also dependent on yang for its creation and generation.

A most important example of yin and yang for Chinese medicine is that of qi and blood. Qi is associated with yang, and blood with yin. Qi generates and circulates blood, while blood carries and nourishes qi. Without qi, there would be no production (a yang quality) of blood. The qi circulates the blood in the body to bring nutrients back to the organs in order to create more blood. Without blood, there would be no "ground" or basis for the qi. Qi would fly off chaotically, and eventually, both would disappear. Therefore, the two promote and complement each other and are inseparable. So, we see that yang's existence depends upon yin, and vice versa. If the relationship of this dependency is lost for any reason, it will lead to solitary yang or single yin failing to grow, or even to a complete separation between yin and yang. Separation of yin and yang implies death for a living being, or the end of a phenomenon.

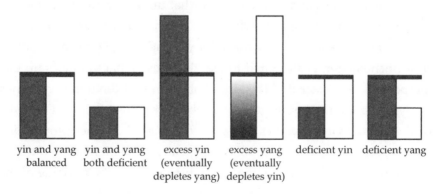

yin and yang balanced | yin and yang both deficient | excess yin (eventually depletes yang) | excess yang (eventually depletes yin) | deficient yin | deficient yang

The Growth and Decline of Yin and Yang (Waxing and Waning)

Yin and yang are in a state of constant change of increase and decrease in order to maintain a dynamic and healthy balance. The growth and decline of yin and yang refers to the quantitative changes or the "amounts" of yin and yang.[1] Balance here means the relative and dynamic balance within a certain range and to a certain degree; it is not a static or an unchanging absolute balance.

Mutual growth and decline

This means that one increases while another decreases and is caused by the opposition and restraint between yin and yang. There are four pairs of the process: yin decreases when yang increases; yang decreases when yin increases; yang increases when yin decreases; yin increases when yang decreases. We can see the growth and yang decline of yin and during one day. In the morning, yang increases while yin decreases; in the afternoon, the yang decreases while yin increases. In the first half of night, yin increases and yang decreases, and in the second half of the night, the yin decreases while yang increases.

Simultaneous growth and decline

This means that one increases or decreases while another increases or decreases at the same time because of the interdependence of yin and yang. There are four pairs of the process: yin increases when yang increases, yang increases when yin increases, yang decreases when yin decreases, yin decreases when yang decreases.

Concretely, in the life of a person with a natural lifespan, yin qi and yang qi grow in the first half of life. In the average person, during the second half of life, both yin and yang are in a state of decline (sometimes equally and sometimes not).

Transformation

The transformation of yin and yang means that under certain conditions, yin and yang may convert into their opposite. The facets of yin and yang exist in all things and phenomena, so the basis for the conversion of yin and yang is intrinsic within them. If a thing or phenomenon is attributed to yin, this means that yin takes up the larger relative proportion. It is clear that this does not mean that the thing or phenomenon contains only yin, but only that its general attribute pertains to yin.[2] For a yin object or phenomenon, as its yin properties grow, the yang aspect declines proportionally. As long as the proportion of the yin component is greater, it is still attributed to yin. If the change of yin grows to the extreme, the yin component and the attribute of the thing

---

[1]   Here, again we must warn against thinking of yin and yang as substances and having quantities or "weight". Yin and yang are both abstractions of functions and properties that cannot be measured except for seeing their "manifestations" of quietness, action, form, and function.

[2]   Anything or phenomenon which contains only a yang or yin component is rarely found. When it does exist it is called "solitary yin" or "solitary yang" but it cannot develop and change. The implication is that solitary yin or yang will soon expire.

or phenomenon then changes into yang. This is the transformation of yin into yang. Obviously, the reverse can occur as well, and there can be a transformation of yang into yin. [1] When the decline or growth of yin or yang reaches its apex, it is at this point that the attribute of the thing or associated phenomena then changes into its opposite. Thus, *The Spiritual Pivot* states, "Extreme cold produces heat, and extreme heat creates cold. "

The transformation of yin to yang or yang to yin can be either gradual or sudden. For example, the alternation of winter and summer in the four seasons in a year is a gradual change, while a sudden rain or hail on a dry summer day is an obvious and dramatic change. A person who is strong as a young adult may become weaker as time goes on; this is a gradual change. A sudden change would involve for example a person who becomes angry and then has a stroke; yang changes to yin very quickly in this case. The more subtle decline or growth of yin or yang is a process of quantitative change by degree. The transformation of yin to yang and vice versa is a qualitative change based on quantitative change.

The Laws of Yin and Yang	
Opposition and Restraint	• Opposition and restraint within a single object or phenomenon, or between different objects • Opposition of yin & yang maintains the balance of health • When yin & yang become unbalanced, disease results
Interdependence	• Neither yin nor yang can exist without the other. Each is a condition for the other's existence. Yin & yang oppose each other, yet depend on each other for existence • Yang tends towards activity (qi) • Yin tends towards nutritive substances (blood/*xuè*, essence/*jīng*, body fluids/*jīn yè*)
Growth and Decline	• Supportive relationship • Yin & yang are not fixed amounts, but always changing and adjusting their relative levels to maintain health • Consumption of yin leads to a (relative) increase of yang • Consumption of yang leads to a (relative) increase of yin • Mutual consumption is a quantitative change process
Transformation	• Yin & yang can transform into each other under certain conditions • Capacity-must have requisite internal and external factors. The time must be right for transformation to occur. Change usually happens at the extreme or peak. Transformation is a qualitative change process based on quantity • Transformation can be a gradual or a dramatic change
(Divisible)	• Yin & yang are infinitely divisible, but always found together. Few things can be called pure yin or pure yang. There is yin within every part of yang, and vice versa

APPLICATIONS OF YIN AND YANG THEORY IN CHINESE MEDICINE

Yin and Yang within the Body

Every part of the body has its own yin or yang attributes, and all organs and tissues of the body can be classified into yin or yang according to their locations,

---

[1] It is said that it is "easier" for yin to become yang than for yang to transform into yin.

functions and properties. The upper half of the body is associated with yang, and the lower half with yin. This means that the head is more yang than the feet. The lateral parts of the body pertain to yang, and the medial (towards the middle) parts to yin. The back of the body belongs to yang, while the front belongs to yin. The superficial aspects of the body (such as the skin) pertain to yang, and the more internal parts to yin.

According to location

As to the organs, there are five solid organs (*zàng*) which belong to yin and the interior because they store substances. There are also six hollow (*fǔ*) organs[1], which pertain to yang and the exterior because they transport and transform substances but do not store them. Among the five yin organs, the heart and lung are located in the upper part of the body, so they do have aspects that pertain to yang (even as they are also yin organs). The liver, spleen and kidney are located in the lower body, so they belong to yin. Among the twelve main acupuncture channels, the pathways running along the lateral side of the limbs pertain to yang[2], while those running along the medial side of the limbs pertain to yin.

According to function

Among the five *zang*-organs, the heart and lung are located in the upper part of the body and belong to yang. The heart, attributed to fire and being in charge of warming, pertains to yang within yang. The lung, attributed to metal and being in charge of purification and descent, pertains to yin within yang. The liver, spleen and kidney are located in the lower part and belong to yin; among them the liver, attributed to wood and being in charge of upward-going, pertains to yang within yin. The kidney, attributed to water and being in charge of storing, pertains to yin within yin. The spleen, attributed to earth, is located in the middle and nourishes the other four viscera (yang organs).

Onset and Transmission of Disease

When the yin and yang of the human body are not in balance, and cannot re-achieve balance by themselves, human body will suffer from disease.

The struggle between upright (*zheng*) qi and pathogenic (*xie*) qi can lead to the imbalance between the yin and yang of human body. Pathogenic qi can be yin or yang while upright qi also consists of yang qi and yin qi. When yang pathogenic qi attacks the human body, yin qi of the upright qi will fight against it; when yin pathogenic qi

---

[1]   The yin organs are called the "*zang*", and the yang organs are called the "*fu*". Therefore, together the organs are referred to as the "*zang-fu*".

[2]   With the exception of the stomach channel.

attacks the human body, the yang qi of the upright qi will fight against it.

Yin and yang imbalances manifest as exuberance of yin or yang, decline of yin or yang, or mutual damage between yin and yang.

Exuberance of yin or yang

Exuberance of yin or yang refers to one part which increases too much during the growth and decline of yin or yang, usually leading to an "excessive disease". Exuberance of yin leads to excessive cold diseases while exuberance of yang leads to excessive heat diseases.

Exuberance of yang will consume or damage yin qi according to the opposition and restraint of yin and yang. Exuberance of yang qi includes exuberance of yang with deficient yin and exuberance of yang without deficient yin.

Exuberance of yin will consume or damage yang qi according to the opposition and restraint of yin and yang. Exuberance of yin qi includes exuberance of yin with deficient yang and exuberance of yin without deficient yang.

Decline of yin or yang refers to one part which decreases too much during the growth and decline of yin or yang, usually leading to deficient disease. Decline of yin leads to deficient heat diseases, while decline of yin leads to deficient cold diseases.

Decline of yang will cause yang qi failing to restrict yin qi, failing to warm and promote, manifesting as cold symptoms.

Decline of yin will cause yin qi failing to restrict yang qi, failing to cool and suppress, manifesting as warm symptoms.

Repelling between yin and yang

Exuberant yin repelling yang refers to excessive yin qi which forces yang qi to float to the outside, developing into internal cold with external heat, manifesting as true cold with false heat.

Exuberant yang repelling yin refers to excessive yang qi which forces yin qi to move outside, developing into internal heat with external cold, manifesting as true heat with false cold.

Mutual impairment between yin and yang

According to the interdependence of yin and yang, when yin or yang declines to a certain degree, the decline of yin will affect yang or the decline of yang will affect yin, and gradually develop into deficiency of both yin and yang.

Yin impairment affecting yang

When yin qi declines to a certain degree, the decline of yin will affect the generation of yang qi, leading to the deficiency of both yin and yang.

Yang impairment affecting yin

When yang qi declines to a certain degree, the decline of yang will affect the generation of yin qi, leading to the deficiency of both yin and yang.

Location of Disease

Chinese medicine holds that conditions located at the surface of the body pertain to yang. Yang diseases then are those more at the surface. When a disease is located interiorly, it belongs to yin. Furthermore, those conditions characterized by heat are yang in nature, and those characterized by cold are yin. No matter how complex the disease or clinical presentation, the principles of yin and yang can always be applied in this manner. In fact, ascertaining whether a disease is a yin or yang condition is the most fundamental aspect of diagnosis.

The Yin and Yang of Substances

When we discuss bodily substances such as qi, essence, blood and fluids, we see that qi is characterized by motion, and thus pertains to yang. Essence, blood and fluids are characterized by relative stillness and form, and therefore pertain to yin. Essence is the basic substance in the human body, while qi, which is derived from essence, is the active power. Essence, which is stored in the organs, is in charge of the interior and thus pertains to yin. Qi is active and moves throughout the body and so belongs to yang. The essence and qi, with their relationship of yin and yang, act to maintain order and stability in the functional activities of the body.

It is important to understand that qi in the body is classified into yin qi and yang qi. Yin qi is characterized by properties of cooling, moistening, quietness, inhibition, and descending. Yang qi is characterized by properties of warming, propelling, excitement, and ascending. Yin qi and yang qi in the body are involved in a circulation of movement where they ascend, descend, exit and enter the organs and other body forms. During this process of motion, yin qi and yang qi maintain the yin and yang balance within the body. They promote the various normal physiological activities through opposition and restraint, mutual grounding and supplementing, growth and decline, and by converting into one another.

Yin and Yang in Signs and Symptoms

To diagnose disease, Chinese medicine uses the following methods of obtaining information from a patient: touching (such as taking the pulse), listening (to the sounds of the breath and the voice), inquiring (asking the patient questions about their condition), looking (inspection of the patient) and olfaction (noticing any smells). The signs and symptoms that are observed from these methods can be separated into yin and yang categories. For example, a bright color of the body belongs to yang, while a dark and dim color belongs to yin. When listening to the voice, a loud volume with a high tone, talkativeness and agitation belong to yang. A feeble voice with a low tone and reticence to speak belongs to yin. Feeble breathing also belongs to yin, while forceful breathing and a loud coarse voice belong to yang. A pulse that is floating, rapid, surging or large belongs to yang, while a deep, slow, thin and small pulse belongs to yin.

Chinese medicine holds that signs and symptoms characterized by excess or hyperactivity pertain to yang. If the signs and symptoms reflect deficiency, weakness or cold, this indicates a yin condition. Viewed in this way, no matter how complex the disease or the clinical presentation, any condition involves the basic principles of yin or yang as expressed within the body.

Yin and Yang of Herbs

The functions of Chinese herbs can also be categorized as either yin or yang. The "four properties" of herbs refers to their four temperature categories: cold, hot, warm and cool. Herbs that act to diminish heat are usually cold or cool (and therefore yin) in nature, such as *huáng lián* (Coptidis Rhizoma) and *zhī zǐ* (Gardeniae Fructus). Herbs that relieve cold are usually warm or hot (and therefore yang) in nature, such as *fù zǐ* (Aconiti Lateralis Radix Praeparata), and *gān jiāng* (Zingiberis Rhizoma).

Yin and Yang of Herbs

Yin Properties	Yang Properties
cool	warm
cold	hot
sour	acrid
bitter	sweet
salty	bland
lowering	lifting
sinking	floating

Herbs have five main "tastes" or "flavors", which are acrid, sweet, sour, bitter and salty. In addition, some herbs are referred to as bland or astringent in flavor. Acrid, sweet and bland pertain to yang, while sour, bitter and salty to yin.

The functional trends of the herbs in the body include lifting, lowering, floating and sinking. In terms of these directional movements of qi within the body, the actions of lifting and floating pertain to yang, while lowering and sinking belong to yin. Understanding the relationships between the yin and yang attributes of the patient's presenting pattern and the yin and yang attributes of the medicinal herbs is extremely important for their successful use.

SUMMARY

This section presents one of the most fundamental and important aspects of Chinese medical theory and practice. Although we tend to look at yin and yang as being qualities (hot or cold, up or down), equally as important are the actions of yin and yang. Every object and every phenomenon has a tendency towards expansion or contraction and movement or stillness. Understanding this is highly relevant when assessing the movement of qi in relation to the internal organs and their proper tendencies. To more fully grasp this concept, it is useful to spend some time each day considering yin-yang theory and how it corresponds with the things or processes that surround you in your daily life experience.

Section 3   Five-Phase Theory
(*Wŭ Xíng Xué Shuō*, 五行学说)

The "five phases" can also be translated as five elements, five agents, five stages, or five movements. The application of the five-phase theory is so broad that any one of these translations can be "correct", depending on the context in which it is used. The five-phase system permeates Chinese culture, such as in *fēng shuǐ* (风水), where the arrangement of objects in a given environment is based on their associations with the five natural elements or phases.

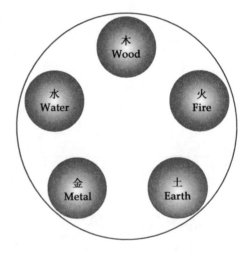

Initially, the five phases referred to the five basic materials as seen in daily life, and the ways in which humans could effectively control their environment through their use. For example, in order to control water, one needs to build dikes or ditches in the earth. Fire is needed to melt metal. Metal can cut wood, and water can extinguish fire. From this understanding of the five phases, the five-phase theory evolved into a universal methodology used to understand, explain and explore the universe, and by extension, the human body.

The importance of the five phases in Chinese medicine has been diminished or elevated depending upon the period in history, styles and themes of geography, and practitioners. At different times it has been either embraced fully or downplayed as "superstition", much as astrology has been viewed in Western history. It has also been suggested that modern Western physiology can explain much of what was described millennia ago by the five phases. However, although modern Chinese medicine's use of the five phases contains certain ambiguities and contradictions, we can still see that a full understanding of Chinese medicine must involve the five phases. This becomes particularly important when one considers how this model acts to fill the spaces left by the relatively simple oppositions of yin and yang. Like yin-yang theory, five-phase theory can be seen as an elegant system that not only describes the functional characteristics of the organs, but also explains the inner connections among them. As practitioners, we find that the five phases can be an extremely useful and holistic paradigm from which to work in the clinic.

Five-phase theory has several practical facets in Chinese medicine. The first involves an illumination of functional relationships between the phases and the *zang-fu* organs. By showing excesses and deficiencies in the organs, we can map and predict their behavior in both disease and health. The second aspect is that the five-phase system is also a way of classifying worldly phenomena into groups, including tastes, seasons, directions, musical notes and smells. Just as everything is either yin or yang, phenomena or objects can be placed into five-phase categories. Five-phase theory can also be utilized as a sophisticated acupuncture treatment protocol that utilizes the "antique" or "element points" at the ends of the hands and feet. If not emphasized in modern traditional Chinese medicine, this acupuncture method remains as a vital part of many other Chinese, Korean and Japanese styles. Additionally, five-phase theory has spawned "five-element schools" which have taken these ancient traditions and developed them for the modern-day patient and practitioner.

In this chapter, we will see that the five phases in the five-phase theory symbolize not only the five materials themselves, but the generalization of their attributes. Note in particular that all of the five phases have directionality associated with them. This becomes vital throughout all of Chinese medicine, and is particularly important in diagnosis and herbal treatment. The properties of the five phases can be seen in pathology as well, and follow closely the functions of the organs as each phase or element is associated with a particular *zang-* and *fu*-organ. Many of the attributes of the organs and their issues will also be seen in the later chapters concerning the *zang-fu* organs. When it comes to actual clinical practice, some of the relationships of the different cycles of elements are more applicable than others; clinicians must not attempt to inappropriately and mechanically fit the patient, pattern and disease into a pre-conceived theory.

THE PHASES

Wood is characterized by bending and straightening. The branches of a tree grow strong and are not easily broken, but are also flexible and are thus able to bend and straighten. The attributions of wood are extended to things or phenomena that have the properties or actions of growing, flourishing, stretching or unfolding.

Fire is characterized by upward flaring and heat. Fire moves upward, and has brightness and light. The attributions are extended to things or phenomena that have the properties or actions of warmth and hotness, upward movement, and brightness.

Earth is characterized by sowing and reaping; this refers to the farming activities of planting and harvesting grain. The attributions are extended to things or phenomena that have the properties or actions of producing, receiving and harmonizing.

Metal is characterized by adaptability. Metal is processed from ores, and as a rigid material, it can be molded by humans to change its shape. Metal can be made to become a mirror, jewelry, a sharp weapon, or a hardened tool. The attributions are extended to things or phenomena that have the properties or actions of harshness, descending, purification and condensing.

Water is characterized by moistening and descending, as water tends to flow downward. The attributions are extended to things or phenomena that have the properties or actions of moistening, going downward, coolness, coldness and storage.

Wood

The nature of wood is to grow, flourish and unfold, but it also can be soft and flexible. The liver likes free activity, governs the free flow of qi, and stores blood. Therefore, the liver is the *zang*-organ attributed to wood. When the movement of liver qi becomes constrained or stagnated, treatment of the liver would be applied to promote the free flow of qi and blood. When liver qi is hyperactive or rising too quickly, the liver should be calmed and softened to normalize the movement of qi. The tendons, eyes, and nails are also associated with wood.

"The east produces wind, wind produces wood, wood produces sour, sour produces the liver, the liver produces the tendons, tendons produce the heart, and the liver rules the eyes. In heaven, this is mystery, in man it is the Tao. On earth it is transformation. Transformation produces the five tastes. The Tao produces wisdom. The profound produces the spirits (*shén*). Of the spirits, in heaven it is wind. On earth, it is wood. Its part of the body is the tendons. Its *zang*-organ is the liver. Its color is green. Its musical note is the 3rd note (*jué*, 角). Its sound is shouting. Its reaction to change is contraction. Its orifice is the eyes. Its taste is sour. It expression is will." —*The Spiritual Pivot*, Chapter 5

Fire

Fire has the properties of warmth and heat, excitement and upward movement. Pathologies of fire manifest as redness with frequent movement and are often, (but not exclusively) in the upper part of the body. It is considered as the most "yang" of the five phases. The heart governs the blood and vessels, beating unceasingly to maintain the body temperature, so the heart is attributed to fire. If a heart disease is caused by a failure of warming, the treatment should be to warm. If a heart disease is due to overactive fire, the internal fire can be restricted by nourishing water. Fire is also associated with the blood vessels and the tongue.

> "The south produces heat, heat generates fire, fire produces bitter, bitter produces the heart, the heart produces blood, and blood produces the spleen. The heart rules the tongue. In heaven, this is heat. On earth, it is fire. In the body, it is the vessels. Its *zang*-organ is the heart. Its color is red. Its musical note is the 4th (*zhǐ*, 徵). Its sound is laughter. Its reaction to change is great grief. Its orifice is the tongue. Its taste is bitter. Its expression is elation." — *The Spiritual Pivot*, Chapter 5

Earth

Earth is a yin-element that has properties of producing and receiving. It functions to transform and transport the essences of food and drink, as well to generate qi and blood. Earth harmonizes the rest of the phases, and is considered by many practitioners to be primary for treating any of the internal organs. When the qi of the earth phase is deficient, it may fail to provide nourishment to the organs. Earth may also play too prominent a role, drawing from the other elements and causing sluggishness and lack of vigor. The spleen and stomach are both attributed to earth, with the *zang* spleen-organ and the *fu* stomach-organ being very closely related as yin and yang partners. Therefore, they are often mentioned together. These two organs together coordinate ascending and descending so that the essential or "clear" substances are transformed and transported (the function of the spleen), while the impure or turbid substances are transmitted downward and discharged (the function of the stomach). Earth is also associated with the mouth and the muscles.

> "The middle produces dampness, dampness produces earth, earth produces sweet, sweet produces the spleen, the spleen produces the flesh, and the flesh produces the lung. The spleen rules the mouth. In heaven, this is dampness. On earth, it is earth. In the body, it is the flesh. Its *zang*-organ is the spleen. Its color is yellow. Its musical note is the 1st (*gōng*, 宮). Its sound is singing. Its reaction to change is belching. Its orifice is the mouth. Its taste is sweet. Its expression is thought." — *The Spiritual Pivot*, Chapter 5

Metal

Metal is considered yin and has the properties of purifying, astringing, adapting, forming and reforming. In order to produce metal, one must heat ore to purify it. The making of tools, jewelry, and swords are all created through the properties of metal. One can also see the adaptable nature of metal in the flexibility of our breathing through the lung, which can change from slow and gentle when resting to strong and forceful during exercise. One can consider tai ji or qi gong practices where the breath and qi are sent to various parts of the body in a structured and orderly manner.

As the normal direction of lung qi is to descend and disperse, lung diseases often involve rebellious movement of qi, which goes upward to cause coughing and/or breathlessness. Lung issues should be treated by purifying and downbearing of the lung qi. The nose, the skin and body hair are also associated with metal. "Heaven" is associated with metal because both reflect that which shines upon it.

> "The west produces dryness, dryness produces metal, metal produces the pungent taste, pungent produces the lung, the lung produces the skin and body hair, the skin and body hair produces the kidney. The lung masters the nose. In heaven, this is dryness. On earth, it is metal. Its part of the body is the skin and body hair. Its *zang*-organ is the lung. Its color is white. Its musical note is the 2nd note (*shāng*, 商). Its sound is sobbing. Its reaction to change is coughing. Its orifice is the nose. Its taste is pungent. Its expression is great grief." — *The Spiritual Pivot*, Chapter 5

Water

Water moistens, goes downward, and stores. The *zang*-organ associated with water is the kidney, which stores essence, governs water, and receives qi. Water issues are therefore those of dampness, fluids and water in a state of either abundance or deficiency. Although the kidney organ is attributed to water, it contains an element of fire as well. (One could visualize this as the pilot light on a gas stove.) This fire in the kidney is called the "ministerial fire" or the assistant to the heart's "sovereign fire". Water and fire issues, being a complementary pair, often occur simultaneously. When water is weak, then fire easily burns out of control and consumes or "boils away" the water. When there is weak fire either from the heart or the kidney, the fluids often leak out of their proper place as in incontinence, diarrhea or edema. The bones, ears and the "two yin" (anus and urethra) are also associated with water.

"The north produces cold, cold produces water, water produces salty, salty produces the kidney, kidney produces bone marrow, marrow produces the liver, and the kidney rules the ears. In heaven, this is cold, and on earth it is water. Of the parts of the body, it is bone. Of the *zang*-organs, it is the kidney. Its color is black. Its musical note is the 5th (*yǔ*, 羽). Its sound is sighing. Its reaction to change is shaking. Its orifice is the ears. Its taste is salty. Its expression is fear." — *The Spiritual Pivot* , Chapter 5

MOTION WITHIN THE FIVE PHASES

The above discussion of the five phases presents them as neat categories related to properties. The following section examines how the phases move between each other to maintain their order. This concept, although seemingly simple, can be rather confusing at first. For this reason, various aspects of five-phase motion are discussed here several times and in slightly different ways.

Objects and phenomena activate and restrict each other in five-phase theory. The motion among the five phases maintains the dynamic balance in nature. There are three specific modes or patterns for the five phases. They are the "generation" cycle (*shēng*, 生), the "restraint" cycle (*kè*, 克) and the "cosmological" (*hé tú*, 河图) pattern. In general, we see that the generation cycle is the normal or functional cycle that proceeds effortlessly in a healthy body. The restraint cycle, based on the generating pattern, maintains the structural integrity of the generation cycle. (The cosmological pattern is considered apart from the generating and restraining patterns.) In a well-functioning body, any deficiency or excess in any one phase or element will be corrected by the balancing actions of other elements that come into play throughout the cycle.

Generation Cycle

Generation here means the promotion and "stimulation" among the five phases. In the generation cycle, wood generates fire, fire generates earth, earth generates metal,

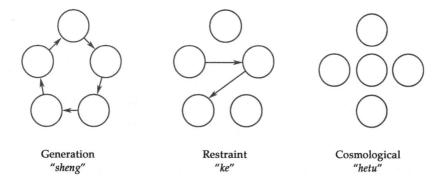

Generation
"sheng"

Restraint
"ke"

Cosmological
"hetu"

metal generates water, water generates wood. There are several ways to visualize the five phases in the generation cycle. Our first method is to visualize or draw a circle with the placement of each element in a specific order around the circle. This "cycle" is always clockwise in the order of wood, fire, earth, metal and water. (It doesn't matter where we begin.) The elements generate each other clockwise, from one element to the next. For example, water generates wood. This cycle is therefore referred to as the "generation cycle."

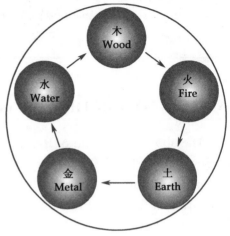

Generation Cycle

The generation cycle is a progression in which wood generates fire, fire generates earth, earth generates metal, metal generates water, and water finally generates wood. The generation cycle, when working correctly, only moves in one clockwise direction.

Five-phase mother-child relations

In the generating relationship among the five phases, each of the five phases/elements has a "mother-child relationship". In the generation cycle, the strength of one phase is passed on to the next phase in the cycle of "mother to child". The "generating" phase is called the "mother" and the "being-generated" phase is called the "child". For example, earth generates metal, so earth is the mother of metal. Because metal generates water, metal is the mother of water (and water is the child of metal). In this way, each of the five phases has a mother-child relationship, and depending on where you begin, each phase acts as a child or as a mother. Given the scenario, any one particular phase can be the mother, while the one that "follows" clockwise will be the child.

Restraint Cycle

In addition to the generation cycle there is the equally important "restraint cycle" (*xiāng kè*, 相克)[1]. Restraint means to restrict and limit. In the restraint cycle, wood restrains earth, earth restrains water, water restrains fire, fire restrains metal, and metal restrains wood. This cycle of relationship creates the shape of a five-pointed star within the circle. If the generation cycle can be visualized as the rubber on the wheel of a bicycle tire, then the restraint cycle can be seen as the spokes on the wheel. The restraint cycle (spokes) connect across the wheel (skipping a phase), which creates a

---

①   In Japanese, the *kè* cycle is called the *"ko"* cycle and is the term often used among Western acupuncturists.

restriction or pressure in both directions. The generation cycle provides the motion to the wheel, while the restraint cycle provides integrity and structure to the circle. Thus, as well as in the bicycle wheel, we can also parallel the generation and restraint cycles with the two main elements of tai ji quan exercises, those of free movement combined with gentle tension. In other words, the restraint cycle keeps the phases from going out of control (and so is often called the "control cycle" and the "restricting cycle"). For example, fire and metal restrain each other to maintain a balance, as seen in the chart.

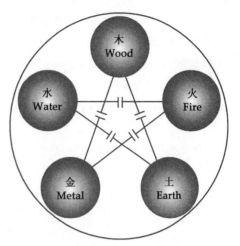

Restraint Cycle

While we talk about the mother-child relationship in the generation cycle, the restraint cycle is different in that it "skips a phase". In the restraint cycle when the balance between two phases is disrupted, the dominant phase might either "over-restrain" or "counter-restrain" on the weaker (subordinate) phase. The restraint cycle prevents any one of the five phases from becoming too large or overwhelming in relation to another. These concepts will be explored more fully explained in the next section. [1]

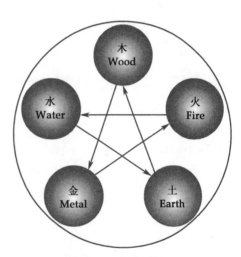

Counter-restraint Pattern

Because all of the phases are interconnected, a healthy body will quickly adjust through the generation and restraint cycles. In fact, this happens frequently every minute and every day. For example, after eating too big of a meal, the earth phase increases and as a result acts to restrict wood, thus affecting the movement of qi, which causes a person to become bloated and lethargic. By activating metal, which controls the descending of qi, wood becomes reactivated. Gentle exercise such as

---

[1] The beauty of this system is that in a relatively healthy body, should one element become deficient or in excess, by following the cycle around, eventually balance will be maintained by the other elements. An example of a self-balancing scenario would be if fire becomes excessive, it will overact on metal causing a deficiency of metal. This deficient metal then can't restrain wood. Wood consequently becomes excess and it over-restrains earth which then becomes deficient. Deficient earth cannot restrain water, which then becomes excess to now restrain the excessive fire.

walking is good for both the lung-metal and the liver-wood phases, while also benefiting spleen-earth. One can imagine any number of daily activities that involve imbalance and subsequent rebalancing of the five phases.

PROBLEMS OF MOTHER AND CHILD IN THE GENERATION CYCLE

In this section, we return to the five-phase patterns of generation and restraint and explore them with a special emphasis on dysfunction. Diseases are seldom the result of a problem with a single organ in isolation. In most cases, multiple organs are involved - the five phases are useful in creating coherence to complex cases.

Generating / Nourishing

In the simple generation cycle, problems can develop between the mother and child. The mother should "nourish" the child, but if the mother phase is weak, then the child may also become weak. For example, water generates wood, and if water is deficient and not able to nourish wood, the result is that both water (the mother) and wood (the child) become deficient. However, if the child is in excess (hyperactive), then it can draw from the mother phase, which leads to an overactive child with a weak mother. This is called "child stealing the mother's qi" or "pulling from the mother".

In treatment there are two simple principles for mother-child problems: "for deficiency, supplement the mother; for excess, restrain the child". Put another way, if an organ is deficient, the mother organ can be reinforced in order to build up the child. If the mother is in excess, restrain/sedate the child.

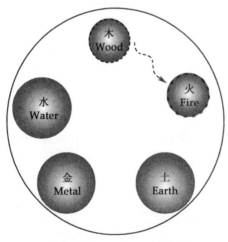

Mother Cannot Nourish Child

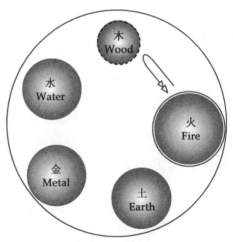

Child Stealing Mother's Qi

Restraint / Over-Restraint / Counter Restraint

While the restraint cycle is a normal mutual restriction of the phases, over-restraint and counter-restraint of the five phases are both abnormal conditions. The order of over-restraint is the same "pattern" of restraint. Counter-restraint is the same "pattern" as that of over-restraint but in the reverse direction.

The causes of over-restraint of the five phases occur in a few ways: either one phase is "too excessive" or another is "too weak" or a combination of the two. Over-restraint due to being "too excessive" means that a strong "dominate" phase over-restricts (overacts) on a weak or weaker "subordinate" phase. This leads to a deficiency or more of a deficiency of the subordinate phase. For example, if wood is too excessive and restricts earth too strongly, it may lead to a deficiency of earth, which is called "excessive wood encroaching upon earth". Another important way in which a phase may overact is when a

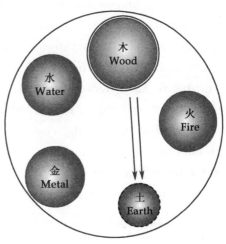

Wood Overacting on Earth

subordinate phase becomes so deficient that it allows the dominate phase to easily overcome it.

The clinical differences between an dominate phase overwhelming and a subordinate phase allowing itself to become overwhelmed are quite subtle, and they may both occur at the same time. One common example involves the wood phase function of controlling the free flow of qi throughout the body. If wood is normal, but earth (which here is the digestive function) is too weak to bear the restraint by wood, wood takes advantage of earth's deficiency and makes it even weaker.

As another example, if the emotions are very strong, the wood phase (which controls the movement of stagnant qi, including the qi of the emotions) will then overwhelm an otherwise healthy earth phase. This explains why a poor appetite or stomach pain appears when we are upset over something. If a person is especially weak in spleen-earth and the earth phase becomes weaker and weaker over time, the result may involve chronic digestive issues. This is called "wood encroaching (over-restraining) on insufficient earth".

Counter-Restraint / Counter-Restriction / Insulting

Counter-restraint is translated as "counter-restriction", "counteracting" or "insulting". Counter-restraint involves the same two phases as in the restraint cycle, but the actions between them are reversed. In this way, wood counter-restrains metal, metal counter-restrains fire, fire counter-restrains water, water counter-restrains earth, and in turn, earth counter-restrains wood. Counter-restraint is also caused by one phase being "too excessive" (dominating) or "too weak" (subordinate). Earth that is too strong may counter-restrain wood. If wood-qi is too excessive, it will not be restrained by metal, but instead it will counter-restrain metal. In

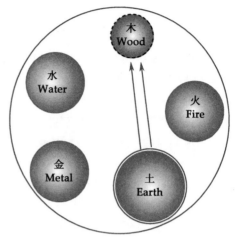

Earth Counter-restraining Wood

the clinic, this can be seen in some lung conditions, which in fact result from excessive anger of the liver-wood phase which then counter-restrains the lung-metal.

Although the five phases offer a tempting set of dichotomies of excess and deficiency, one should not apply them mechanically. In the clinic, some cases fall easily into five-phase theory while others may require either advanced theory or other systems for diagnosis and treatment.

FIVE-PHASE APPLICATIONS IN CHINESE MEDICINE

Five Phase Attributions

	Wood	Fire	Earth	Metal	Water
Flavor	sour	bitter	sweet	acrid	salty
Color	green	red	yellow	white	black
Transformation	germination	growth	harmonize	reaping	storage
Climate	wind	heat	dampness	dryness	cold
Direction	east	south	middle	west	north
Zang-organ	liver	heart	spleen	lung	kidney
Fu-organ	gallbladder	small intestine	stomach	large intestine	urinary bladder
Body Part	tendons	vessels	muscles	skin	bone
Opening	eyes	tongue	mouth	nose	ears
Voice	shouting	laughter	singing	crying	moaning
Fluid	tears	sweat	saliva	mucous	spittle
Associated Pulse	wiry	surging	moderate	floating	deep
Season	spring	summer	late-summer	autumn	winter
Emotion	anger	over-joy	thinking	sadness	fear

Five *Zang*-Organs

The five *zang*-organs correspond to the five phases, and their functions are explained according to the properties of the five phases.

Wood pertains to ascending, extending, and softening. The liver corresponds to wood to extend and unblock, and has the functions of softening and of storing blood.

Fire pertains to warmth, excitement, and ascending. The heart corresponds to fire to circulate blood and to warm the body.

Earth pertains to generating, bearing and containing. The spleen corresponds to the transportation and transformation of food and water to generate qi and blood.

Metal pertains to bending, killing, consolidating, descending, and changing. The lung corresponds to metal and consolidates, descends, and disperses.

Water pertains to moistening, moving downwards, and storing. The kidney corresponds to water to store essence, control water and to receive qi.

Based on the generation cycle and restraint cycle, there are promotion and restriction relationships among the five *zang*-organs.

Since wood generates fire, liver (wood) stores blood to assist the heart (fire), and unblocks to assist heart (fire) to circulate blood. Since fire generates earth, heart (fire) yang warms spleen (earth), to assist the generation and transformation of the spleen.

Since water restrains fire, kidney (water) can restrain the heart (fire) so as to not be too strong. Since heart (fire) restrains metal, heart (fire) can restrain the lung (metal) so as to not excessively clear and descend.

Each phase is "being generated, generating, being restricted, and being un-restricted". These relationships keep the five phases in a dynamic balance.

Chinese Herbs

Chinese herbs are associated with "the five colors" (green, red, yellow, white and black) and "the five flavors" (sour, bitter, sweet, acrid and salty). These five colors and flavors are also attributed to the five *zang*/yin-organs according to five-phase theory. The associated colors correspond with which organ channels the herbs will enter, and the flavors tell us the herb's direction of movement. Green and sour correspond to the liver, red and bitter to the heart, yellow and sweet to the spleen, white and acrid to the lung, and black and salty to the kidney. For example, *shí gāo* (Gypsum Fibrosum) is white in color and acrid in flavor, and it enters the lung channel. *Dān shēn* (Salviae Miltiorrhizae Radix et Rhizoma) is bitter in flavor and red in color, and it enters the heart channel. Sweet is associated with the spleen, and is sometimes called the blending of all the flavors, as happens with well-chewed food. Sweetness benefits the spleen, and the herbs associated with the spleen are often common foods. Throughout the world, meals often end with a bit of sweet food to help the digestion such as small piece of fruit, chocolate, or a full dessert.

In addition to the five colors and flavors, herbs are also associated with four properties (cold, heat, warm and cool) and directions (lifting, lowering, floating and sinking).

Acupuncture Points

Located near the ends of the legs and arms, there are five special acupoints on each organ channel, one for each of the five phases. Depending on different clinical conditions, these points can be selected according to the five-phase cycles of generation, over-restraint and counter-restraint. For example, Kidney 10 (KI 10, *yīn gǔ*) is a "water-point" often used to strengthen yin-fluids; it is an especially powerful point as it is also located on a channel also associated with water (kidney), that is, a water-point on a water-channel. This point is useful for treating the ministerial fire as mentioned above. Conversely, Liver 2 (LV 2, *xíng jiān*) is a fire-point that can be used to drain fire from the liver. We can see this as "subduing fire by draining wood" or "draining the child to subdue the mother".

Mental and Emotional Issues

Emotional activities are also associated with each of the five *zang*/yin-organs, which generate and restrain emotions according to the five phases. In the clinic, the generating and restricting relationships of emotional activities can be used in order to treat many emotional conditions.

Disease Mechanisms

Generation cycle: mother disease affecting child, child disease affecting mother.

Mother disease affecting child: since water generates wood and liver pertains to wood, kidney (water) in this case is the mother *zang*-organ, and the liver is the child *zang*-organ. When kidney disease affects liver, it is called mother disease affecting child.

Child disease affecting mother: since wood generates fire and liver pertains to wood, and heart pertains to fire, the liver in this case is the mother *zang*-organ, and the heart is the child *zang*-organ. When heart disease affects the liver, it is called child disease affecting mother.

In general, mother disease affecting child is mild, while the child disease affecting the mother is more severe.

Restraint cycle: over-restricting, counter-restricting.

Over-restricting can cause disease in two ways: the first is when the *zang*-organ is excessive and over-restricts another *zang*-organ. The second is when one *zang*-organ is deficient, and another *zang*-organ over-restricts it. As examples, excessive wood over-restricting earth (excessive liver qi over-restricting spleen) and deficient earth over-restricted by wood (deficient spleen over-restricted by liver).

Counter-restricting can cause disease in two ways: the first is when one *zang*-organ is excessive, and counter-restricts another *zang*-organ. The second is when one *zang*-organ is deficient, and is counter-restricted by another *zang* organ.

In general, when over-restricting occurs, the disease is severe, and when counter-restricting occurs, the disease is mild.

Preventive Principle

Since the disease of one *zang*-organ can affect other *zang*-organ according to the generation and restraint cycles, during treatment, the diseased *zang*-organ should first be treated by preventive methods to avoid it affecting the other *zang*-organs. In general, "the excess of one tends to affect the other, and the deficient one tends to be affected". The liver in excess tends to over-restrict the spleen and counter-restrict the lung; the spleen or lung in deficiency tends to be affected by the liver. When treating such diseases, tonifying the lung and spleen can avoid affects on the liver.

Therapeutic Principle

Therapeutic principle is also based on the generation cycle and restraint cycle.

Generation cycle

In deficiency tonify the mother; in excess purge the child.

1) In deficiency tonify the mother: when one *zang*-organ is deficient, tonify that *zang*-organ as well as its mother *zang*-organ.

The major principles are based on this:

Nourishing water to moisten wood, also known as nourishing kidney to moisten liver, is usually applied to treat deficient kidney yin combined with liver yin deficiency or causing liver yin deficiency.

Replenishing fire to nourish earth, that is, warming kidney fire to tonify spleen yang, is usually applied to treat spleen yang deficiency leading to kidney yang deficiency. Fire usually pertains to heart, but in "life-gate theory" the fire that warms the body refers to the life-gate fire, or kidney yang.

Banking up earth to generate metal, that is, tonifying spleen to supplement lung qi, is usually applied to treat deficient spleen and stomach failing to nourish lung leading to deficient lung and spleen.

Mutual generation between metal and water, that is, tonifying yin of lung and kidney, is usually applied to deficient lung failing to nourish kidney yin or deficient kidney failing to nourish lung yin, leading to both deficient lung and kidney.

2) In excess purge child: when one *zang*-organ is excessive, purge that *zang*-organ as well as its child *zang*-organ.

The major principles are based on this:

Purging fire to clear wood, that is, clearing heart fire to clear liver fire, is usually applied to excess heart fire stirring up liver fire, or liver fire flaming up and stirring up heart fire, leading to excessive fire of the heart and liver.

Purging earth to clear fire, that is, purging the undigested and accumulated food in the spleen and stomach to clear heart fire, is usually applied to accumulation in the spleen and stomach, turbid qi failing to move downwards, the accumulation transforming into fire, the stomach fire flaming up, causing heart fire to flame up, resulting in excessive fire of the heart and stomach.

Restraint cycle

Suppressing the strong and assisting the weak. Suppressing means to suppress the hyperactive *zang*-organ, and is usually applied in over-restricting or counter-restricting due to one organ which is hyperactive; assisting the weak means to assist the hypoactive *zang*-organ, and is usually applied in over-restricting or counter-restricting due to one organ being hypoactive.

The major principles are based on this:

Suppressing earth and control water, that is, tonifying spleen and promoting urination, is usually applied to treat spleen deficiency failing to transport, with the overflowing of water and dampness, manifesting as edema.

Assisting metal to balance wood, that is, tonifying lung yin and clearing lung fire to treat liver fire attacking lung, also known as tonifying lung and purging liver, is usually applied to treat lung yin deficiency with liver fire flaming up to attack the lung.

Purging south and tonifying north, that is, purging heart fire and nourishing kidney water to treat heart and kidney failing to communicate, is also known as purging fire and nourishing water, and is usually applied to treat deficient kidney yin and excessive heart fire, fire and water failing to communicate, or heart or kidney failing to communicate.

📖 Supplement: Cosmological Pattern (*Hé Tú*, 河图)

There is a third pattern of the five phases most often referred to as the "cosmological" pattern. What is remarkable about this pattern is that the earth phase is in the middle or "earth-centric". In this model, the elements also do not move in a circle, but rather they move to their complementary pairs, left and right and up and down. This gives us a very useful tool for understanding the directionality and movement of qi and can be very helpful in diagnosis and treatment.

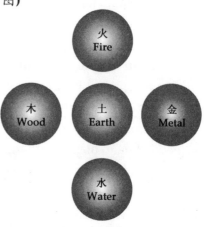

Cosmological Pattern

In the cosmological pattern, the earth is in charge of the surrounding four seasons of the year. The liver is attributed to wood, located in the east, and corresponds to spring. The heart is attributed to fire, located in the south, and corresponds to summer. The lung is attributed to metal, located in the west, and corresponds to autumn. The kidney is attributed to water, located in the north, and corresponds to winter. The season associated with the earth phase is sometimes seen as the transition or harmonizing period that lies in between each of the changing seasons. Other ancient texts attribute earth to the "late summer" period that occurs between summer and fall.

> Understanding the four directions (north, south, east, and west) in the cosmological pattern may be a bit confusing for students. One convenient image can be visualized within the very heart of China. The emperor's palace (now called the Forbidden City) sits in the middle of Beijing. If one were the ruler of China, you could sit in the palace chair and look south through the gates to Tiananmen Square and your empire. Behind you would be a small man-made hill, strategically situated to the north. Each morning you would watch the sun rise on your left (wood) and see it pass upwards and to the south (fire) and then finally set in the east (metal). The emperor or empress is viewed as the center of world; thus at the end of the day, the warmth of the sun would pass behind you to the north (water), and the temperature would become cold.

Based on this we can say that wood-qi moves upward and spreads from the left, like the early morning sun. Metal-qi descends and contracts, like the setting sun on the right. The sun (fire) activates the warmth and movement of the daytime, and the night (water) becomes quiet and restful. Fire is therefore thought of as being "in front" and water as "behind". Although this may seem rather removed from medicine, this model is actually used quite frequently in clinical practice. For example, many practitioners find that liver (wood) issues often predominate on the left side of the body, and that lung (metal) issues tend to manifest on the right.

The spleen is attributed to earth, which is located in the middle of the cosmological pattern; the middle position serves to identify and control the four directions. The spleen transports the essence of food in order to nourish the four other *zang*-organs. The earth is in charge of the four seasons, so if spleen qi functions well, the organ-qi will be abundant through all four seasons so that the healthy qi of the whole body can resist invasion by pathogenic qi.

Phase	Organ	Direction	Season
火 Fire	heart	south	summer
木 Wood	liver	east	spring
土 Earth	spleen	middle	late summer
金 Metal	lung	west	autumn
水 Water	kidney	north	winter

SUMMARY

This chapter section on the five phases contains a vast amount of information with many practical implications in the practice of Chinese medicine. The list below summarizes some of the most relevant points:

- The five phases may be translated as five movements and/or five elements; each translation may be appropriate, depending on the context.
- Disease in any one of the five *zang*-organs may affect the other four *zang*-organs by involvement between the mother- and child-phase, or through over-restraint and counter-restraint cycles.
- According to the generating law of the five phases, the therapeutic principles simply involve reinforcing the mother-phase in deficiency-type conditions, and reducing the child-phase in excess-type conditions.
- According to the restricting law of the five phases, the therapeutic principles involve inhibiting the excess phase and supporting the weaker phase.
- In clinical treatment of the five *zang*-organs, Chinese herbs are selected according to five-phase attributes, properties and flavors.

Students at this point should be able to complete this chart, draw five-phase charts, and identify the generation and restraint cycles as well as the cosmological pattern.

	Wood	Fire	Metal	Earth	Water
Flavor					
Color					
Transformation					
Climate					
Direction					
Zang-organ					
Fu-organ					
Direction					
Body part					
Opening					
Voice					
Fluid					
Emotion					
Associated pulse					
Season					

Chapter 2

Essence, Qi, Blood, Fluids and Spirit

Introduction

In the human body, essence (*jīng, 精*), qi (气), blood (*xuè, 血*) and fluids (*jīn yè, 津液*) are called the "essential substances" of human life. These are the basic materials for the actions of the *zang-fu* organs, channels and collaterals, and the overall functioning of the body. Essence, qi and spirit, are collectively referred to as "the three treasures", "three mysteries" or the "three gems".

In the body, essence, qi, blood, fluids and spirit are on a continuum with essence/*jīng* as the densest form of qi and spirit/*shén* as the most rarified.[①]

3 Treasures

Section 1   Human Essence

In ancient Chinese philosophy, essence is an invisible and ever-moving foundational substance that constitutes the entire universe. In Chinese medicine, essence is more specifically related to human life, and is generally thought of as being fluid-like in that it flows between the organs in which it is stored.

> In the ancient dictionaries of China, *jīng* was once defined as rice of the highest quality that had been carefully selected and considered as the most "elite" of all substances.

Essence in Chinese medicine has a variety of meanings, including the essence in the narrow sense, in the broad sense and in the general sense. Essence is initially

---

① In Chinese medical theory, it should be stressed that spirit is the ultimate product of essence, qi, blood, and fluids, yet also influences the same.

defined as reproductive essence with function of producing offspring, which is called essence in the narrow sense, and is also the initial concept of essence in Chinese medicine. From the point of view of liquid essence, blood, fluids, innate essence, foodstuff essence, reproductive essence, and visceral essence all belong to the scope of the broad sense of essence. However, in terms of the formation and function of a specific substance, there is a difference between the essence and the blood or fluids in concept. In general, the concept of essence is limited to the innate essence, foodstuff essence, reproductive essence and visceral essence, not including blood and fluids. Essence in Chinese medicine usually refers to the general sense.

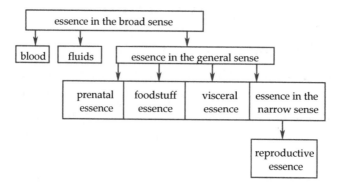

Wiseman and Feng define essence qi as "any essential element of the body (blood, qi, fluid, essence); specifically the acquired essence and the essence stored by the viscera and indissociable from the essential qi that is stored by the kidney and used in reproduction."[1]

"Blood, vessels, *yíng*, qi, essence and the spirit are all stored by the five *zang*-organs." —*The Yellow Emperor's Inner Classic*

Human essence is created from prenatal/congenital and postnatal/acquired essence. Prenatal/congenital essence is inherited from the "reproductive essence" of the parents.[2] It is this material that constitutes the embryo, and as such, serves as the foundation of human life. After the birth and throughout life, postnatal/acquired essence is extracted from the water and food that has been ingested. The postnatal qi is absorbed by the organs (particularly the stomach and spleen) and then distributed to the other organs. The human body is therefore founded upon congenital essence,

---

[1]   Nigel Wiseman, Ye Feng. *A Practical Dictionary of Chinese Medicine*. Taos: Pradigm Publiations; 1998. p. 96.

[2]   *Jīng zǐ* (精子) translates literally as essence-child, one of the Chinese words for semen.

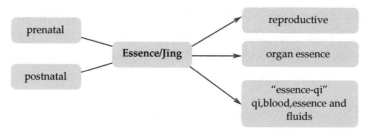

Essence/Jīng in Chinese Medicine

which is constantly supported by acquired essence throughout the life of the person.

The part of essence that is stored in the organs is called organ-essence. Organ-essence moistens and nourishes the organs while also producing organ-qi which acts to activate and regulate the organs, channels and collaterals. The essence in the organs encompasses qi, postnatal essence, blood, and fluids.

There is another conception of essence called "essence-qi". Essence-qi incorporates blood, fluids, prenatal/congenital essence, food-essence, reproductive essence, and organ-essence. The essence-qi within a specific organ will differ in the amount of qi, blood, fluids and essence present, depending upon that organ's specific function.

METABOLISM AND ESSENCE/ *JĪNG*

Essences are for the most part stored in the *zang*/yin-organs and the "extraordinary organs", while not as much in the *fu*/yang-organs. Therefore, we have heart-essence, liver-essence, spleen-essence, lung-essence, and kidney-essence. These essences and the qi, blood, and fluids present within the organs can also transform into one another in order to further promote organ function.

As stated above, the five *zang*-organs all store essence, but for many reasons, essence is most strongly associated with the kidney. During the formation of the fetus, congenital essence is stored in the kidney, and therefore is the main component of kidney-essence. The proportions of congenital essence and acquired essence as contained in the kidney are different from that of the other four *zang* organs. Kidney-essence is primarily comprised of congenital essence, while the essence of the other *zang-fu* organs is mainly composed of acquired essence. Because congenital essence is primarily stored in the kidney, the kidney is called the foundation of the congenital constitution.

During the developmental stages of the fetus, some congenital essence is stored in the other *zang-fu* organs, tissues, and orifices. Through the transporting function of spleen qi, acquired essence is constantly taken to the various *zang-fu* organs and tissues, where they become organ-essence. The kidney not only stores essence like the other four *zang*-organs, but also accepts surplus essence from them. The acquired essence supplies the other organs, while at the same time, the other organs transport their surplus acquired essence back to the kidney. Therefore, all the *zang-fu* organs store both congenital essence and acquired essence in various proportions.

The Release of Essence and *Yuan* Qi

There are two forms of essence that are released from the organs. The first is the essence that is stored in the *zang-fu* organs, which moistens and nourishes these organs while also transforming into qi that is required for activating and regulating the organ functions. When coming from the kidney-organ, essence is converted into *yuan*/original qi (元气) which then moves through the *sanjiao* organ system for distribution to the other *zang-fu* organs and tissues. Clavey writes, "Kidney *jīng*, which is yin, produces *yuan* qi through the vaporizing action of kidney yang." [1] The *yuan* qi acts to promote and stimulate the functions and activities of the body, and in doing so is considered the driving force of a human life. Indeed, "*yuan* qi" is a vernacular Chinese term for "vitality"[2].

A second concept involving the "release of essence" is narrower, regarding that which has been transformed into the reproductive essence[3] that is released during sexual activity. The release of semen is obvious in men, but there are different discussions of the possibilities for women. One view is that essence is released during a woman's sexual activity, particularly during vaginal fluids and orgasm; another is that menstruation releases essence, and a third view is that essence is released during childbirth. Many of these concepts conform to the idea that women's essence is held closely within the blood. Chinese medicine and Taoist culture both emphasize that for both men and women essence must not be "wantonly" discharged, thus there are various prohibitions and even exercises for preserving essence within the body. [4] There can also be "essence stagnation", a condition where the free flow of essence is repressed.[5]

---

[1] Steven Clavey. *Fluid Physiology and Pathology in Traditional Chinese Medicine*. Vol. 2. London: Churchill Livingston; 2002. p. 25.

[2] Wenlin electronic dictionary

[3] (*shēng zhí zhī jīng*, 生殖之精) reproductive essence

[4] Taoist essence-retaining practices for men are common, but if done incorrectly can cause difficulties in the reproductive structures. As well, some Taoist practices aim to stop women from producing menses.

[5] Although the loss of essence through sexual activity can be easily visualized and contemplated, we often speak of the loss of *jīng* through many lifestyle activities. Any extreme activity or emotion will eventually damage the kidney, and so eventually damage the *jīng*. Narrow thought and behaviors and addictions will also drain *jīng* as the lifestyle is directed towards one obsessive behavior and away from balance. Substance abuse has the added element of taxing the body systems. Methamphetamine use is the most dramatic of these, as it quickly causes deterioration of the "sea of marrow" (the brain) also causing dental loss as well as destroying the organ systems. Yet, emotions such as constant anger can also eventually consume *jīng* as it is pulled from the kidney to the liver. Even over-joy of the heart will cause exhaustion, where the search for it can damage the heart as well as the *jīng*.

Essence and *Tiān Guǐ*

Reproductive essence is derived from congenital essence through assistance from the acquired essence of food and water. At fourteen years of age for females and sixteen for males, a special substance, *tiān guǐ*[①](天癸) reveals itself. The kidney-essence, stimulated by *tiān guǐ*, then converts into reproductive essence. Under the stimulation of *tiān guǐ* and with the supplementation and nourishment from food-essence, a part of the congenital essence within the kidney transforms into reproductive essence. At this time, men and women are able to generate offspring.

Concerning young women, *The Yellow Emperor's Inner Classic* states, "At age 14, *tiān guǐ* begins to be produced which ensures active functioning of the *chong mai* and *ren mai*, thus she starts to menstruate and is able to conceive." *Tiān guǐ* cannot help but be compared to reproductive hormones in modern science yet it is uncertain that for women if there is a direct correspondence to ovulation, menstruation or actual menstrual blood that is being described. Whatever the answer, these processes are related to *tiān guǐ*.

FUNCTIONS OF HUMAN ESSENCE

Organ-essence moistens and nourishes the body. With ample organ-essence, all of the *zang-fu* organs, tissues and orifices of the body can maintain their normal functions. If the congenital essence is weak or the production of acquired essence becomes disordered, then the organ-essences will also become deficient and thus fail to sufficiently nourish the body, which leads to functional interruptions and decline. For example, insufficient spleen-essence leads to malnutrition or a decline of qi and blood, while insufficient lung-essence leads to respiratory disorders. Impaired kidney-essence can lead to both mental and physical retardation in children, or premature aging in adults. Kidney-essence also generates marrow which acts to nourish the bones, teeth, and the brain.

PATHOLOGIES OF ESSENCE

Essence/ *Jīng* Deficiency

Reproductive essence is obviously central to producing offspring, where weak

---

① *Tiān* is the word for heavenly, and *guǐ* is last of the 10 heavenly stems or suns that are said to revolve around the earth. *Guǐ* is associated with yin, water and the kidney. *Tiān guǐ* thus has the poetic implication of a cycle coming from heaven that is being renewed.

reproductive essence can lead to infertility or result in the birth of a child with weakened prenatal essence. In Chinese medicine, mental retardation and genetic abnormalities are considered to be a result of weak reproductive essence.

The kidney is the main organ for storing essence, a most important consideration in cases of essence deficiency. Kidney-essence deficiency has many signs and symptoms including male and female infertility, listlessness, tinnitus, amnesia, physical weakness and premature senility. When kidney-essence fails to generate marrow, there will be loosening of the teeth, dizziness, and both physical and mental weakness in both children and adults.

The spleen generates postnatal essence; therefore, problems with essence deficiency also lie with the spleen. A shortage of postnatal essence can create deficiency-type conditions manifesting with a sallow lusterless complexion, dizziness, confusion, and a lack of energy.

Essence/ *Jīng* Loss and Obstruction

Chinese medical texts emphasize that problems associated with essence often result from excessive essence loss and/or essence stagnation. Loss of "genetic essence" (sperm and seminal fluid[①]) will inevitably cause a loss of kidney-essence and food-essence, which then results in "essence loss" or "essence desertion". Treatment generally involves supplementation of kidney qi and essence. The other type of essence loss involves massive losses of food-essence through extreme dieting, bulimia, purging and/or poor digestion which results in shortness of breath, fatigue, lassitude, a sallow complexion, insomnia, and poor memory, etc. Treatment generally involves supplementation of the spleen qi, which will then supplement the essence. Essence exhaustion[②] is a more serious form of essence loss that can result in qi exhaustion or be the result of qi exhaustion; in these cases, the main principle of treatment is to strengthen and benefit qi.

Essence stagnation is an ejaculation disorder in men due to stagnation of semen in the seminal duct. This can result from sexual overactivity, over-control of ejaculation through Taoist exercises, frustration due to sexual abstinence, injury to the kidney by fear, blood stasis, stagnation due to internal damp-heat, or surgical scars. When deficiency leads to kidney qi failing to activate, or when liver qi fails to govern the free flow of qi due to constraint, there can be stagnation with obstructive ejaculation. The main clinical manifestations of essence stagnation are obstruction of ejaculation or inability to ejaculate accompanied by pain in the seminal duct, heavy downbearing

---

①   There is a modern debate about whether male *jīng* consists of only sperm or all of the seminal fluids and whether vasectomies, for example, can conserve *jīng*.

②   (*jīng tuō*, 精脱) essence exhaustion

sensations in the testes and lower abdomen, varicocele, back pain, dizziness, etc. According to the diagnosis, the treatment principles can include supplementing qi, soothing liver qi, invigorating blood and dissolving stasis, or dispelling phlegm and eliminating dampness in some cases.

Section 2   Qi

BASIC CONCEPT OF HUMAN QI

Qi moves continually through the body to promote and regulate the human metabolism. Qi is also transformed by essence, which forms the material basis for functional activity, while qi is the active force which promotes and regulates the physical functions of the organs. Essence is the origin of human life, and qi is the vehicle for its maintenance. From the point of view of yin and yang attributes, essence has a tangible fluid state, is stored in the *zang*-organs, and belongs to yin. Qi is in comparison more intangible and in constant motion, therefore belonging to yang.

When the movement of qi ceases, human life comes to an end. No matter the source, any kind of qi that disturbs the body is called a pathogenic (*xie*) qi. The opposite of pathogenic qi is the *zheng*/upright qi, which can be conceived of as the sum of all forces that protect the body against pathogenic qi.

The qi in humans is derived from prenatal/congenital qi and the postnatal qi as transformed from food-essence, as well as from the qi extracted from the air inhaled by the lungs. An adequate amount and quality of qi therefore also depends on a complex coordination of the various *zang-fu* organs.

The kidney stores congenital prenatal essence, and is supported by acquired postnatal essence. Congenital essence is the main component of kidney-essence, where the *yuan*/original qi that is transformed from congenital essence is the fundamental component of a person's qi. Thus, the function of the kidney in storing essence is absolutely essential for the production of qi. When the essence stored in the kidney is abundant[①], qi will also be sufficient. If the kidney fails to store or there is a loss of essence, this will result in the decline of qi.

The spleen and stomach function together to complete the digestion and absorption of water and grain. Food-essence is conveyed from the middle *jiao* to the heart and lung through the ascending function of spleen qi, where it is then transformed into blood and fluids. The generation of qi then has three sources:

---

① (*zú*, 足) full, ample

congenital essence, postnatal food-essence, and air. The spleen and stomach transform food and water into refined essences, and then into qi for distribution to the *zang-fu* organs and the rest of the body. Therefore, the spleen and stomach are called the source of qi production. When the spleen and stomach cannot absorb food-nutrients due to dysfunctions of the spleen and stomach, the qi production of the whole body will also become compromised.

The lung governs qi and is in charge of the generation of *zong*/pectoral qi which plays a very important role in the process of qi generation. On one hand, through its respiratory function, the lung governs respiratory qi by inhaling fresh qi into the body and exhaling turbid qi to the outside. On the other hand, the lung combines the inhaled fresh air with the food-qi as transformed by the spleen. This process results in the formation of *zong* qi. *Zong* qi accumulates inside the chest and penetrates into the heart vessels in order to move the qi and blood. It then flows upward into the respiratory tract to promote breathing, and also downward to an area below the navel called the *dān tián* in order to supplement the *yuan*/original qi.

QI MOVEMENT/DYNAMIC (*QÌ JĪ*, 气机)

Qi movement is classified in four ways: ascending, descending, exiting and entering. All distribution of congenital qi, postnatal food qi, and inhaled fresh air rely on qi movement. Essence, blood, and fluids depend upon the constant movement of qi to moisten and nourish the whole body. The functions of the *zang-fu* organs, channels and collaterals, body structures and orifices also rely on this movement. All phenomena such as inhaling and exhaling, sweating, digesting food and discharging feces and urine are embodiments of qi movement. The movement of qi is fundamental to life itself, and once its movement ceases, the life of the body comes to an end.

The characteristics of the *zang-fu* organs cause unique movements of qi. In general, organ-qi that is in the upper part of the body flows downward, while organ-qi in the lower portion flows upward. Yang-organ qi flows downward and yin-organ qi flows upward, with yin qi and yang qi acting upon each other in a great number of complex ways.

For example, the heart and lung are located in the upper part, so their visceral qi flows downward. The liver and kidney are situated in the lower part, hence their visceral qi flows upward. The spleen and stomach are in the central area, then according to the yin or yang attribute they respectively belong to, the spleen as a *zang*-organ belonging to yin flows upward, the stomach as a *fu*-organ belonging to yang flows downward; subsequently, the spleen and stomach can connect the upper part with the lower part between the visceral qi, acting as the hub for ascending and descending motion. In terms of the six *fu*-organs as a whole, they convey and digest foodstuff instead of reserving them, and function well when their qi freely flows downward. As for relations among *zang-fu* organs (viscera), all of the visceral qi movement such as the lung governing exhaling and the kidney governing receiving qi; the liver qi tendency to ascend and the lung qi tendency to descend; the spleen qi governing ascent of the clear, and the stomach governing descent of the turbid; and the interaction between heart and kidney, show the unity of ascending and descending among qi of *zang*-organs or between *zang*-organs and *fu*-organs. And as to one single *zang*- or *fu*-organ, it also shows the unity of ascending and descending within itself, such as dispersing and descending of the lung qi, and separating the lucid from the turbid by the small intestine.

Lung qi, in general, moves downward, however it also disperses outward to the surface of the body to nourish the skin. As a metal-organ, its qi can change to fit the circumstances of the inside and outside world. For example, when exercising, its qi is important to access the legs for running, and the arms for lifting weights. Because kidney is a water-organ, kidney qi is often hidden and stored, yet it remains available for use. Liver qi should move both upward and in a spreading-outward direction. The liver also moves subtly across to the spleen to aid that qi upward. As a wood-organ, liver qi can be compared to a tree or bamboo that moves upward and outward, yet it is firm but flexible when it needs to bend. This combination of firmness and flexibility reflects the dual nature of the liver. Heart qi can be seen as dominating in all directions and influencing over all that it rules. Yet the heart has a number of "administrators", which are the other *zang-fu* organs. They bring information (qi) to the heart, which then determines how it is to be used. As a fire-organ, its qi has the tendency to move upward, while to maintain balance, the heart's upward movement is kept in check by the kidney-water.

The motion of spleen qi is upward and toward the flesh of the extremities. The spleen is interiorly/exteriorly paired with the stomach, and stomach's qi movement is normally downward. The respective downward and upward movement of the stomach and spleen is vital for the production of the postnatal qi. The spleen and stomach also act together to harmonize the rest of the body's qi (as both are earth phase organs).

Qi which counterflows contrary to its usual direction is sometimes called "rebellious qi", most obviously seen in vomiting when stomach qi moves upward, or with coughing due to lung qi counterflow. Liver qi can also counterflow, where instead of moving upward and outward, it moves laterally to the stomach, causing stomach pain and otherwise inhibiting the harmonizing actions of the earth phase.

Qi can also become constrained or stagnated. Qi "constraint" (*yù*, 郁) usually involves the qi of organs, most often seen in patterns of liver qi constraint. "Stagnation" (*zhì*, 滞) usually involves the qi only, and is often a more limited process. However, *yù*/constraint is also a Chinese term for emotional depression (as well as constraint of other processes and substances). This reinforces the Chinese conception that emotions and the spirit are both based on qi. Within many Chinese texts, "constraint" and "depression" are used interchangeably and are thus best understood according to the context[1].

QI TRANSFORMATION (*QÌ HUÀ*, 气化)

Qi transformation refers to various changes resulting from qi movement (*qì jī*, 气机), although the application of qi transformation is usually seen within the context of fluids and essence. For example, we say that kidney-essence becomes kidney qi and that food-essence becomes spleen qi. Steven Clavey quotes a modern textbook to define qi transformation as "making one type of substance into many types of substances, or making many types of substance into one type of substance."[2] In a mixture of biomedical and Chinese contexts, qi transformation can be seen as metabolic processes that involve essence, qi, blood, and fluids.[3] Qi transformation is both a material transformation as well as a process of converting energy.

Qi transformation is a simple concept that names one of the most important and complex processes of the body. It also helps to explain processes that may seem amorphous or mysterious when following Chinese medical thinking. For example, this idea allows the practitioner to distinguish between substances and processes in order to precisely pinpoint the role of yin qi and yang qi in the transformation of fluids into qi and back again. The maintenance of the *zang-fu* organs and all of the body systems depends upon qi transformation, and qi transformation depends upon a well-functioning *zang-fu* organ system.

FUNCTIONS OF QI

Warming, Cooling, Propelling and Regulating

In Chinese yin-yang theory, the qi of the body can be divided into yin qi and yang qi. Yin qi has cold, cool, and containing properties, and yang qi has warm, hot, and active properties. Yang qi stimulates and promotes the growth of the body,

---

[1]   *The Practical Dictionary* (Wiseman) translates *yù* (郁) as "depression".

[2]   Clavey quoting the *Zhōng Yī Jī Chǔ Lǐ Lùn Xiáng Jiě* (中医基础理论详解)

[3]   Although they are not traditional Chinese medical concepts, biomedicine posits that hormones can initiate a cascade of energetic processes, and that exercise can facilitate the production of bone.

reproductive functions, and the functions of the *zang-fu* organs and channels and collaterals. It also promotes the generation and distribution of essence, blood, fluids, and mental activities. Yin qi is that which slows down, gathers, regulates, and calms these same activities.

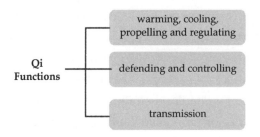

Yin qi and yang qi have opposite effects, and their natures restrict each other to maintain balance. If yin qi is deficient, it cannot restrain yang qi. Over time, the relative excess of yang will consume too much of the yin substances and deplete fluids. This can cause a number of issues including hot flashes, night sweats, insomnia and mental agitation.

Conversely, if yang qi is deficient, it cannot move yin qi, thus yin qi will be in relative excess, where the yin-aspects of quietude and inhibition can lead to hypo-functioning of the *zang-fu* organs. There may be decreased generation and metabolism with impaired circulation of essence, qi, blood, and fluids. Signs and symptoms of yang qi deficiency include mental depression, phlegm-dampness accumulation, fatigue, edema, lack of sexual desire and infertility, among others.

The warming function of qi refers to the yang qi action of generating heat in the body which maintains normal body temperature while warming all the organs, orifices, and channels and collaterals. Essence, blood, and fluids are also supported by the warming action of yang qi.

Yin qi cools and moistens the organs, orifices, and channels and collaterals in order to prevent overactivity and excessive heat that would affect the essence, blood, and fluids. When yin qi becomes deficient, the cooling action decreases, thus leading to patterns of deficiency-type heat. Manifestations include a low-grade fever, night sweats, and a rapid and thready pulse.

On the other hand, when yang qi is deficient, heat production will decrease, thus leading to patterns of deficiency-type cold with weakened activities of the *zang-fu* organs and decreased metabolism of essence, blood, and fluids. Manifestations include an aversion to cold, cold limbs, reduced libido and sexual function, slow physical movement, and a reduced body temperature.

Defending and Controlling

When pathogenic qi invades the body, it is not easy to maintain health if the *zheng*/upright qi is weak. Qi not only protects the body surface from the invasion of external pathogens, but also serves to eliminate pathogens that have already invaded the body. When the pathogenic qi invades the body, the *zheng* qi attempts to drive it outward. Therefore, the normal defending functions of qi should prevent the invasion of pathogenic qi. The functional ability of *zheng* qi determines the frequency, development, severity, and prognosis of diseases.

The "controlling function of qi" means that qi can consolidate and govern materials such as blood, fluids, and essence in order to avoid their abnormal loss. For example, the failure of qi to control blood inside the vessels can cause bleeding. The qi must also control the secretions and excretions of sweat, urine, saliva, and gastric fluids. The failure of qi to control fluids can cause spontaneous perspiration, frequent urination, urinary incontinence, excessive salivation, vomiting, diarrhea, etc. Finally, it is said that this controlling function also limits the secretion of semen in order to prevent various forms of "inappropriate release" such as in spermatorrhea or premature ejaculation.

Qi Transmission

Qi can both create and transmit information within the body. Any information transferred between the interior of the body and the outside environment depends on the invisible but ever-present qi as a carrier. The condition of the organ-essence and qi corresponds on the body surface to different *zang-fu* organs. Information is transmitted between the internal *zang-fu* organs through the passages of the channels and collaterals. This ability for qi to transmit through the channels and collaterals is what allows the body to respond to treatments such as acupuncture, moxibustion, and massage. All these and other external therapies are all carried out by the conduction of qi. Therefore, qi is a carrier of information, as well as a mediator between the *zang-fu* organs and all the other body structures. However, qi transmission is also what allows pathogenic qi to penetrate into the body through the channels.

CLASSIFICATION OF HUMAN QI

Yuan Qi, *Zong* Qi, *Ying* Qi and *Wei* Qi

Qi distributes through every part of the body but has different names according to its generation, distribution, and functional characteristics. In terms of its generation, qi is classified as *yuan*/original qi when it comes from prenatal/congenital and postnatal/acquired essence. In terms of distribution, it is classified as *ying* qi when it circulates inside the vessels, and *wei* qi when it circulates outside the vessels. The combination of food-qi and qi from the air accumulates in the chest and is called *zong*/pectoral qi. Qi in the *zang-fu* organs is called organ-qi, and when distributed in the channels and collaterals it is called channel-qi.

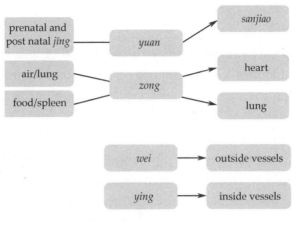

Classifications of Qi

Original / *yuan* qi (*yuán qì*, 元气)

1) Generation and distribution

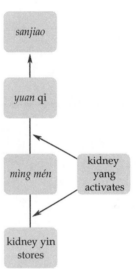

Yuan qi[1] is generated by congenital essence in the kidney. From there it is distributed by the *sanjiao* to all parts of the body. *Yuan* qi runs in the interior to the *zang-fu* organs, and in the exterior to the flesh and skin surface. Although some books may refer to *yuan* qi as being stored in the kidney, one could also conceptualize it as being stored in the kidney as a "potential" until it passes through the *mìng mén*, where it is then activated by kidney yang and distributed throughout the body via the *sanjiao*.

2) Physiological functions

There are two aspects of the physiological functions of *yuan* qi. The first is to promote and regulate growth, development, and reproductive functions. The second is to promote and regulate the activities of the *zang-fu* organs, channels and collaterals, body structures, sense organs, and the orifices.

Yuan qi can be divided into *yuan*-yin and *yuan*-yang, which influences both the yin and yang of the whole body. For example, *yuan* qi can perform the "yang" actions of promotion, activation and warmth and the "yin" function of calming, inhibiting, and cooling. The balance between water and fire, or yin and yang in the *mìng mén* maintains the *zang-fu* organs in a healthy state of "calm yin and sound yang". In short, all life activities are carried out under the promotion and regulation of *yuan* qi, which is the driving force for life activities. So loss of *yuan* qi or an imbalance between *yuan*-yin and *yuan*-yang will bring about any number of disorders.

---

[1] Original qi is also called "true qi" in the Inner Classic, and called "source qi" in *The Classic of Difficult Issues* (*Nàn Jīng*, 难经). Whatever the name, all are connected to prenatal (congenital) qi.

Zong qi (*zōng qì*, 宗气)

Zong/pectoral qi[1], as a combination of air and food qi, is a qi that accumulates in the chest which belongs to the category of postnatal acquired qi. Its formation directly relates to the abundance of human qi. The place in the chest where *zong* qi accumulates is called the "sea of qi".[2]

1) Generation and distribution

Zong qi comes from two sources. The first is from food-qi derived from food-essence transformed and transported by the spleen and stomach, and the second is from the air inhaled by the lung. The normal functions of the spleen and stomach to transform and transport, as well as the normal function of the lung to dominate qi and control respiration, are directly related to the generation and abundance of *zong* qi.

After accumulating in the chest, *zong* qi flows in three ways. The first is from the lung to move upwards through the respiratory track, the second is to pour into the heart and vessels, and the third is to run downwards in the *sanjiao* to the *dān tián* just below the navel.[3]

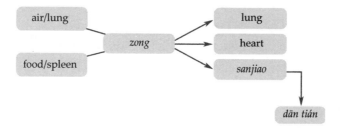

2) Physiological functions

The three main physiological functions of *zong* qi are to promote respiration, move blood and qi, and nourish the prenatal/congenital qi. *Zong* qi moves upward through the respiratory tract, propelling the movements of the lung. Therefore, it is also related to the breath, voice, and speech. When *zong* qi is plentiful there is an even breath, clear speech, and a rich voice. Otherwise, there would be short and weak breathing, unclear speech and a low voice.

Zong qi also pours into the heart vessels, assisting it to promote blood circulation. Therefore, the power and rhythm of the heart and blood circulation are both

---

①   *Zong* qi (宗气), in various English language books is called center qi, chest qi, ancestral, gathering qi, governing qi, and pectoral qi.

②   Also called *dàn zhōng* (膻中).

③   *The Spiritual Pivot* also points out that *zong* qi flows downward from sea of qi to *qì jiē* (气街, a point in the groin area), and then down to the foot.

associated with *zong* qi. When *zong* qi is sufficient, there is a strong and regular pulse, and when insufficient, the pulse can be rapid, irregular, or weak.

The *xū lǐ* (虚里)[①] is an area below the left nipple, at the pulsation area of the heart apex; the pulse at this position indicates the state of *zong* qi[②]. With plentiful *zong* qi, the pulsation is normal, but if overly rapid and forceful it suggests a serious deficiency of *zong* qi. If the pulsation disappears completely, it means that *zong* qi is on the verge of expiry.

By propelling respiration and blood circulation, *zong* qi influences a variety of physiological activities. For example, it affects circulation of blood and qi, temperature, movement of the limbs, the strength of the voice, and speech.

In addition, as a form of postnatal/acquired qi, *zong* qi has an important function in supporting *yuan* qi. Through the *sanjiao*, *yuan* qi runs from the lower parts of the body to the upper, and spreads over the chest to support the *zong* qi. *Zong* qi distributes from the upper to the lower parts of the body, and accumulates below the umbilicus at the *dān tián* where it supports congenital and acquired qi. Through the actions of *zong* qi, congenital qi combines with acquired qi to generate the qi of the whole body.

Ying qi (*yíng qì*, 营气)

Ying qi is a kind of qi that is rich in nourishment which circulates inside the vessels; it is also the most important component of blood. *Ying* qi is often translated as "nutritive qi".

1) Generation and distribution

Ying qi comes from the food-essence that is transported and transformed by the spleen and stomach. When refined food-essence is transformed into food-qi, the thick and nutritious part turns into *ying* qi, which then runs within the vessels to circulate throughout the body.

2) Physiological functions: generating blood and nourishing the body

Ying qi and body fluids pass into the vessels together where they transform into blood. Together they should maintain a constant and adequate volume of blood. *Ying* qi flows through the body within the vessels to nourish the organs, tissues, limbs and bones.

The two physiological functions of *ying* qi to transform blood and nourish the body are interrelated. When *ying* qi becomes deficient, this will cause a deficiency of blood and further decrease the functions of the *zang-fu* organs and tissues in the body due to inadequate nutrition.

---

① Pronounced more or less like "shoe lee".
② This likely corresponds with the apical pulse found at the 5th intercostal space.

"The qi that is superficial and does not follow the vessels is the *wei* qi. The essential qi that moves in the vessels is the *ying* qi." — *The Yellow Emperor's Inner Classic: Basic Questions* (*Huáng Dì Nèi Jīng-Sù Wèn*, 黄帝内经·素问)

Ying qi is seen as a part of blood. While *ying* qi and blood are often combined and called "*ying*-blood", an advanced view reveals some subtle differences between them. *Ying* has functional activities and can more easily transform into fluids. *Formulas and Strategies* says, "The term *ying*, furthermore, is generally associated in the medical literature with the spleen and heart, while *xue* (blood) is more often associated with the liver and other aspects of the sea of blood in the lower *jiao*, that is, the *chong mai* and the womb. This makes sense as the liver and sea of blood store blood (emphasizing its substantive nature), whereas the heart and spleen exert functional control over the blood (producing qi, governing it)."[1] The extent to which the nutritive *ying* qi and *yuan* qi are involved in the production and exchange of nutrients is left to be more fully explored.[2]

Wei qi (*wèi qì*, 卫气)

Wei/defensive qi circulates outside the vessels, and its functions are those of protection and defense. Because it is seen as protecting the body from pathogenic invasion, it is often also translated as "protective qi". In comparing their properties, distribution and functions, *ying* qi belongs to yin, and *wei* qi to yang.

Wei qi is produced from the refined food-essence that is transported and transformed by the spleen and stomach. When refined food-essence is transformed into food-qi, the active and floating parts turn into *wei* qi. It circulates outside the vessels without being confined by the vessel system, circulating both outward to the skin and muscles and inward to the *zang-fu* organs in the chest and abdomen. *Wei* qi defends the body from external pathogens, warms the body, and controls and adjusts the opening of the "striae and interstices" (*còu lǐ*, 腠理) or the area just in and below the pores and skin.

---

[1] Dan Bensky, Randall Barolet. *Formulas and Strategies*. Seattle: Eastland Press; 1990. p. 352.

[2] In *Applied Channel Theory in Chinese Medicine*,"... there is a circular flow of nutritive and source qi occurring along the pathways of the twelve channels. There is an almost multidimensional aspect to these two movements." Ju-Yi Wang, Jason D. Robertson. *Applied Channel Theory in Chinese Medicine: Wang Ju-Yi's Lectures on Channel Therapeutics*. Seattle: Eastland Press; 2008. p. 440.

> The defensive qi circulates, linking above and below as if in an endless circuit. —*The Systematic Classic of Acupuncture and Moxibustion*

Wei qi also warms the body to maintain a constant body temperature. When *wei* qi is deficient and fails to warm, a patient may have cold-type diseases caused by the invasion of yin-pathogens as coldness and dampness. However, when *wei* qi is blocked and cannot disperse, this can result in heat-type diseases with yang excess.

Wei qi regulates the opening and closing of the skin and pores to regulate sweating. This regulative function has both containing and activating actions. Through the normal secretion of sweat, a relatively constant temperature is maintained. When *wei* qi is weak, the normal opening and closing of the pores and skin is affected. Manifestations include an inability to sweat, profuse sweating, or spontaneous sweating, depending on the afflicting pathogen.

There are both similarities and differences between *wei* qi and *ying* qi. Both come from the food-essence that is transported and transformed by the spleen and stomach. *Ying* qi belongs to yin, and *wei* qi to yang. Since the yin and yang of the body must remain coordinated, only when the harmony between *ying* qi and *wei* qi is maintained can a normal body temperature and normal sweat secretions be maintained.

Zheng Qi (*Zhèng Qì*, 正气)

Zheng/upright qi is a simple yet important concept that is so encompassing that it is often overlooked. *Zheng* qi may be seen as the body's overall resistance to disease and a collection of all types of anti-pathogenic qi in the body. *Zheng* qi has no direct or specific connection to the organs in Chinese medical physiology, yet it is involved in the background of any bodily dysfunction. The mention of *zheng* qi often comes up when discussing complex, chronic and serious diseases such as HIV/ AIDS or cancer. A lack of *zheng* qi is that which allows diseases to overwhelm the body.

Organ-Qi and Channel-Qi

After qi is distributed to the *zang-fu* organs or channels-collaterals, the qi in the *zang-fu* organs is called "organ-qi", and the qi in channels and collaterals is called "channel-qi". Organ-qi is transformed from organ-essence, so it can be considered a very fine material which is invisible and runs endlessly to promote and regulate the functions of the *zang-fu* organs. It can also be said that organ-qi is a kind of qi with different structures and functions based on which organ is involved. Organ-qi is a driving force to promote and adjust the physiological functions of the *zang-fu* organs and keep their functions as normal as possible.

Qi in the human body can be divided into yin qi and yang qi, so the organ-qi transformed from it also has properties of yin and yang. Organ-yin qi is the part of qi with properties of cooling, calming and inhibition. The organ-yang qi is the part of qi with warming, propelling, and activating properties. Under normal circumstances, organ-yin qi balances with yang qi to maintain orderly motion and harmony of the organ-qi.

Channel-qi is a very fine material which senses, carries, and transmits various stimuli and information. The therapeutic effects of acupuncture, moxibustion, massage, and cupping need channel-qi movement in order to reach the disease.

QI DISORDERS (PATHOLOGIES)

Qi disorders have two aspects. The first involves qi deficiency or a shortage of qi resulting in qi not being sufficiently generated, or because the qi has been consumed over time. The second kind of qi disorder involves functional impairment or abnormal qi movement involving patterns of qi stagnation, qi counterflow, qi sinking, qi obstruction /block, or qi desertion.

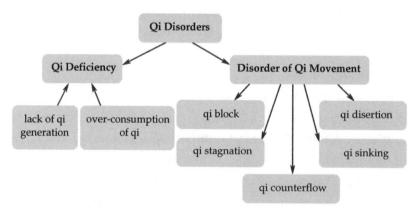

Qi Deficiency (*Qì Xū*, 气虚)

Qi deficiency is a pathological state involving a shortage and/or under-functioning of qi. Qi may fail to be sufficiently generated as a result of congenital endowment, improper care after birth, or organ dysfunctions (particularly of the lung, spleen, and kidney). Qi deficiency may result from malnutrition and/or over-consumption of qi through lifestyle choices or prolonged disease.

Qi deficiency typically presents with fatigue, dizziness, spontaneous sweating, a greater susceptibility to the common cold, a pale complexion, a pale tongue, and a weakened pulse. Patients with a deficiency of *yuan* qi may show slowed growth and/

or impaired reproductive function. Patients with a deficiency of *zong* qi may have palpitations and shortness of breath.

According to the theory of qi dividing into yin and yang, qi deficiency can involve predominant signs of deficient yin qi or deficient yang qi. Yin qi deficiency manifests deficiency-type heat symptoms due to the declined cooling and moistening actions of yin qi. Yang qi deficiency manifests deficiency-type cold symptoms due to the declined warming actions of yang qi. When neither heat nor cold manifestations are predominant, the condition is simply referred to as qi deficiency. Manifestations of general qi deficiency such as listlessness and lassitude can appear patterns of yin qi deficiency or yang qi deficiency.

Kidney qi comes from kidney-essence, of which the main component is the prenatal/congenital essence. Kidney yin and kidney yang are both derived from the kidney qi, thus serving as the root of other organs' yin qi and yang qi. This is stated as "without the kidney yin qi, the yin qi of five *zang*-organs cannot be nourished", and "without the kidney yang qi, the yang qi of five *zang*-organs cannot be replenished". With a longstanding deficiency of yin qi and yang qi, both kidney yin and kidney yang are affected; thus the saying, "prolonged illness involves the kidney".

Disorder of Qi Movement

Disorders of qi movement include patterns of qi stagnation, qi counterflow, qi sinking, qi block, and qi desertion. These conditions arise due to the abnormal ascending, descending, exiting and entering of qi.

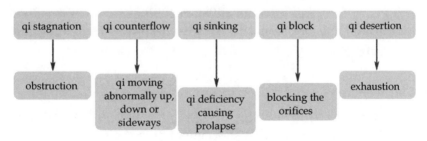

Qi Movement Disorders

Qi stagnation (*qì zhì*, 气滞)

Qi stagnation is state of obstructed or stagnated qi flow in a particular part of the body. Qi stagnation can be associated with excess internal phlegm or dampness, food accumulation, blood stasis, heat constraint, *zang-fu* organ impairment or emotional depression. Any of these can impact the flow of qi and lead to a localized stagnation of qi movement that lead to functional disturbances of the *zang-fu* organs as well as the channels and collaterals. Qi stagnation is usually considered to be an excess-type pattern, although stagnation can result from patterns of deficient qi failing to move qi and blood. Manifestations of qi stagnation usually include distention, fullness and pain, chest distress, cough, and/or shortness of breath, as well as possible related signs of blood stasis or phlegm-fluid retention.

Qi stagnation has various clinical signs, but the most common characteristics simply involve a dull, achy discomfort. When qi stagnation combines with blood stasis, the result is a sharper pain, such as from over-exercise, while a stabbing pain is often attributed to qi stagnation due to cold.

Qi counterflow (*qì nì*, 气逆)

Qi counterflow describes qi that flows opposite to its normal direction of movement, for example rising when it should be descending, or moving abnormally in a lateral direction as in the case of liver qi overacting on the spleen and stomach. Qi counterflow can result from pathogenic invasion, obstruction of turbid phlegm, or qi deficiency, as well as excessive emotions or improper diet. Qi counterflow most often occurs in the lung, stomach, and liver. Manifestations may include cough, nausea and vomiting, headache, a feeling of distention in the head, and irritability.

Generally speaking, qi counterflow is considered as an excess pattern, although it may also be the result of deficiency. For example, lung qi counterflow with cough and wheezing may be caused by the lung qi failing to descend with kidney qi failing to receive qi. When deficient stomach qi fails to maintain the stomach's descending function, stomach qi counterflow may result. Acid reflux associated with nausea or poor appetite during times of high stress is an example of liver qi counterflow affecting the stomach; in five-phase theory, this is called "wood overacting on earth".

Qi sinking (*qì xiàn*, 气陷)

Qi sinking is a further development of qi deficiency and spleen qi deficiency in particular. The pathology lies in a shortage of qi in the upper parts of the body, and a sinking of qi in the middle *jiao*. Generally a result of spleen qi deficiency with a failure to send food-essence upward, shortage of qi in the head or upper *jiao* creates malnourishment of the head and eyes with dizziness, confusion, or tinnitus.

The sinking of middle-qi occurs when due to deficiency, the spleen qi cannot maintain the relatively fixed positions of the *zang-fu* organs. Various organ prolapses result, such as gastroptosis (stomach), nephroptosis (kidney), metroptosis (often uterus), and proctoptosia (rectum). Such conditions are not uncommon in older people and in women after childbirth.

Qi block or obstruction (*qì bì*, 气闭)

Qi block or obstruction refers to a blockage of the clear orifice (brain) and a loss of consciousness due to a disturbance of qi. Qi block results from emotional over-excitement, external pathogens, or turbid phlegm, any of which can block the flow of qi. Although the conditions for qi block may build over time, generally speaking, the qi block itself occurs suddenly. Although usually the patient will revive spontaneously without treatment, prolonged blockage may be fatal.

Qi desertion/exhaustion (*qì tuō*, 气脱)

Qi desertion is a sudden pathological state of exhausted vital functions due to a massive loss of qi or failure of qi to contain itself within the body. Qi will follow fluids and blood outward in cases of profuse sweating, bleeding or loss of fluids from vomiting or diarrhea. Deficiency and prolonged consumption of *zheng* qi in a chronic disease may also result in qi desertion with a pale complexion, continuous sweating, closed eyes and an open mouth, general paralysis, urinary and fecal incontinence, and a faint or large weak pulse with no root.

The pathomechanisms of qi desertion, yin collapse, and yang collapse all involve a great loss of qi. When qi desertion results from a sudden loss of yang qi, this is referred to as yang collapse. When qi desertion is caused by a sudden loss of yin qi, this is referred to as yin collapse. Yang collapse displays cold manifestations such as cold sweating and reversal cold of the limbs. Yin collapse shows heat manifestations such as profuse sweating with warm skin, restlessness, and a racing, rapid pulse.

A condition without obvious manifestations of either cold or heat along with exhaustion of vital functions is simply called qi desertion. All forms of qi desertion and collapse are critical conditions.

Section 3   Blood (*Xuè*, 血)

GENERATION OF BLOOD

Blood is generated from food-essence and kidney-essence through the processes of qi transformation and the functions of the spleen, stomach, heart, lung and kidney.

The basic material for blood generation is food-essence

The spleen and stomach receive and transform water and grain while also refining and transporting the essential substances. The refined substances become *ying* qi and body fluids which then pass into the vessels and engender blood. Therefore, the *ying* qi and body fluids derived from food-essence not only generate blood, but are also its main components. The spleen and stomach are called the "source of qi and blood production". Thus, weakened spleen and stomach function can lead to blood deficiency.

Kidney-essence is also a basic material for blood generation

Treatise on the Origins and Manifestations of Various Diseases (*Zhū Bìng Yuán Hòu Lùn*, 诸病源候论) states, "The kidney stores essence, from which blood comes", and that "essence and blood mutually supplement and transform into each other". The essence-qi in the kidney should be plentiful to supplement the generation of blood, while kidney-essence can also transform into liver blood.

The kidney activates the functions of the spleen and stomach, which then generates blood. If kidney-essence is inadequate or the kidney fails to store essence, the production of blood will be decreased. Therefore, patterns of blood deficiency are often treated by supplementing the kidney and enriching essence. It should be remembered that in Chinese medicine, both marrow and bone are closely related to the kidney.

The heart and lung also play an important role in the process of blood generation

Ying qi and body fluids transformed by the spleen and stomach are transported upward to the lung and heart, where they combine with the qi inhaled by the lung. Under the action of heart qi, both are then infused into the heart vessels to form "red blood".[1]

FUNCTIONS OF BLOOD

Xue is translated as blood, which in Chinese medicine has broader implications than the blood of biomedicine in that the *xue*/blood acts to nourish and moisten the body while also generating the spirit. Blood is transformed from food-essence, thus providing the nutrients necessary for nourishing and moistening the tissues and *zang-fu* organs. The functions of blood are reflected in the spirit, complexion, flesh, skin, hair, sensory functions, and even body movement. With deficient blood and impaired nourishing and moistening, signs and symptoms include a pale complexion, dry skin, lusterless hair, and numbness or weakness of the limbs and muscles. In addition, blood deficiency is often implicated in cases of constipation, insomnia, fatigue, and

---

① This process is the function of *zong* qi.

menstrual disorders.

The spirit is in the blood

Blood is the material basis for mental activities in that mental activity depends upon the nourishing function of blood. When the blood and qi are plentiful, the mind can be clear, have the ability to work long hours, have good judgment, agile thinking, and clear speech. On the contrary, when there is blood deficiency or abnormal blood circulation, there can be emotional or mental disorders such as mental fatigue, forgetfulness, anxiety, insomnia, confusion, restlessness, fright, or even delirium and coma.

The responses of the organ-essence and qi to external stimuli can produce different emotional activities. The seven emotions include anger, joy, grief, thinking, sorrow, fear, and fright, and are all emotional experiences responding to outside stimuli. *The Spiritual Pivot* states, "Deficiency of heart qi leads to sorrow, and excessive heart qi leads to endless laughing." *The Spiritual Pivot* states that "An excess of blood leads to anger, and deficiency of blood leads to fear."

The generation of spirit is not only based on vital substances, but the spirit also has the ability to command and control these same substances to maintain normal metabolism in the body. Organ-essence and qi generate the spirit, and the spirit regulates the physiological functions of the *zang-fu* organs by governing the organ-essence and qi. Under normal circumstances, mental activities based on the essence and qi of the *zang*-organs also act to regulate the circulation and movement of organ-qi. So it is said, "The five *zang*-organs store the five spirits" and "The five *zang*-organs dominate the five emotions". Some types of specific mental activities can also regulate the *zang-fu* organs in order to assist recovery from physical disorders.

BLOOD CIRCULATION

The normal circulation of blood in the vessels is influenced by multiple factors, including the functions of several *zang-fu* organs. Blood belongs to yin, which has calming and cooling properties; therefore, blood depends on the warming and propelling actions of qi. When the activating and warming function of yang qi weakens, the speed of blood circulation reduces; however, without the calming, cooling and moistening functions of yin qi, the blood may move too quickly. Therefore, yin qi and yang qi must remain coordinated to maintain normal blood circulation.

The vessels are the passageways for blood circulation, where qi acts to contain the blood within the vessels. The qi functions of propelling and containing must also remain coordinated to support the normal circulation of blood.

BLOOD DISORDERS

There are three types of blood disorders. The first is blood deficiency, which results from insufficient generation or overconsumption of blood. The second condition is blood stasis, and the third is bleeding.[1]

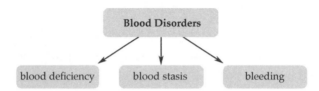

Blood Deficiency (*Xuè Xū*, 血虚)

Blood deficiency involves a shortage of blood and/or its nourishing action. It should be emphasized that blood deficiency is defined more as a deficiency of the nourishing and functional properties of blood, rather than a deficiency of the quantity of blood.[2] Blood deficiency can occur for several reasons, such as in cases where new blood is not being generated, or because of heavy bleeding. A lack of spleen qi or dietary deficiencies may create insufficient generation of blood, while internal dryness and heat as well as chronic disease can result in the consumption of blood.

The heart governs the blood and vessels, and the liver stores blood, so signs and symptoms of both heart blood and liver blood deficiency are most common. Manifestations of heart blood deficiency with blood failing to nourish the heart include palpitations, insomnia, profuse dreaming, forgetfulness, and a thready and choppy or intermittent pulse. Liver blood deficiency manifestations include dry eyes, blurred vision, numbness of the hands and feet, and impaired joint movement. When liver blood is deficient, this can lead to disharmony of the *chong mai* and *ren mai*, manifesting with scanty menstruation, delayed menstruation, or amenorrhea (lack of menses).

---

[1] Some texts define only two kinds of blood disorders: those due to deficiency and those due to blood movement disorders (including both stasis and bleeding).

[2] Therefore, an often asked question is if blood deficiency is the same as anemia in biomedicine. The answer is that while there are some overlaps, there are innumerable blood deficiency conditions that would not show as anemia in a blood test.

Blood Stasis (*Xuè Yū*, 血瘀)

Blood stasis[1] is a state of impaired blood circulation that can result from qi deficiency, yang deficiency, yin deficiency, qi stagnation, turbid phlegm, blood cold, or heat in the blood.[2] Blood stasis patterns can present with obstruction, stagnation, or coagulation of blood which may be a general disorder or a more specific disorder localized in part of the *zang-fu* organs, channels and collaterals, body areas or orifices.

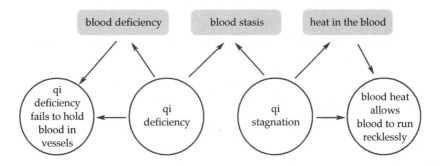

Normal blood circulation depends on heart, lung, liver and spleen functions, the propelling and controlling actions of qi, the smoothness of the vessel system, as well as the temperature of both internal and external environments. Any of the factors listed above that create normal circulation of blood, but when disordered, can lead to the formation of blood stasis. After it forms, blood stasis not only diminishes the nourishing function of blood, but it also can create new diseases.

"Blood is the mother of qi." Once blood stasis forms, qi stagnation becomes increased as well, thus it is also said that "blood stasis is always accompanied by stagnation of qi". Furthermore, "Qi is the commander of blood", so any stagnation of qi can also disturb the circulation of blood, locally or generally. A vicious cycle consequently develops in which blood stasis causes qi stagnation and qi stagnation causes blood stasis. For instance, if surgical trauma damages the blood vessels and causes bleeding, qi stagnation manifests in a local area with swelling and pain.

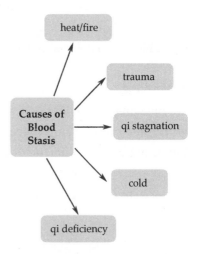

---

① In this section we will try to adhere to the concept that blood stasis is a larger process than static blood which is more specific.

② Gunter Neeb. *Blood Stasis*. London: Churchill Livingstone; 2007. p. 15.

Stasis occurs as the viscosity and thickness of the blood affects normal circulation. If there is turbid phlegm in the blood or the blood itself is too thick, the resulting sluggish or stagnated circulation can lead to stasis. Invasion of yin-pathogens or internal cold can also cause a prominence of yin-cold which constrains and obstructs the vessels, also causing slow blood circulation and blood stasis. Additionally, trauma to the body often causes stasis as well as bleeding.

Blood stasis is a condition or pattern where there is a loss of the nourishing functions of blood. Over time this can also seriously affect the flow of qi and blood in the body. When the organs fail to be nourished, the abnormal functioning that results will inevitably affect the production of fresh blood. As examples, a patient with prolonged blood stasis may have dry skin, lusterless hair or abnormal menses.

Blood stasis can affect the functions of the heart, liver, and vessels, leading to abnormal blood circulation systemically or in a local area. If there is blood stasis in the heart, blockage of the heart vessels results in chest *bi* and heart pain. Static blood in the liver can block the liver vessels resulting in an obstructed flow of qi and blood. Blood stasis can damage the vessel system and blood might extravasate the vessels, leading to "static blood" and the appearance of dark purplish blood mixed with clots. When blood stasis blocks the channels, the smooth flow of qi and blood becomes impaired, leading to dark purplish lips, purplish areas on the skin, petechia on the tongue, and a pulse with a choppy quality. More seriously, blood stasis and static blood are often implicated in the formation of tumors and other benign and malignant cancers.

The concepts of "static blood" and "blood stasis" are discussed in detail in Chapter 4. Blood stasis can be described as a pathological condition or pattern while static blood is a specific pathological product.

Bleeding

Bleeding can be defined as any blood that leaves the vessels, whether contained within the body or not. Bleeding can be caused by a number of factors that overlap including either deficiency or stasis. The causes of bleeding include qi deficiency, blood stasis, traumatic injury, and blood heat, much of which has been described above. There are also special conditions such as heat that forces blood to flow

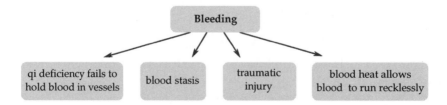

"recklessly" out of the vessels, or otherwise impair the vessels.

Deficient qi failing to contain blood

Deficient qi failing to contain blood can be result of the failure of (spleen) qi to control blood which then results in blood leaving the vessels. We often see this pattern in middle-aged and elderly people who bruise easily or develop spontaneous bruising on the skin. Additionally, children with spleen weakness are often prone to nosebleeds. The signs and symptoms of qi deficiency also include coughing of blood, purpura (discoloration of the skin), bloody stool, bloody urine, and profuse vaginal bleeding. At the same time, signs of qi deficiency include fatigue, a weak pulse, and a pale tongue.

Bleeding due to blood stasis

This type of bleeding means that blood leaves the vessels as a result of stasis. Bleeding due to blood stasis is a bit counter-intuitive to diagnose, and a thorough understanding of the condition is required. Treatment can be problematic in that treatment methods that move static blood are required despite the serious loss of blood caused by the bleeding.

Traumatic injury

Involving car accidents, knife wounds and the like will obviously cause bleeding and may lead to blood stasis and static blood, especially when blood remains within the body outside of the vessels.

Blood heat

Blood heat is a pathological state in which heat enters the blood vessels which then accelerates the blood flow. Excess heat expands the vessels, which then leads to bleeding, commonly caused by an invasion of heat into the *ying-* and blood-levels.[1] In addition, blood heat may also be caused by blood-level accumulation of internal fire induced by the five emotions, or by yin deficiency with exuberant fire.[2]

The clinical manifestations of blood heat are characterized by both heat signs and bleeding. In addition to general heat signs and symptoms, there is often redness of the skin, eyes, and tongue with agitation or restlessness and an abnormal pulse. In extreme cases there can be coma, delirious speech, and mania.

---

[1]   (*xuè fēn*, 血分) blood-level

[2]   (*yīn xū huǒ wàng*, 阴虚火旺) yin deficiency with extreme fire, defined in the Wiseman Practical Dictionary as "effulgent yin vacuity fire".

Section 4   Fluids (*Jīn Yè*, 津液)

BASIC CONCEPT OF FLUIDS

Jīn yè refers to all fluids within the body, including those inside the structures of the *zang-fu* organs. With the exception of the essence stored in the *zang-fu* organs and the blood circulating in the vessels, all other types of normal fluid substances are usually referred to as *jīn yè*.

Jīn yè is a collective term for thin fluids (*jīn*) and thick fluids (*yè*). *Jīn*-fluids scatter on the surface of the skin, flesh and orifices, go into the vessels, and have a moistening function. *Yè*-fluids are more viscous and sticky. They enter the joints, organs, brain, and marrow where they act to nourish and lubricate.

Jīn yè is derived from water and food received, then generated by the functions of the spleen and stomach and other *zang-fu* organs. The stomach governs the reception and decomposition of food and water, and absorbs the refined parts of them to create the "clear". The small intestine separates the clear from the turbid, absorbing the food-essence and a large amount of water, then sending the food residue to the large intestine. The large intestine governs the liquid by absorbing water from the food residue and thus turns it into stool. The clear food-essence and water absorbed by the stomach, small intestine and large intestine are conveyed upward and scattered to the whole body through the transporting function of spleen qi.

FLUIDS AND THE ORGANS

The transportation and distribution of fluids mainly relies on the coordination of the functions of the spleen, lung, kidney, liver, and *sanjiao*.

Spleen

One of the most important functions of the spleen is to transport and distribute body fluids, and this happens in several ways. The first is to transport the fluids (using spleen qi) up to the lung. The lung qi then diffuses and descends to scatter the fluids over the entire body. Another spleen qi function is to direct fluids directly to the *zang-fu* organs. In addition, fluids in the gastrointestinal tract can pass directly into the bladder through the *sanjiao* by the actions of spleen qi.

Lung

The lung governs diffusion-dispersion and purification-descent, and acts to free and regulate the waterways. After receiving fluids transferred by the spleen, the lung diffuses and disperses fluids to the body surface. Additionally, the lung qi sends the fluids downward and inward to the lower parts of the body and to the *zang-fu* organs. The lung also transforms turbid fluids coming from the *zang-fu* organs and sends them to the kidney and urinary bladder. For these reasons, the lung is called the "upper source of water", and this process is referred to as the "lung governing water movement".

If lung qi fails to diffuse-disperse and purify-descend, the waterways will become blocked, the movement of fluids will be constrained, and as a result there may be the formation of internal phlegm or edema. After being transmitted to the skin by the purifying and downbearing functions of the lung qi, the fluids are transformed by qi to form sweat which is then discharged through the pores of the skin. In addition, some water content is removed from the system through the process of exhalation.

Kidney

The kidney is a water-organ which plays a major role in the metabolism of body fluids due to the kidney qi function of regulating and promoting fluid metabolism. The generation, distribution and excretion of fluids all depend on the stimulation of kidney yang to warm and vaporize[①] fluids, while kidney yin both cools and moistens. If kidney qi is deficient, the normal transmission and distribution of fluids will be affected. The kidney also plays an important role in the transforming of fluids. Through the descending action of the lung qi, turbid fluids from the *zang-fu* organs are transported downward to the kidney, where it is again processed by kidney qi. In this action, the clear part is reabsorbed and sent upward for transformation, while the turbid part is sent downward to the urinary bladder to be transformed into urine for excretion. Therefore, kidney action of ascending the clear upward and descending the turbid is vital for maintaining the normal transformation of body fluids.

Liver

The liver governs the free flow of qi. Normal qi movement is required in order to maintain the waterways and normal fluid distribution, so when the liver fails to maintain the free flow of qi and stagnation results, the transmission and distribution of fluids is often affected. This can lead to the accumulation of water as seen in patterns of phlegm-fluid retention, edema, goiter, a swollen abdomen, and other conditions.

Sanjiao

The *sanjiao* is the passageway for the circulation of water and *yuan* qi throughout

---

① (zhēng, 蒸) vaporize, steam

the body. When the *sanjiao* is unobstructed, the smooth transmission and distribution of fluids is maintained. Obstruction of the *sanjiao* passages leads to fluid accumulation that can lead to a variety of diseases. It is said that most fluid disorders involve issues of the *sanjiao*.

The transmission and distribution of fluids depends on the kidney qi actions of evaporation and regulation, the spleen qi functions of transportation and transformation, lung qi diffusion-dispersion and purification-descent, the freeing function of liver qi, and the free flow of the *sanjiao* waterways. The normal transmission and distribution of fluids is the result of coordinated cooperation among the physiological functions of multiple *zang-fu* organs, so fluid metabolism and distribution can be seen as a comprehensive reflection of overall physiological activity within the body.

FUNCTIONS OF *JĪN YÈ*/FLUIDS

The main functions of *jīn yè*/fluids are to moisten and nourish, supplement blood, and nourish the vessels. *Jīn yè* contain nutrients with strong nourishing functions. The moistening and nourishing functions complement each other. Although we say that the two cannot be separated, we make the distinctions that the *jīn*-fluids are thinner in quality, so its moisturizing effects are more obvious. *Yè* is thicker and more dense, so it is more associated with nourishment. Because of these differences between *jīn* (liquids) and *yè* (humors), we can distinguish pathological damage to the *jīn*-fluids and those of the *yè*-fluid desertion. However, both are generally considered as being similar substances that complement and transform into one another, so they are most often referred to together simply as *jīn yè*/fluids.

Fluids that are distributed on the surface of the body act to moisten the skin, hair, and flesh, while those that enter more deeply into the body will nourish and moisten the *zang-fu* organs. *Jīn*-fluids nourish and moisten the nose, head, mouth, ears and other orifices, while *yè*-fluids infiltrate the bones, bone marrow, spinal cord and brain marrow. The *yè*-fluids also move within the joints to maintain their flexibility.

In addition, fluid metabolism plays an important role in yin-yang regulation while also maintaining a balance between internal and external environments. During hot weather or when there is a fever present, body fluids will be transformed into sweat in order to dissipate heat. During cold weather or when the body has a low temperature, body fluids are prevented from leaving the body surface. Through the interactions of the *ying* qi and *wei* qi, a relatively constant body temperature is maintained. *Wei* qi controls the opening and closing of the pores, thus abnormal sweating is often attributed *ying-wei* disharmony.

DISORDERS OF FLUID METABOLISM

Fluid metabolism depends on the functional coordination of several *zang-fu* organs, among which the lung, spleen, *sanjiao* and kidney play key roles. Disorders in the generation, transportation, and excretion of fluids include shortage of fluids (deficiency) and stagnation of fluids (excess).

Shortage of Fluids

The shortage of fluids involves a series of dry and astringent symptoms and therefore have reduced moistening and nourishing functions. The causative factors are consumption of fluids by heat pathogens, vomiting, diarrhea, profuse sweating, frequent urination, large areas of burns, or the shortage of fluid generation. In addition, weak organ functions or the consumption of fluids in chronic disease may also result in the shortage of fluids.

Clinically, the signs and symptoms have two facets. The first are manifestations appearing following damage to the *jīn*[1] such as sunken temples, dry mouth and tongue, and dry skin that has lost its elasticity, no tears while crying, little urination, listlessness, and cramping. Other manifestations due to the desertion of *yè* include a thin body figure, withered skin and hair, tremors of the hands and feet, trembling muscles, chapped lips, and a "mirrored", glossy, and red tongue with no or little coating.

Generally speaking, damage to *jīn*-fluids involves a loss of water where the thicker *yè*-fluids are not always affected. Therefore the damage to *jīn* is a loss that does not always develop into a desertion of *yè*. Loss of *yè*-fluids not only also involves the concurrent loss of *jīn*-fluids, but also and more importantly, a loss of essential nutritive substances. Any damage to *yè*-fluids also damages *jīn*-fluids; therefore, in terms of the severity of a condition, desertion of *yè*-fluids is more serious than damage to *jīn*-fluids.

Stagnation of Fluids

Stagnation of fluids is a pathological state in which fluids cannot be transported and distributed normally and thus circulate slowly or stagnate in a particular part of the body. The disturbance of the distribution and excretion of fluids may lead to stagnation of turbid dampness, retention of phlegm and fluid, and retention of water.

Turbid dampness stagnation[2] commonly results from spleen qi deficiency. Because dampness is not considered to be a "clear" or useful fluid, it is often described as "turbid". Decreased transformation and transportation of fluids affects

---

① Some texts will translate *jīn* as fluids and *yè* as humours.
② (*shī zhuó kùn zǔ*, 湿浊困阻) turbid fluids blocked

normal distribution, thus leading to an accumulation of turbid dampness that blocks the free flow of qi in the middle *jiao*. Manifestations include chest distress, stomach cavity *pǐ* (痞, blocked sensation), nausea and vomiting, distending sensations in the abdomen, loose stools, and a greasy tongue coating.

Phlegm and fluid retention[1] mainly involves the lung, spleen-stomach, *sanjiao* and heart. Dysfunction of the spleen and lung leads to retention of fluids which in turn coagulate into phlegm. Phlegm can move along with the flow of qi within the channels and collaterals or stay within the *zang-fu* organs.

Water retention[2] is caused by dysfunctions of the lung, spleen, kidney, and liver. The liver qi fails to promote the flow of qi which slows the movement of fluids and disturbs normal fluid metabolism. For example, fluids lodged in the chest and ribsides is called pleural fluid retention, or pleural effusion.[3] Stagnated in the skin or body can also manifest as edema or ascites among many other conditions.[4]

The differences between phlegm, turbid dampness and water retention (pathological fluids) often are subtle and overlap both in texts and in the clinic. Generally (although not always), phlegm is thick and turbid in nature, whereas retained water is more thin and clear in nature. (Other fluid issues regarding phlegm and fluid retention are discussed in detail in Chapter 4.)

Section 5   Interrelationships of Essence, Qi, Blood, Fluids

Essence, blood, and fluids depend upon and supplement one another. Compared with qi, essence, and blood, fluids are relatively more yin in nature. Both essence and blood are generated from food-essence, which are transformed mainly through the actions of spleen qi. These liquid substances act together to moisten and nourish the entire body, while also playing a part in the generation of spirit. Essence, blood, and fluids mutually transform and supplement each other through the actions of qi as they convert into and nourish each other. They also influence one

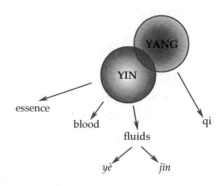

---

①   (*tán yǐn níng jù*, 痰饮凝聚) phlegm and fluid concentration or retention
②   (*shuǐ yè zhù liú*, 水液潴留) water fluids remain stored or retained
③   (*xuán yǐn*, 悬饮) pleural effusion
④   (*yì yǐn*, 溢饮) subcutaneous fluid retention

another pathologically. This relationship demonstrates the theory that "essence and blood come from the same source" and "fluids and blood are from the same source".

QI AND BLOOD

As the two main fundamental substances in the body, qi and blood depend upon and promote one another. Qi pertains to yang, and blood to yin. Their relationship can be summarized as "qi is the commander of blood, blood is the mother of qi".

The concept of qi commanding the blood includes three facets: qi generating blood, qi circulating blood, and qi containing blood.

"Qi generating blood" has two meanings

First, qi is the driving force that generates blood. Secondly, *ying* qi flows into the blood vessels and then transforms into blood. Therefore, the abundance of qi creates the active generation of blood. When qi is deficient, the generation of blood is decreased and the result is blood deficiency. Therefore, when treating blood deficiency, treatments that nourish blood and supplement qi are often used together.

The circulation of blood is inseparable from the propelling actions of qi

The smooth circulation of blood depends on the propelling actions of heart and lung qi, as well as the smooth flow of liver qi. Blood stasis results either when deficient qi fails to nourish the blood, or when qi fails to move the blood due to qi stagnation. Furthermore, disorders of qi can cause frenetic blood movement, also leading to conditions such as "blood ascending with qi counterflow" or "blood descending and qi sinking". Therefore, when treating blood circulation disorders, treatments that supplement and move qi are often used together.

"Qi containing blood"[①] implies that the normal circulation of blood inside the vessels depends on the containing function of qi

Ample spleen qi acts to control the blood inside the vessels in order to prevent it from leaving the vessels. However, when spleen qi is insufficient, the blood fails to be controlled, often leading to various bleeding conditions associated with "qi failing to control blood" or "spleen failing to control blood". For these conditions, the principles of treatment are to strengthen the spleen and supplement qi. In critical cases with severe bleeding, a large dose of qi-supplementing herbs are employed to contain the blood along with herbs that specifically stop bleeding (hemostatics).

---

① (*qì néng shè xuè*, 气能摄血) qi contains blood

Blood pertains to yin, and qi to yang

The coordination and balance between yin and yang and qi and blood is essential to good health. Therefore, adjusting the relationship between qi and blood is a fundamental approach to treatment.

The statement "blood is the mother of qi" has two aspects in that blood both nourishes and carries qi. Abundant qi also depends on the moistening and nourishing functions of blood, whereas blood constantly provides nutrients for the generation of qi. Therefore, sufficient blood leads to sufficient qi. If the blood fails to provide any part of the body with adequate nutrients, dysfunctions or deficiencies of qi may also result. Insufficient qi can also lead to blood deficiency and/or blood stasis. Qi in the vessels attaches itself to the blood so that it can be carried throughout the body by the blood. For this reason, patients with blood deficiency most often also present with signs of qi deficiency.

Patients afflicted with uncontrolled bleeding can also lose a considerable quantity of qi, which in severe cases may lead to a condition called "qi desertion following blood loss".

ESSENCE AND QI

Qi promotes generation of essence and controls essence

Essence stored in the kidney is based on innate essence, and depends upon constant supplement of acquired foodstuff essence. Only when the spleen and stomach qi is sufficient and coordinated in ascending-descending, and function normally, can the refined essence from water and grain be well transported and absorbed so as to supplement the visceral essence, and, after utilization, the surplus part of the visceral essence pours into the kidney to nourish and support the innate essence, becoming part of kidney-essence. Thus, the generation of essence depends on the sufficiency of qi. Qi cannot only promote generation of essence, but also can control essence to keep it from undue loss. This is the embodiment of the controlling function of qi. Therefore, deficiency of qi will cause decrease of essence generation, or essence deficiency and loss of essence because of failure of qi to control. So the therapeutic methods of supplementing qi to generate essence or supplementing qi to control essence are often used clinically.

Essence transforms into qi

Essence in the body can transform into different kinds of qi under the promotion and stimulation of qi. Essence in *zang-fu* organs can transform into qi of *zang-fu* organs, innate essence stored in the kidney can transform into original qi, and foodstuff essence can transform into foodstuff qi. Essence is the root of qi production, so sufficient essence keeps human qi in abundance for distributing into *zang-fu* organs and channels-collaterals to make qi in them sufficient. Sufficient visceral essence results in abundant visceral qi, so that the physiological functions of *zang-fu* organs, body constituents and orifices are well promoted and regulated. Therefore sufficient essence makes sound qi, and deficient essence makes qi declined. In clinic, patients suffering from essence deficiency or loss of essence often manifest symptoms of qi deficiency.

ESSENCE AND BLOOD

Essence is one of the basic materials required for the generation of blood. The kidney stores essence, from which the blood is created, and the liver stores the blood. As essence generates blood, blood can also transform into essence; thus it is said that "essence and blood are from the same source".

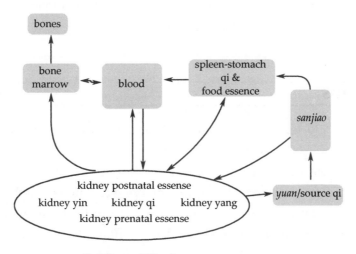

Essence and Blood

Furthermore, the essence-qi of the *zang*-organs is also involved in the transformation of blood as associated with each respective organ. The essence-qi in the organs, or organ-essences, merge[①] in the vessels to produce blood: the essence-qi of the liver takes part in the production of liver blood, and the essence-qi of the heart produces heart blood. Regarding the spleen, the food-essence transformed and absorbed by the spleen is transformed into *ying* qi, while the more refined and clear parts transform into fluids which enter the vessels and become blood. Because kidney-essence distributes to and supports the essence-qi of all the organs in the body, only with sufficient kidney-essence can these various transformations between essence and

---

① (*róng rù*, 融入) merges, blends

blood occur.

Problems

Food-essence is also a main source of blood generation, where kidney-essence depends on constant supplementation as provided by the acquired essence. At the same time, blood can transform into essence in order to supplement and nourish the essence in the kidney. Therefore, abundant blood ensures sufficient essence, while a shortage of blood can lead to an insufficiency of essence.

The kidney is the organ primarily associated with the storage of essence, and the process of kidney-essence transformation into blood is most significant. Kidney-essence transforms into blood, and blood nourishes the hair, so the hair is said to be "the exterior manifestation of the kidney" as well as "the extension of the blood". Blood deficiency due to kidney-essence exhaustion may result in hair loss or withered hair along with other manifestations of kidney deficiency such as soreness of the lower back and knees, scanty menses, scanty semen, a lusterless complexion, dizziness, tinnitus, mental fatigue, forgetfulness, delayed menstruation, and infertility.

QI AND FLUIDS

Regarding qi and fluids, qi pertains to yang and fluids to yin. The relationship between qi and fluids is very similar to that of qi and blood. The generation, distribution, and release of fluids all depend on the functions of qi, whereas normal qi function also depends on the moistening and carrying functions of fluids.

Qi controls the release and excretion of fluids in order to maintain a relatively constant amount of fluids in the body, and the containing function of qi prevents undue loss of fluids. For example, *wei* qi controls the opening and closing of the sweat pores in order to avoid excessive fluid loss, and kidney qi controls the lower two yin-orifices (urethra and anus) to avoid excessive fluid discharge. When qi becomes deficient, there may be excessive sweating, spontaneous sweating, and incontinence. For this reason, qi-supplementing methods are often used in cases of excessive fluid loss.

Jīn-fluids and *yè*-fluids are two bodily substances that carry qi. Outside of the blood vessels, qi attaches itself to the fluids; if this were not to occur, the qi would instead float

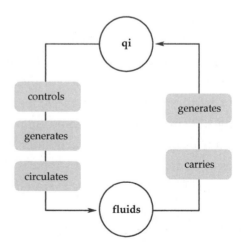

outward and disperse. Because of this relationship, loss of fluids will inevitably cause a loss of qi. For example, in summerheat patterns, not only are body fluids consumed, but qi also leaks outward with sweat. This gives rise to signs of qi deficiency such as shortness of breath, unwillingness to speak, and fatigue. With profuse sweating, heavy vomiting, or diarrhea, a great loss of fluids will lead to a severe loss of qi, referred to as "qi desertion with heavy loss of fluids". Therefore, in clinical practice, one must use with caution when applying diaphoresis (sweating), emesis (vomiting), and purgation (defecation) methods, as their overuse may lead to more severe or complex conditions.

Problems

Because fluids are the carrier of qi, normal fluid metabolism also ensures the smooth flow of qi. When the circulation of fluids is blocked, this often leads to a stagnation of qi flow called "qi stagnation with fluid retention"; when complicated by "failure of qi to move water", a vicious cycle is often produced with a rapidly

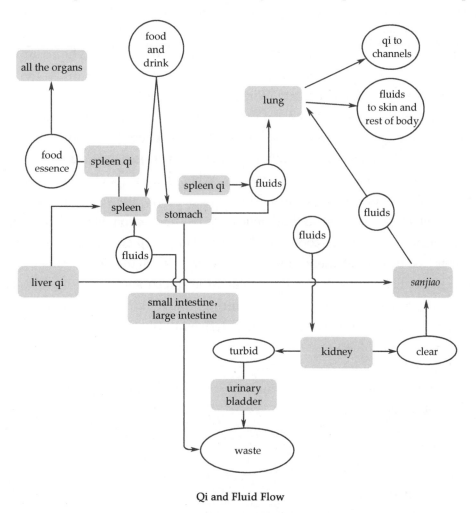

Qi and Fluid Flow

deteriorating condition. Much more about fluids will be discussed in Chapter 4.

FLUIDS AND BLOOD

Blood and fluids both moisten and nourish, and both are transformed from food-essence. The blood and fluids inside and outside of the vessels are also the basis for mutual transformations between fluids and blood.

Fluids and blood can convert into and nourish each other. Fluids are transformed from food-essence in the middle *jiao* and then brought to the upper *jiao* through the actions of spleen qi. There, through the actions of the heart and lung, fluids seep[①] into the vessels. Inside the vessels, fluids transform and become a component of the blood.

Fluids also convert into sweat. As fluids that scatter over the surface of the skin, they can also penetrate into the minute collaterals where they transform into and supplement the blood. Fluids can also seep out of the vessels in order to supplement any shortage of fluids in the body or to moisten and nourish the *zang-fu* organs, tissues and orifices as needed.

Fluids regulate the concentration or density of blood. When the blood concentration increases, fluids will seep into the blood vessels to dilute the blood and supplement the blood capacity. When the surface of the body is dry, the fluids will seep out of the vessels to moisten the surface. Because of this interplay between the outside and inside of the vessels, the body can regulate the blood concentration in response to physiological and pathological changes. This helps maintain a normal blood volume and the fluidity of the vessels. When there is a deficiency of blood in the vessels, fluids outside of the vessels will flow back into the vessels to supplement the blood which can give rise to fluid deficiency. For this reason, blood deficiency and fluid deficiency often appear concurrently. This relationship of mutual transformation is summarized by the statement, "blood and sweat are from the same source".

When the diet is poor or the functions of the spleen and stomach are weak, or because of profuse sweating, heavy vomiting, diarrhea or serious burns, fluids outside the vessels can become severely deficient. Then not only will fluids be unable to enter the blood vessels to supplement and generate blood, but fluids in the vessels will seep outward to supplement the shortage of fluids outside of the vessels. This scenario may lead to shortages of blood, thickening of the blood, and impaired blood circulation.

---

①   (*shèn chū*, 渗出) seep out

Section 6   Spirit (*Shén*, 神)

Spirit can be understood in both a broad sense and a more narrow sense. In the broad sense, spirit refers to the vital activities of life and all of their external manifestations. In the narrow sense, it refers to mental activities such as consciousness, thought, and emotion. Essence, qi, blood, and fluids comprise a material basis for the generation of spirit, and thus spirit cannot exist independently apart from these substances. The organs and orifices and body structures are all filled with essence, qi, blood, and fluids. Propelled and regulated by organ-qi, the spirit is what is expressed through the complexion, eyes, speech, facial expression, responses, behavior, psychological activity, emotions, sound, breath, and pulse.

The spirit resides in the heart *zang*-organ. *The Yellow Emperor's Inner Classic* refers to the heart as the "monarch-organ", and "the master of *zang-fu* organs". It is also said that "a brilliant monarch (spirit) ensures the harmony of the *zang-fu* organs", and furthermore that "a monarch (spirit) who is unclear endangers the twelve officials (other organs)".[1]

The concept of the "souls" or "spirits" as described below is found in many Asian religions which predate Taoism. Spirituality and religious thought are not often explored in modern medical literature, but the concept of the "five spirits" does remain relevant to mainstream Chinese medical thought.

In Chinese medicine, spirit can be classified into five divisions including the spirit (*shén*, 神), ethereal soul (*hún*, 魂), corporeal soul (*pò*, 魄), thought (*yì*,意) and will (*zhì*, 志), with each spirit stored in a particular *zang*-organ.

The Yellow Emperor's Inner Classic: Basic Questions states that the heart stores the *shén* (spirit), the liver stores the *hún* (ethereal soul), the lung stores the *pò* (corporeal soul), the spleen stores *yì* (thought), and the kidney stores *zhì* (will). When essence, qi, blood, and fluids are abundant and the functions of the *zang-fu* organs are normal, the spirit will remain sound. When these essential substances are disordered, the spirit will also

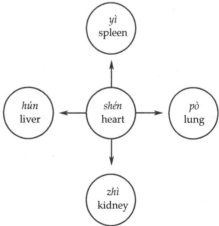

---

[1]   (*zhǔ bù míng zé shí èr guān wēi*, 主不明则十二官危) When the master is unclear he endangers the twelve officials.

become disordered. Furthermore, when the essence-qi of the five organs becomes deficient, the five spirits also fail to be generated and supplemented.

The *shén* can be seen as the ruler of the other spirits, or as an accumulation of them. The *hún* and *pò* are paired, as are the *yì* and *zhì*. The *hún* is yang, associated with wood and is expansive in its motion. It is characterized by creativity and imagination. The *pò* is yin, metal, associated with the lung, and as such is more constrained and thus associated with bodily processes. The *hún* can conceive of creative projects, but it takes the *pò* to implement them into the material world.

The *hún* is associated with collective consciousness, and is said to leave the body at night in dreams. The *pò* is more concrete and predictable, and thus enjoys the rhythms and certainties of physical life. A simple comparison might be to look at scholarly thought as *hún* and physical exercise as *pò*. Yet as it takes the power of *pò* for the scholar to actually sit down and complete a project, the *hún* is also required to create and maintain the physical health of the body. In simple terms, the strong *hún*-type person with a weak *pò* is characterized as a "dreamer" with fantastic ideas but without the ability to actualize their projects. The strong *pò*-type person with a weak *hún* is the "exercise freak", "health nut" or anorexic that may not see the limitations of extreme diets and physical behaviors and thus goes beyond what is actually healthy.

Internal and external information is first sensed and transmitted into the heart where it is perceived, but not yet "processed" by the *yì*. Rossi quotes Zhang Jie-bin, "When a thought is first born, the heart has a direction, but it is not yet stabilized, this is called *yì*."[1] The process of maintaining the memory of these appearances to form the cognition of things is the *zhì* associated with the kidney. *Zhì*, although often translated as "will", is also closely associated with memory. *Yì* which is repeated turns into *zhì*, so *yì* and *zhì* are also classified as a complementary pair.

Beyond the five spirits, there are other somewhat lesser used terms that remain present in the medical literature. On the basis of *zhì*, the process of repeatedly pondering, analyzing and comparing is called ideation (*sī*, 思). Based on ideation, the process of considering the near to far future is called contemplation (*lǜ*,虑). Finally, based on the above, what dominates an individual's behavior to respond appropriately to circumstances is called wisdom or intelligence (*zhì*, 智).[2]

The concepts of spirit in Chinese medicine and ancient philosophy share influences in their formation and development, yet there is clearly a strict distinction between them. While the *hún* and *pò* are culturally engrained as associated with ghosts and spirits, modern Chinese texts often stress that the spirit in Chinese medicine is

---

①   Elisa Rossi. *Shen*: *Psycho-emotional Aspects of Chinese Medicine*. London: Churchill-Livingstone; 2007. p. 64.

②   Eisenstark, D. Addictions, Recovery and the Five Spirits. Journal of Chinese Medicine. Oct 2010; 94.

dependent on material for its production, thus avoiding any sense of metaphysics. [1]

Some Western practitioners who are making an effort to introduce "spiritual psychology" into diagnosis and treatment may find these concepts useful. Yet practitioners would also be wise to be careful to distinguish their role as adjunctive, and also as quite separate from psychotherapy. In *Transforming Emotions with Chinese Medicine*, Zhang Yan-hua states that the doctor is more of an advisor than psychiatrist; "a Chinese TCM doctor does not pose him or herself as an expert in emotions, but as a wise person who has accumulated practical wisdom through life and professional experiences ... the TCM doctor very often forges a connection with the patient by transforming the 'patient's problem' into shared human conditions..." [2]

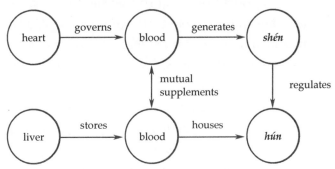

Heart, Liver, Blood, *Shén* and *Hún* Relations

RELATIONSHIPS AMONG ESSENCE, QI AND SPIRIT

Essence, qi and spirit, are called the "three treasures" of the human body. Essence and qi can transform into each other, while both essence and qi act to generate and support the spirit. In turn, the spirit can control both essence and qi.

The endless circulation of qi also promotes the generation of essence. The essence stored in the kidney is based on congenital essence, but it also depends upon constant supplementation from the postnatal or acquired essence. Only when the spleen and stomach qi are abundant[3] and functioning normally can the refined essences of water and grain be well-transported and absorbed so as to supplement the essence-qi of the organs. The surplus of essential organ-qi pours into the kidney to nourish and support the congenital essence, thus becoming part of kidney-essence. So the generation of essence depends on a sufficient supply of qi in the body.

Qi not only promotes the generation of essence, but it also can control the essence

---

[1] For further reading about spirits within the medical context see *The Psychological Significance of Yuanshen and Shishen* by Lifang Qu and Mary Garvey. Journal of Chinese Medicine. Oct 2009; (91).

[2] Yanhua Zhang. *Transforming Emotions with Chinese Medicine*. New York: SUNY Press; 2007. p. 125.

[3] (*chōng zú*, 充足) adequate, sufficient, ample

to prevent its undue loss; this is the embodiment of the controlling function of qi. Therefore, a deficiency of qi will lead to decreased generation of essence, where the failure of qi to control essence can give rise to a loss of essence. For these conditions, the respective principles of treatment are to supplement qi to generate essence and to supplement qi to control essence.

Essence in the body can transform into different kinds of qi. Essence can transform into the essential qi of the *zang-fu* organs, congenital essence stored in the kidney transforms into *yuan*/original qi, and food-essence can transform into food-qi. Essence is the root of qi production, so sufficient essence maintains an abundance of qi for distribution into the *zang-fu* organs and the channels and collaterals. Sufficient organ-essence results in abundant organ-qi so that the functions of *zang-fu* organs, body parts, and orifices are well-promoted and well-regulated. Therefore, sufficient essence supports qi, and deficient essence leads to qi deficiency. Patients with essence deficiency or loss of essence often show concurrent signs and symptoms of qi deficiency.

Both essence and qi are the fundamental materials for the generation of spirit, where the spirit depends on the nourishment of essence and qi to function normally. Sufficient essence is said to maintain the spirit-brightness, whereas an insufficiency of essence leads to fatigue of the spirit. In short, the spirit is the master of all life activity, where essence and qi and blood and fluids are all fundamental materials for the generation of spirit. Because the spirit is not independent of the physical body, the spirit resides among the bodily constituents.

Essence, qi and spirit have a dynamic relationship where essence is the material basis for spirit, while the spirit has the power to promote the movement of qi and to govern essence. The functional activities of *zang-fu* organs, body constituents, and orifices, as well as the metabolism of such vital substances as essence, qi and blood, must all be adjusted and dominated by the spirit.

The spirit is the master of the body, while the body houses the spirit. When there is an abundance of essence and qi, the spirit is peaceful and calm; however, when the spirit is disturbed, essence will be lost and qi will decline. Thus the statement, "the presence of spirit indicates a favorable prognosis, and loss of spirit indicates a poor prognosis."

CASES

This chapter contains a vast amount of material, yet it is vital that students understand these essential processes and substances. Below are a few brief case studies that can be explored with a teacher to help students begin to sort out the processes associated with the substances.

1. Your patient is a 50-year-old man with recurrent episodes of bronchitis with thick yellow sputum and tiredness. He lives in a city that is often cold and foggy. He drinks 2 to 3 beers every day, and does not smoke cigarettes. He writes for a living, and although he takes daily walks his lifestyle is mainly sedentary. His tongue has a thick yellow coating, and his pulse is slippery.

2. Your patient is a 42-year-old woman who had recently broken up with her boyfriend of 5 years. Since that time she has had a time concentrating and eating. She cannot sleep more than 3 hours without waking up and after that she often can't get back to sleep. She claims she is not upset by the breakup since she initiated it, but does admit she finds her co-workers very annoying recently. She works full time as a physical fitness trainer and often exercises after work. Despite having gone off birth control 4 years ago, she hasn't had a menstrual period in 6 years. Her tongue is red with no coating, and her pulse is wiry and thready.

3. Your patient is a 38-year-old man who comes in for pain in his shoulders. He has been to chiropractors and massage therapists, which help for a few days or hours. He works at a job he doesn't like, working long hours with computers. He doesn't make eye contact as he talks to you, and is vague about when the physical symptoms began. His tongue is large with a thick greasy coating and contains many teeth marks. His pulse is slippery. He also complains of insomnia and constipation.

Chapter 3

Organ Manifestation (*Zàng Xiàng*, 藏象)

In Chinese medicine there are five yin organs, six yang organs and 6 "extraordinary" organs. Chinese medicine views the internal organs not only as physical structures, but also according to the theory of visceral/organ manifestation (*zàng xiàng*, 藏象) which studies the organs' functional interconnections as well as the essential qi-blood-fluids associated with them. There are also associations between the organs and other body structures and openings (orifices), as well as relationships between the organs and the natural and social environments. The following chapter looks at each of the organs and their many interconnections.

INTRODUCTION TO THE ORGANS

In Chinese medicine, "organs" refers to the five yin *zang*-organs (liver, heart, spleen, lung and kidney), the six yang *fu*-organs (gallbladder, stomach, small intestine, large intestine, bladder and *sanjiao*), and the extraordinary *fu*-organs (brain, marrow, bone, vessel, gallbladder and uterus). Throughout history, the distinction between the pericardium and the heart has often been indistinct, but the pericardium is now considered not as an organ, but an attachment to the heart.[1]

The character *zàng* (藏) suggests hiding and storing and *xiàng* (象) implies an "image", "manifestation", external appearance, similarity or resemblance. The connotation of *"zàng xiàng"* (visceral/organ manifestation) therefore creates an inseparable relationship between *"zàng"* (internal organ) and *"xiàng"* (outward manifestations). *Zàng* is the core of *xiàng*, while *xiàng* is the outward manifestation of the internal *zang*-organs. Chinese medicine understands both internal organ function and organ pathology also in accordance with their outward manifestations; therefore, we have statements such as "the organs inside the body present themselves to the outside", and "one can understand the internal organs by observing their outside

---

[1] Within the channel and collateral system however, the pericardium has its own channel, making for six acupuncture yin-channels.

presentations".

Zàng should be seen as conceptually different from the strictly physical organ. *Zàng* is the combination of the physicality of its structure and its functions. Therefore, *zàng* implies functional processes based on the framework of physical structure. For example, when we say "the heart stores the spirit" it does not mean that the spirit is held in the center of the chest as if within a bag. However, physical damage or dysfunction to the heart-*zang* will often create a spirit disorder, just as spirit disorders have the potential to eventually damage the structure of the heart-*zang* itself. In fact, even in a spirit disorder in which there is no physical damage to the heart, the condition is still viewed as a heart disorder.

The theory of "organ manifestation" holds that the various components of the body are structurally inseparable, functionally interdependent, metabolically coordinated, and pathologically interactive. The channels system links the five *zang*-organs to the other six-*fu* organs, the five sense organs, the "nine openings"[1], the four limbs and the hundreds of bones, so as to form an organic whole.

In addition, the physiological activities of the five *zang*-organs are also closely related to what we see as psychological activity. For example, we say that "the liver stores the ethereal soul (*hún*, 魂) and anger is its emotion; the heart stores the spirit (*shén*, 神) and joy is its emotion; the spleen stores thought (*yì*, 意) and thinking is its emotion; the lung stores the corporeal soul (*pò*, 魄) and sorrow is its emotion; the kidney stores the will (*zhì*, 志) and fear is its emotion". The physiological and psychological functions and the pathological changes of any organ cannot be separated from the other functions that the organ possesses.

There are many statements in Chinese medicine which overlap with those of biomedicine, while others may seem strange from the biomedicine perspective. We have statements such as "the heart governs the blood and vessels", "the lung controls breathing", "the stomach is the reservoir of food and drink", and "the large intestine conveys and transforms waste". In addition, there are expansions of these concepts such as "the heart stores the spirit", with an example being that a person's heart beats faster when frightened. In clinical practice, physicians noticed that supplementing the kidney organ-system promotes the healing of bone fractures; therefore, we have the concept that "the kidney dominates bone". Because there is muscular loss in a patient with spleen deficiency, we have the concept that "the spleen governs the muscles".

---

[1]   The nine openings are those of the eyes, ears, nose, mouth, anus and urethra.

CHARACTERISTICS OF THE FIVE *ZANG*-ORGANS, THE SIX *FU*-ORGANS, AND THE EXTRAORDINARY *FU*-ORGANS

The five *zang*-organs are internal organs with compact tissue structures which are considered as relatively solid. Inside of the organs is "essence-qi" (*jīng qì*, 精气) (sometimes called essential qi), which is made up of *jīng* (essence), fluids, qi, and sometimes blood. The *zang*-organs both generate and store the essence-qi. The Chinese ancients believed that essences are the basic substances for creating and maintaining the human body. Essence is thus extremely precious and should not flow out[①] of the body; rather it should be stored and moved about within the body. This reference to essence-qi flowing outward refers to conditions with excessive blood loss as in menstrual bleeding, or from excessive sweating, or from excess sexual activity.

The essence-qi stored in the five *zang*-organs moves continuously so that it may function at any given moment without interruption. Because essence-qi is vital, having a full supply of essence-qi is always desirable. [②]

The six *fu*-organs are the internal organs which receive, contain, digest and decompose food and water while also transporting and excreting waste. The six *fu*-organs are hollow by nature, often in the form of tubes or pouches. They are described as "discharging without storing" and can be "full of food, but should not be stagnated or obstructed". *Fu* (腑) means storeroom or granary, where things must be imported, exported, and in constant circulation as if in a successful and well-running market. The food and water in the six *fu*-organs should only stay temporarily, and need to be circulated constantly to help in digestion and transportation. If food and water stagnates in one of the six *fu*-organs, it will not only reduce its transformation of substances into essence-qi, but also lead to transportation disorders; this creates food retention and urinary difficulties among other conditions. So, the six *fu*-organs should transport and transform food and water without storing. We say then that the six *fu*-organs function well when their qi flows smoothly and (for the most part) downward.

One major statement is that "disorders of the *zang*-organs mainly involve deficiency, while those of a *fu*-organ involve excess". Supplementation is most often the method used in patients with deficiencies of the *zang*-organs, while drainage is more often the method used in patients with excess-type disorders of the *fu*-organs.

The extraordinary *fu*-organs are eight organs which are different from those discussed above. They are structurally similar to the six *fu*-organs in that they are hollow, yet they are also able to hold or store essence and other material substances;

---

① (*bù xiè*, 不泻) not flowing
② (*mǎn ér bù néng shí*, 满而不能实) full but cannot be excessive

in this way they are similar to the five *zang*-organs.

ORGAN-ESSENCE, -QI, -YIN AND -YANG

Organ-essence is a part of the overall essence. It is that which nourishes the organs, and is the material basis for their functions. Actually, the essences of the five *zang*-organs and the overall essence are the same material. They are named differently only because they are in the organs. As well, they are classified into five functional systems because of the different shapes and structures of the organs. Heart-essence exists mainly in the form of heart blood, liver-essence in the form of liver blood, lung-essence in the form of fluids, spleen-essence is the essence of food and water, and kidney-essence comes from the combination of pre-natal (innate) essence and post-natal (acquired) *jīng*/essence.

Organ-qi is an extremely refined substance that has been transformed from the organ-essence which circulates constantly throughout the body. It can also be considered as the distribution of the overall qi in and around the organs, and as the functional force for the *zang*-organs.

Organ-yin and organ-yang are aspects of the organ-qi. The aspect that cools, constrains, moistens, inhibits, and calms organ function is called organ-yin. This might be seen in biomedical terms as that which slows down the body's metabolism. The aspect that warms, activates, and propels is called organ-yang. Organ-yang promotes organ function, and can be seen as that which speeds up the metabolism. These two aspects of yin and yang organ-qi, under normal conditions, mutually coordinate and harmonize so as to maintain the stability and order of all the functions of the organs.

Section 1   Five *Zang*-Organs (and Pericardium) (*Wǔ Zàng*, 五脏)

For the *zang*-organs especially, these pairings are often seen as various ways to see "levels" or "stages" of the disease according to the organs and their functions. The *taiyin* "stage" is seen as the first stage or the yin stage most related to the outside of the body. Depending on the theoretical framework, the *shaoyin* system serves as the "pivot" leading to the deeper *jueyin* level or stage[①]. The influential book, *Treatise on Cold Damage (Shāng Hán Lùn*, 伤寒论) (which is greatly concerned how pathogens

---

① Bensky et al refer to the levels as "warps". (Volker Scheid, Dan Bensky, Andrew Ellis, Randal Barolet. *Formulas and Strategies*. 2nd ed. Seattle: Eastland Press; 2009.)

penetrate into the body) puts the *taiyin* of the yin stages as the most exterior, then the *shaoyin*, with the most interior level being the *jueyin*.

hand		lung
taiyin		
foot		spleen

What follows is a general summary of the six levels or stages and their associated internal organs. Note that we do not include here a complete list of pathological signs and symptoms, as this information is generally provided in classes devoted exclusively to *zang-fu* organ pathologies.

hand		heart
shaoyin		
foot		kidney

hand		pericardium
jueyin		
foot		liver

◆ *Taiyin* — **Lung and Spleen**

The *taiyin* is the opening of the interior of the body to the outside environment. We see this as the lung and skin contact the air, and as the spleen contacts food. Both the lung and spleen are linked to the distribution of fluids throughout the body. The spleen is related to the stomach (*yangming*) and the lung to the bladder (*taiyang*) and we will find that these two *fu-yang* organs have definite relations to fluids as well. The pairing of the spleen with the lung sets off the process of producing the vital substances of qi, blood and fluids which are the fundamental substances required for proper functioning of the body and its systems.

In addition, the *taiyin* system has a sense of rhythm that it likes to maintain. Breathing from the lungs likes to be smooth and regular, and the spleen enjoys a consistent feeding pattern. We know how uncomfortable we can become when breathing is disrupted through a cough or asthma. As well, biomedicine tells us that maintaining a consistent blood sugar level is dependent on a regular schedule of meals given at the same time every day. These are two processes that depend on the outside environment of air and food, which through the actions of the *taiyin*, become well-ordered once inside the body.

LUNG (*FÈI*, 肺)

Main Physiological Functions of the Lung

The main functions of the lung are to govern and control respiration[1], govern water movement, connect the vessels, and govern the management and regulation of the qi of the entire body. The lung not only is the basis of the overall qi of the body,

---

[1] (*zhǔ qì sī hū xī*, 主气司呼吸) govern qi and control respiration

but also assists the heart to circulate blood. In this regard, the lung is compared to a government's "prime minister", the person who reports to and carries out the commands of the emperor or "monarch" (the heart). In addition, the lung is the "issuer of management and regulation"; this means that the lung is the organ that begins the process of carrying out the "orders" of the heart, by communicating them to the rest of the organs. The lung is also said to "link with the hundred vessels" as the lung qi pushes the heart blood throughout the vessels (*mài*, 脉)[1]. In this way, the lung acts as the governor for all of the body's qi.

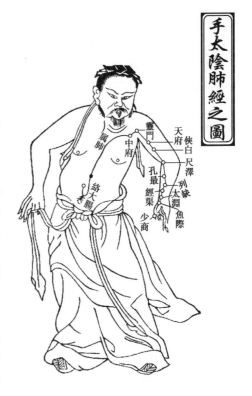

The lung qi acts and moves in several different ways by purifying and moving downward, upward, and outward. The lung takes in clear qi (fresh air) from the exterior and exhales the turbid. The upward and outward movement of lung qi is called "diffusion and dispersion"[2]. Diffusion refers to qi moving out of the lung with exhalation, while dispersion is its outward movement to the surface of the body.

The diffusion and dispersion of lung qi distributes qi and fluids upward and outward in three ways. The first is by exhaling turbid qi from the lungs, and this is self-evident. Next the lung conveys the fluids and a part of food-essence (received from the spleen) up to the orifices of the head and face, and also outward to the skin, hair, and the general body surface. The third aspect is the dispersing of *wei* qi (defensive qi) to the skin, hair and body surface to warm, nourish and moisten the flesh, skin and the body surface. The *wei* qi controls the opening and closing of the pores that secrete the sweat, a form of metabolized fluids. If the lung qi cannot diffuse and disperse because of an exteriorly-contracted condition of pathogenic wind-cold, this will result in breathing disturbances, chest distress, gasping, coughing, aversion to cold, and the expectoration of phlegm; also because the pores are closed, there will be no sweating.

The "purification and descent" function of lung qi acts to distribute qi and fluids

---

①   The "vessels" are like blood vessels, but with a broader connotation. However, in this section one can use the blood vessels as an appropriate image.

②   (*xiàng shàng xiàng wài*, 向上向外) upward and outward

downward and inward, and also manifests in three ways. The first is through the inhaling of air-qi which is then sent down to the rest of the body. [This is an aspect of *zong* qi, which is formed through combination of the inhaled air and the qi of digestion created by the spleen.] The second way is through the distribution of fluids and essence that are transported downward and inward to the other organs for the purposes of nourishment. Ye Tianshi, in *Handbook of Clinical Case Histories* (*Lín Zhèng Zhǐ Nán Yī Àn*, 临证指南医案) in 1746 writes about the lung: "Its nature is to be clear and aloft, and its functional quality is to expand downwards, purify and descend, and be in charge of all descending movement within the body."[1]

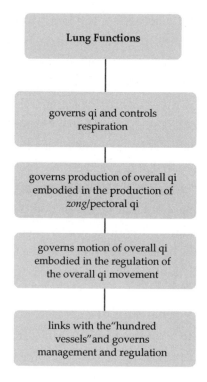

The last aspect of purification and descent is the conveying of turbid or impure fluids from the organs into the kidney and bladder where it is turned into urine and discharged out of the body. If the lung qi fails to purify and descend, this will lead to shallow and short breathing with panting or coughing due to "qi counterflow", sometimes accompanied by constipation and/or difficult urination.

The coordinated motions of lung qi in diffusion-dispersion and purification-descent maintains free and even respiration, thus making for a normal exchange of qi in and out of the body. As mentioned earlier, the even and rhythmic actions of the lung are an important feature of *taiyin* actions. In *Applied Channel Theory in Chinese Medicine*, Wang proposes that this interchange of the "clear and turbid" takes place at all levels within the vessels as well. "Lung function is therefore thought to be everywhere in the body–wherever vessels can be found. Either at the cellular level or within the lung organ itself, *taiyin* lung function is associated with the separation of clear and turbid qi from the external environment."[2]

The lung dominates qi

Apart from governing the qi of the breath, the lung is said to "dominate the qi" of the organs and tissues of the whole body. This produces and circulates the overall qi

---

[1]   http://www.itmonline.org/5organs/lung.htm

[2]   Wang Ju-yi, Jason D. Robertson. *Applied Channel Therapy in Chinese Medicine: Wang Ju-Yi's Lectures on Channel Therapeutics*. Seattle: Eastland Press; 2008. p. 79.

of the body. The production of this qi mainly is embodied in the production of *zong* qi (pectoral, gathering, ancestral qi). After production, the *zong*/pectoral qi goes up the respiratory tract to the throat to promote the respiration of the lung, as well as to penetrate into the heart vessels to help the heart to circulate blood. It then moves downwards through the body to reach the *dān tián* (丹田) (an area below the navel, or "between the kidneys"), in order to supplement the prenatal/congenital qi. Therefore, the production of *zong*/pectoral qi relates to the strength and condition of the entire qi of the body. If the function of the lung in governing the overall qi becomes disordered, this will lead to qi deficiency, shortness of breath, a lower voice with weak breathing, apathy, weakness, as well as an overall impairment in the flow of qi within the body.

The lung governs water movement

"The lung governs water movement" means that the lung acts to promote and regulate the distribution of fluids in the whole body through the dispersion, purification, and descending of the lung qi. This is also called the "freeing and regulating of the waterways". As mentioned earlier, through the diffusion and dispersion of lung qi, the lung sends fluids from the refined essences of the spleen to the orifices in the head and face and outward to the skin, hair and pores. The lung also changes the fluids into sweat, which is then released out of the body through the pores. Through the purification and descent of lung qi, the lung sends the fluids and the thicker and less-refined parts of essence received from the spleen downward to nourish the other organs. This same lung qi also sends down the impure or turbid fluids from the organs to the kidney and bladder. From the bladder, the fluids are released as urine.

When external pathogens invade the lung, this may lead to a lung qi failure to diffuse and disperse; this will affect fluids being distributed outwardly, sometimes causing edema of the skin. If dysfunctions of other organs affect the lung and cause failure of lung qi to descend, this can also lead to coughing, shortness of breath, difficult urination and/or edema.

The lung governs management and regulation

"The lung links with the many vessels and governs management and regulation." This passage refers to the process where the blood of the whole body flows into the lung via the vessels, where through respiration there is an exchange between the turbid qi in the body and the fresh air. After flowing into the heart, blood passes through the lung where it becomes rich in qi following this exchange of turbid and clear. As the blood becomes rich in qi, the dispersion and descending actions of lung qi then convey the blood through the vessels to reach the whole body.

The diffusion and descent of lung qi plays a key role in the process of blood circulation. On one hand, through respiratory action, the lung regulates the qi movement of the whole body so as to promote blood flow. On the other hand, *zong/*pectoral qi "penetrates into the heart vessels" to promote blood flow. When lung qi is vigorous, the overall qi will move freely and smoothly, the pectoral qi will be abundant, and the normal blood flow is maintained.

If the lung qi becomes deficient, or if it moves sluggishly, it will fail to assist the heart in the circulation of blood, leading to "unsmooth" blood flow or stagnation/stasis[①]; symptoms may include palpitations, chest distress, cyanotic lips and tongue, etc. If the heart blood fails to flow freely, it will in turn affect the diffusion of lung qi, resulting in cough.

We say that the lung governs the management and regulation of the whole body because qi, blood and fluids are the "essential substances" that constitute and maintain the life activities of the whole body. Blood and fluids belong to yin, which depends upon the propelling actions of yang qi. "Qi is the commander of blood", meaning that it acts to move, control and produce body fluids which includes blood. It is through this management and regulation of qi, blood and fluids that the lung also manages and regulates the whole body.

Physiological Characteristics of the Lung

In the five-phase theory, the lung corresponds with metal. It is said that "the lung serves as the canopy". The word canopy (*huá gài,* 华盖) refers to the covering of the vehicle in which the emperor rides, thus serving to protect him. In the human body, the lung is situated at the highest point in the chest, and thus "covers" all the organs. The lung is also associated with "heaven" because heaven too covers all beneath it like a canopy. "Heaven" is associated with metal because it is reflective, and ancient mirrors were made of highly polished metal. Like the metal of armor, the lung *wei* (defensive) qi protects the body surface and the organs from invasion of external pathogens. Furthermore, to create metal, one needs to melt down unrefined ore. The refined portion becomes purified and the unwanted parts are eliminated.[②]

"The lung is the delicate organ" is another common statement regarding the lung. The lung is light in weight, containing holes, and is delicate like lace. Because of its highest position and its connection with the outside, the lung is the first organ to be invaded by exterior pathogens. Furthermore, the lung connects outwardly with the skin and body hair, so that pathogenic invasion of the skin and hair by

---

①   (*yū,* 瘀) stasis
②   Thanks to Lorraine Wilcox, Facebook correspondence May 2011.

exterior pathogenic wind, cold, dryness and dampness may also internally affect the lung. Any upset of the lung, or any foreign object in the lung can cause coughing or other lung disruptions. For example, even a slight amount of dust or dry air entering the lung can cause coughing. The herbal treatment for exterior pathogens entering the lung uses herbs that are light in quality and have diffusing and dispersing actions. This is expressed as "remedies for treating disorders of the upper should be light, like a floating feather".

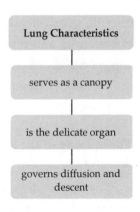

Lung Structure, Openings, Emotions, Secretions and Seasons

The lung is associated with the skin in structure, and its outward appearance is in the body hair

The skin, along with its body hair and sweat glands, comprises the exterior of the whole body, and is dependent upon the warming, moistening and nourishing functions of *wei* qi and fluids. The lung therefore prevents external pathogens from entering, regulates fluid metabolism, regulates body temperature, and assists respiration. The lung has a mutually-dependent relationship between it and the skin and the body hair.

The relationship of the lung to the skin with its body hair has two aspects. The first aspect is that by diffusion and dispersion of lung qi, the lung disperses *wei* qi to the skin to warm, nourish and moisten the flesh, skin, and surface of the skin, as well as to control the opening and closing of the pores in order to prevent invasion by exterior pathogens. Secondly, by diffusion and dispersion the lung also distributes fluids and a part of food-essence upward and outward to the skin, hair and the pores for moistening and nourishment. If the lung-essence or qi becomes deficient, this will lead to insecurity of the *wei*-exterior, which manifests as spontaneous sweating or a predisposition to the common cold. Due to the relationship between the lung and the skin, the skin will also fail to be moistened, manifesting as dry skin and withered body hair[1]. For this reason, many dermatological conditions, such as eczema, are treated by addressing the lung.

The condition of the skin and body hair can in turn influence the functions of the lung. This also has two aspects. The first is that the skin can diffuse lung qi so as to regulate respiration. The second is that as the skin is invaded by pathogens, the illness may be transmitted inward to the lung. For example, when the body surface is invaded by cold, the *wei* qi is restrained, and symptoms appear such as aversion

---

① We often see this in heavy smokers.

to cold, fever, head and body pain, lack of sweating, and a tight pulse. If there are complications of cough and panting, this indicates impairment of the lung itself by the pathogens.

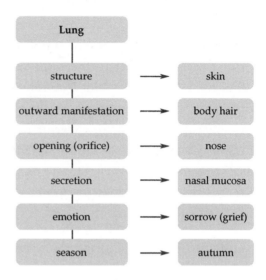

The opening of the lung is the nose and the throat is the gate of the lung

The nose is directly related to the lung, so the nose is called the opening of the lung. The nose functions of exchanging air and smelling both depend on the diffusion and dispersion of lung qi. When lung qi diffuses normally, the actions of the nose will be even, and smelling is acute. If the lung qi fails to diffuse, this leads to nasal stuffiness, disturbed breathing and impaired smelling.

The throat is situated at the upmost end of lung system; it is the gate of breathing and the voice. The throat depends upon the lung qi and the nourishment of the lung fluids. When lung qi is vigorous and the lung-fluids are sufficient, the throat is well nourished, the breathing is free, and the voice is deep and rich. If the lung qi and fluids are impaired, there will be a hoarse voice or a lack of voice altogether.

The lung is associated with nasal mucous

Nasal mucous moistens the nasal cavity. The mucous is transformed from the lung-fluids and it spreads over the nasal cavity through the diffusing action of lung qi. When the lung qi and fluids are sufficient and flow normally, mucous moistens the nasal cavity and should not leak out. When the lung is invaded by pathogenic cold, lung qi fails to diffuse and the lung fluid becomes blocked, causing watery nasal discharge. If lung heat is excessive, this will result in a yellowish turbid nasal discharge. When pathogenic dryness invades the lung, there will be a dry nose with pain.

The lung is associated with sorrow (grief)

Both sorrow and grief are normal emotions, with sorrow generally associated with external stimuli and grief more often associated with the interior of the body. However, over-sorrow or grief will consume qi, impair lung-essence and qi, or affect lung diffusion and descent. On the other hand, when lung-essence or lung qi becomes disordered, the body will have less tolerance for unwanted stimulation thus developing a greater potential for long-term emotional sorrow or grief.

The Yellow Emperor's Inner Classic (*Huáng Dì Nèi Jīng*, 黄帝内经) has an interesting passage concerning atrophy syndromes (*Discussion on Atrophy Syndromes, Wěi Lùn, 痿论*) that can be compared to multiple neuritis or myasthenia gravis with atrophy of the limbs. One cause of *wei* syndrome comes from the lung. "When there is heat in the lung, the lobes of the lung will become withered and the skin and hair will become weak; when the case is severe, there will also be flaccidity of the feet." It continues with a passage that links this condition with the emotions: "The lung governs the qi of the organs and is the canopy for the heart. When one's desires can not be satisfied and one is very disappointed, heart fire will then scorch the lung and cause the fluids of the lung to become dry, also causing flaccidity of the feet."[①]

The lung corresponds to autumn-qi

The lung and autumn seasons both correspond with metal. In autumn, it is cool; the trees and plants wither and their leaves fall, similar to the nature of lung qi purification and descent. Therefore, the lung corresponds to the autumn-qi. When the qi of autumn constrains and cools, it reduces the growth of summer-qi. In the body, the purification and descent of lung qi restrains the heart fire, which naturally flames upward. In the autumn, the body's qi and blood need to be gradually brought inwards so as to conform to the autumn-qi.

The lung is a delicate organ, prefers moisture, and is averse to dryness. Therefore, dryness is more likely to impair the lung qi and fluids to result in dry cough with no expectoration, a dry nose and mouth, and dry skin. Herbs that direct qi downward and moisten dryness are often prescribed during the autumn season.

The flavor associated with the lung is acrid

The flavor of acrid is also called pungent; because of its rising and dispersing nature, this flavor acts to open the lung.

Lung Fluid, Lung Qi, Lung Yin, and Lung Yang

The lung fluid, coming mainly from the fluids and the light lucid part of foodstuff essence transported by the spleen to the lung, depends upon the diffusion-dispersion and purification-descent of the lung qi to go up to moisten the orifices in the head and face, and to go down to the viscera to moisten them. The deficiency of the lung fluid clinically manifests as dry cough with no expectoration, or a little sticky sputum, dry mouth and throat, coarse skin, withered and thin hair, and/or a

---

① *The Yellow Emperor's Inner Classic.* Beijing: China Science and Technology Press; 2002. p. 214.

hoarse voice.

The lung qi is the part of general qi in the lung. The lung qi has the functions to propel and regulate breathing of the lung and water metabolism. Lung qi deficiency signs and symptoms include weak coughing and panting, shortness of breath, and difficult breathing which becomes worse with exertion. There may also be clear thin sputum, a low voice, a pale complexion, listlessness, fatigue, or spontaneous sweating, fear of wind, a predisposition to the common cold, a light red tongue with a white coating, and a forceless pulse. The proper treatment is to supplement and boost lung qi, *Liù Jūn Zǐ Tāng* (Six Gentlemen Decoction, 六君子汤) and a modification of the formula *Bǔ Fèi Tāng* (Supplementing the Lung Decoction, 补肺汤) can be used. Note that herbs contained in this formula also supplement the kidney which is said to "grasp" the lung qi. The spleen is also supplemented with herbs such as *rén shēn* (Ginseng Radix et Rhizoma, 人参).

The lung yin is the aspect of the lung qi that cools, moistens, purifies and descends. When lung yin is deficient, this implies that the fluids of the lung have been diminished and that there is dryness. The common signs and symptoms of lung yin deficiency include physical emaciation, afternoon fever, heat in the five centers (chest, palms and soles), night sweating, a red tongue with a scant coating, and a thready rapid pulse. These are all signs of yin deficiency. More severe symptoms may include coughing of blood following damage to the (blood) vessels. The treatment for the above is to nourish lung yin with formulas such as *Shā Shēn Mài Dōng Tāng* (Glehnia and Ophiopogon Decoction, 沙参麦冬汤) and *Bǎi Hé Gù Jīn Tāng* (Lily Bulb Metal-Securing Decoction, 百合固金汤).

The lung yang is the aspect of the lung qi with the actions of warming and diffusion-dispersion. The common symptoms of lung yang deficiency are weak cough and panting, expectoration of a large amount of frothy sputum, pale complexion, listlessness, low voice, shortness of breath, no thirst, enlarged tongue with white, moist and glossy coating, and a slow or moderate pulse. The treatment method is to warm and supplement lung yang, dissolve phlegm, and relieve panting. Modified *Xiǎo Qīng Lóng Tāng* (Minor Green Dragon Decoction, 小青龙汤) may be chosen as the herbal formula.

SPLEEN (*PÍ*, 脾)

The spleen and stomach are closely connected physically and physiologically, in particular in regards to digestion and absorption functions. Because of this, the concepts of the spleen and stomach are used in combination to describe the digestive function.

The spleen and stomach are situated together in the middle of the body, and are the major organs for digesting food and absorbing and transporting essence. The spleen and stomach are then called the "officials of the granary". A granary is a storage place for grains, usually kept dry and off the ground to prevent food from rotting. The spleen and stomach are the officials, dictating when the grains should come in and leave. The pair is also called as "the foundation of acquired constitution" because the spleen and stomach function to help the production and supplementation of essence, qi, blood and fluids. Perhaps more than any two organs, the spleen and stomach are discussed together, and their actions are referred to as "middle qi".

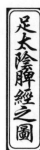

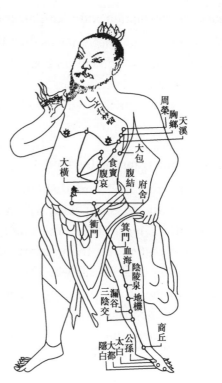

Main Physiological Functions of the Spleen

The main functions of the spleen include governing "transformation and transportation" and controlling blood. Transformation in this context refers to the changing of water and food (grain) in the stomach into food-essence (grain-essence) and fluids (water-essence). The term transformation (*huà*, 化) will be discussed again in a later chapter in greater depth; however, at this point we can say that transformation refers to one bodily substance being changed into another such as when food and water are transformed into essence. Following the transformation, the resulting "acquired" essence is then transported to the organs and the rest of the body.

The second main function of the spleen is controlling blood, which means that the spleen acts to hold the blood within the vessels.

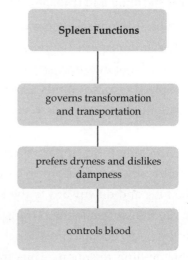

Governing transformation and transportation

This function of the spleen means that the spleen functions to transform the water and grain taken in into foodstuff essence (grain essence) and fluids (water essence), and then absorb them to transport to the viscera of the body. It is generally divided into two sides of the physiological process, namely transforming and transporting food and water.

Transforming and transporting food

After being received and decomposed by the stomach, the food becomes chyme or partially digested food which is sent down to the small intestine for further digestion. The chyme in the small intestine, under the action of the spleen qi, is further digested and then separated into two parts called the "clear" and the "turbid". The clear is absorbed by the small intestine and then transported by spleen qi to the other four *zang*-organs, where it is transformed into essence, qi, blood and fluids used to moisten and nourish the organs, tissues, orifices and limbs. Thus we have the saying, "the spleen transports the body fluids for the stomach". The role of spleen qi in transformation and transportation ensures that the essence, qi, blood and fluids of the whole body are sufficiently moistened and nourished. If the transformation and transportation of spleen qi becomes under-active, food digestion and absorption and the transportation of food-essence become impaired. One will have symptoms of abdominal distention, diarrhea, poor appetite, weight loss, and anemia. The treatment methods include strengthening the spleen and boosting qi.

Transforming and transporting water

The spleen is the center or hub to the actions of the water metabolism of the body. Spleen qi transports the fluids digested and absorbed by the stomach, small intestine, and the large intestine, as well as the water reabsorbed through the actions of kidney qi. Spleen qi raises fluids upward to the lung, where they are then transmitted and distributed to the whole body through the diffusing and descending actions of the lung.

The lung is the upper source of water, the kidney is the lower source of the water, and the spleen is situated in between the two. The spleen transports fluids upward to the lung and downward to the kidney and bladder. If spleen qi functions abnormally in the transformation and transportation of water, this will lead to retention of water in the body, edema, or production of pathological products of water-dampness and phlegm-fluid retention. (Thus the saying, "the spleen is the origin for the production of phlegm.")

The physiological function of the spleen in Chinese medicine is a comprehensive functional system that includes the majority of the digestive system functions described in modern medicine, but it is also related to many functions of the nervous, immunological, and endocrine systems. Many people feel that the actual spleen pictured in the ancient drawings is actually that of the pancreas. In any event, the spleen in Chinese medicine must be assessed on its own terms.

Qi is the commander of blood

Chinese medicine states that "qi is the commander of blood". This means that the spleen qi has the function of containing and controlling the blood circulating in the vessels. Only when qi is plentiful can it control the blood. The spleen qi is the part of the overall qi of the body, so the actual mechanism for the spleen function of controlling blood is the controlling action of qi. When the qi is abundant overall, spleen qi is also abundant with sufficient qi function to control the blood. As a result, the blood can be kept within the vessels and will not escape (extravasate). If the spleen becomes weak and thus fails to transform and transport, this will lead to a shortage of qi, and thus the blood is uncontrolled; the result may be bleeding. However, this kind of bleeding is different from the kind of bleeding where blood is forced out of the vessels by internal heat in the blood. Bleeding caused by deficient spleen qi failing to control blood is usually seen in the lower parts of the body, and includes types of menstrual bleeding conditions. Furthermore, bleeding in the digestive tract, nosebleed, and purple spots on the skin all can result from spleen qi failure to control blood. When treating this kind of disorder, herbs that supplement qi and strengthen the spleen are often more effective than those herbs which stanch bleeding (hemostatics).

Physiological Characteristics of the Spleen

The spleen is characterized by ascent

The spleen qi ascends, and through this motion can transport "clear" food and water-essence upward to the heart and lung. This lifting action is also responsible for maintaining the relative positions of the internal organs within the abdominal cavity.

Sending up the clear

The "clear" refers to the nutritive aspects of food-essence. The spleen and stomach are both located in the middle, acting as the central hub of the overall ascending and descending movement of qi within the body. Comparatively speaking, the spleen qi ascends while the stomach qi descends, making for an opposite yet complementary dynamic. Thus the saying, "The spleen functions well when its qi ascends, while the stomach functions well when its qi descends." If spleen and stomach ascending and descending becomes disordered, this will on one hand result in failure of the clear qi to ascend, combined with issues of dizziness, loose stools, diarrhea and so on. On the other hand, when stomach qi fails to send the turbid downward, it may rise upward or remain in the epigastric area to result in abdominal distention and fullness.

Clinically, for a patient with symptoms of poor appetite, abdominal distension, and diarrhea, accompanied by dizziness, vertigo, and listlessness; or for a patient suffering from symptoms of undersupply of cerebral blood flow, Chinese medicine believes that this is spleen qi deficiency with failure of the clear qi to ascend. So for treatment, the remedies of strengthening the spleen and boosting qi to lift should be taken, and the formulas such as *Yì Qì Cōng Míng Tāng* (Qi-Boosting Intelligence Decoction, 益气聪明汤) or *Bǔ Zhōng Yì Qì Tāng* (Center-Supplementing and Qi-Boosting Decoction, 补中益气汤) may be used. Since the ascending of the spleen qi and the descending of the stomach qi are interdependent, for a disorder of failure of the spleen qi to ascend, the medicinals (herbs) of stomach-qi lowering may be properly added.

Lifting the internal organs

The spleen function of lifting the internal organs refers to the ascending motion of spleen qi that maintains the relative stability of the positions of the internal organs, thus preventing their sinking or prolapse. For example, it is not uncommon to have a prolapse of the rectum in old age, or prolapse of the vagina following childbirth. Some hernias can be also categorized as a prolapse. Chinese medicine holds that all the clinical disorders with prolapsed internal organs are caused by sinking of the middle qi. For these conditions, herbal formulas such as *Bǔ Zhōng Yì Qì Tāng* (Center-Supplementing Qi-Boosting Decoction) can be used to lift the abnormally sinking qi.

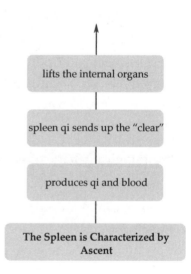

lifts the internal organs

spleen qi sends up the "clear"

produces qi and blood

The Spleen is Characterized by Ascent

The spleen prefers dryness and is averse to dampness

The spleen prefers dryness and dislikes dampness, while the stomach prefers moisture and is averse to dryness. This characteristic of the spleen is inseparable from its function of transporting and transforming fluids. When spleen qi is plentiful, the transportation and transformation of water will be normal, with water and fluids spreading normally through the body. Dryness of the spleen without encumbrance by water-dampness or phlegm is one of the important conditions required for the spleen qi to ascend normally. If the spleen qi becomes deficient and weak and its ability to transport and transform water is affected, this will result in water-dampness or phlegm-fluid retention. In this case, the dampness is created internally. This internal water-dampness in turn encumbers the spleen qi, leading to spleen qi failure to ascend and spleen yang decline; this pattern is called "encumbrance of the spleen by dampness". In addition, an exterior invasion of pathogenic dampness from the environment can also encumber the spleen qi and hinder its ascending action; in this case, the dampness comes from the exterior. Clinically, the encumbrance of the spleen by the dampness manifest with heavy sensations in the head and body, somnolence, abdominal distention and distress, poor appetite, and diarrhea, among others. In addition to drying and eliminating dampness, proper clinical treatment must be applied at the same time to supplement the spleen and boost qi.

Relationships of the Spleen with the Orifices, Emotions, Secretions, and Seasons

The spleen is associated with the flesh and governs the four limbs

The flesh covering the body depends upon the food-essence and fluids that are transformed and transported by the spleen and stomach for moisture and nourishment. If the spleen and stomach are not functioning properly, this impairs the production of food-essence and fluids. Because the spleen governs the four limbs, the activities of the limbs depend upon the nourishing and moistening of food-essence and fluids transported by the spleen and stomach. If the spleen fails to transform and transport, the limbs fail to receive nourishment, leading to a weakness and impairment of the limbs, etc. In the view of Chinese medicine, various kinds of atrophy are due to spleen qi deficiency with impaired transformation and transportation and subsequent under-production of qi and fluids. In the treatment of limb disorders due to the spleen failing to transform and transport, the primary treatment method is to strengthen the spleen and boost qi.

The opening of the spleen is the mouth

The appetite and sense of taste are directly related to the transformation and transportation of spleen qi. The mouth, being at the uppermost end of the digestive tract, directly receives food which is then chewed to allow reception and decomposition by the stomach. The spleen channel "reaches the root of the tongue collaterals (related to the acupuncture channels) over the lower surface of the tongue". The largest functional area of the spleen and stomach on the tongue surface is in the central part, where there are the most taste buds. Therefore, the spleen is closely related with appetite and taste. When spleen qi is abundant[1], the appetite will be good and food will have a normal taste. If the spleen fails to transform and transport and internal turbid-dampness is produced, there may be a poor appetite, and strange greasy or sweet tastes in the mouth or tastelessness.

The spleen's outward appearance is in the lips

The color of the lips can directly reflect the condition of spleen-essence and qi. When spleen qi is sufficient and qi and blood are abundant, the lips are lustrous. If the spleen fails to transform and transport and the qi and blood are deficient, the lips become pale and lusterless.

The spleen is the source of qi and blood production; so as spleen qi becomes deficient, a deficiency of qi and blood will result. Along with inspection of the complexion, an important part of diagnosing blood deficiency is to observe the color of the lips. To treat a patient with blood deficiency, it is important to supplement qi and strengthen the spleen in order to promote the production of blood.

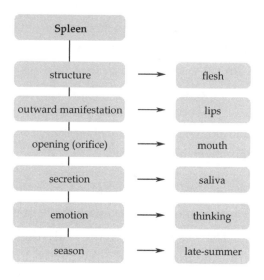

The spleen is associated with the saliva

"Saliva" (*xián*, 涎), is the clear and thin part of what we associate in English with saliva[2]. It is produced and transported by the spleen-essence and qi. Saliva protects the oral mucosa and moistens the oral cavity to assist in the chewing and digestion of food. When spleen-essence and qi are sufficient, the saliva is produced in appropriate amounts and not in excess. If the spleen and stomach are not coordinated, or the spleen qi fails to control, this will lead to an abnormal increase of saliva production, creating an overflow of the saliva out of the mouth. If spleen-essence is deficient and fluids are lessened, or when the spleen qi fails to transport the fluids, there will be reduced saliva with a dry mouth and tongue.

---

① (*chōng zú*, 充足) adequate, sufficient
② Another fluid, "spittle", is associated with the kidney.

The spleen is associated with thinking in emotion

Thinking[①] is a normal activity, which within limits, does no harm to the body. However, excessive thinking, pensiveness, or pursuing an unfeasible goal will affect the normal physiological activity of the spleen. This can impact the qi movement and lead to qi stagnation or "qi knotted"[②]. In modern life, many intellectual workers and students[③] often suffer from impairment of qi and blood because of so much thinking, although irregular dietary habits also impair spleen qi transformation where the source of qi and blood production is also affected. As a result, they may have a poor appetite, tiredness, shortness of breath, a pale complexion, lips and tongue, and early whitening of the hair. For treatment, one should employ methods that strengthen the spleen, boost qi, and nourish blood.

The activity of life depends upon nourishment from the food-essence and fluids produced by the spleen and stomach. The functions of the heart, lung, liver and kidney all depend on the support of spleen qi and the essential substances produced by the spleen and stomach. When the spleen qi functions well, the other four *zang*-organs will function normally so that the body will remain healthy and not predisposed to illness.

The spleen corresponds to late-summer qi

The season associated with the spleen has many complicated aspects. In general, it is said that "late-summer" is the period from the summer solstice to the beginning of fall. The moisture of late-summer is conductive to the growth of plants, but if the dampness becomes overactive, this can adversely encumber the spleen. If a person has a weak spleen, she or he will be more predisposed to invasions by exterior pathogenic dampness. Furthermore, dampness commonly invades the body in combination with pathogenic heat, so there are often conditions of combined dampness and heat such as an un-surfaced fever, heavy feelings of the limbs, gastric distress, poor appetite and digestion, and diarrhea. Note that some sources view the seasonal correspondence with the spleen, as an earth-phase organ in the cosmological five-phase arrangement, as existing during the transitional period of eighteen days, in between each of the other four seasons.

---

① (sī, 思) thought

② Here the word for knotted is *qì jié* (气结) which suggests qi which is stagnated but also with a "physical" component. One example is "plum pit qi", where stress produces a feeling of a foreign body (like a plum pit) in the throat.

③ Chinese texts often emphasize these persons as teachers and "intellectual workers". However modern society has many people having to plan and strategize their lives. Even driving a car or using a computer requires a large amount of "thought" in this sense.

Spleen Essence, Spleen Qi, Spleen Yin, and Spleen Yang

The spleen essence comes from blending of *jīng*/essence stored in the spleen and the food-essence absorbed by the spleen. The four limbs and flesh all depend upon the spleen to transport essence and qi to the rest of the body for nourishment. The spleen qi is transformed from the spleen-essence to activate and regulate the spleen's functional activities. A case of spleen qi deficiency commonly leads to abdominal distention that becomes worse after meals, poor appetite, loose stools, either body thinness or edema, obesity, tiredness, apathy, listlessness, shortness of breath with a reluctance to speak, a pale tongue with a white coating, and a moderate or weak pulse. One treatment approach would be to supplement and boost spleen qi with the herbal formula, *Shēn Líng Bái Zhú Sǎn* (Ginseng, Poria and Atractylodes Macrocephalae Powder, 参苓白术散).

Spleen yin is the part of spleen qi associated with cooling, moistening and calming actions. Pathologically, spleen yin deficiency is often combined with stomach yin deficiency with manifestations including great hunger or hunger but with no desire to eat, epigastric upset, abdominal distention after meals, fatigue, dry red lips, a low fever, heat in the five centers (chest, palms and soles), a red tongue with a scant coating, and a thready and rapid pulse. In a discussion on spleen yin deficiency, Yan Shi-lin writes, "When the body's external structure is deprived of nourishment, this manifests with emaciation and lack of strength in the limbs" and "When spleen yin is depleted, fluids are insufficient and therefore cannot enrich the large intestine below. This can manifest with dry and rough stagnant stools, and in serious cases, with constipation."[1] For treatment, a formula that supplements the spleen and nourishes the stomach such as *Yǎng Wèi Tāng* (Stomach-Nourishing Decoction, 养胃汤) is indicated.

Spleen yang is the part of spleen qi associated with warming and activating actions. Pathologically, spleen yang deficiency often leads to cold pain of the epigastrium and abdomen which responds well to warmth and pressure, loose stools or diarrhea with undigested food, edema, difficult urination, or profuse clear thin leukorrhea in women. There may also be a fear of cold with cold limbs, a bland taste in the mouth without thirst, a pale and enlarged tongue with teeth-marks, and a deep and slow forceless pulse. The treatment principle is to supplement and boost spleen yang, using formulas such as *Lǐ Zhōng Tāng* (Normalizing the Middle Decoction, 理中汤) or *Fù Zǐ Lǐ Zhōng Tāng* (Aconite Normalizing the Middle Decoction, 附子理中汤).

Other types of spleen conditions also exist, often involving combined patterns of

---

① Yan Shi-lin. *Pathomechanisms of the Spleen*. Taos: Paradigm Publications; 2009. p. 193.

spleen-dampness or spleen-heat, etc.

◆ *Shaoyin* — Heart and Kidney

Shaoyin involves the interaction of fire and water. In five-phase theory, the heart is the organ associated with heat and fire, while the kidney corresponds with water. However, the kidney also contains fire which was inherited from the "first yang" of the prenatal *jīng*. The heart, as a fire-organ, can easily gather too much heat, especially when it is not balanced by sufficient kidney-water. The water from the kidney reaches the heart and other organs by being "steamed" upward by the kidney's fire. Kidney-fire can also be seen as a "pilot light" that acts to maintain the fire of the heart. When kidney fire is low, as in yang deficiency patterns, the heart will itself cease to burn as brightly, possibly resulting in heart yang deficiency.

The heart and kidney also form the important axis of the kidney *jīng*/essence and heart-*shén*/spirit. Serious mental illness is often expressed in Chinese as "精神病"(*jīng shén bìng*) or essence-spirit illness, and a severe lack of vitality is literally expressed as "no *jīng shén*". Although we usually think of the body, organs and the mind as separate entities, in Chinese medicine, the mind, body, and spirit are very much seen as one.[1]

HEART (*XĪN*, 心)

The heart is primary to the governance of all life activity, and is thus considered as the "sovereign"[2] of the human body. To emphasize this key position, the heart is likened to an emperor, and therefore called "the ruler of the five *zang* and six *fu*".

Main Physiological Functions of the Heart

The main physiological functions of the heart are to generate and promote blood circulation and govern life activity while also playing a key role in maintaining consciousness within the body. The first function is called "governing blood" and the second is called "storing the spirit"[3]. Chinese medicine believes that the food-essence produced by the spleen and stomach contains "grain-qi" and "grain-essence". The grain-qi from food-essence, after being sent upward to the heart and lung, integrates with the air inhaled by the lung to become *ying* qi (one of the major components of blood). Then, under the warming actions of heart yang, *ying* qi and grain-essence

---

[1]　Yanhua Zhang. *Transforming Emotions in Chinese Medicine*. Albany: State University of New York Press; 2007. p. 38.

[2]　"Sovereign" here refers to the highest government or system (*zùi gāo tǒng*, 最高统); also monarch (*jūn zhǔ*, 君主).

[3]　(*cáng shén*, 藏神) store the spirit

change into red-colored blood. [1]

Chinese philosophers and physicians in ancient times compared the heart with the sun in that both are red in color and warm in quality, and also because they both promote growth and development. Thus, the sun-like energy of the heart is yang in nature. Chinese medicine states that the blood requires the activating actions of yang qi. If heart yang becomes deficient, this impairs the generation of new blood which can result in a clinical pattern referred to as "heart blood deficiency". Signs and symptoms include heart palpitations or skipped heartbeats with a pale complexion, a pale tongue, and a weak pulse.

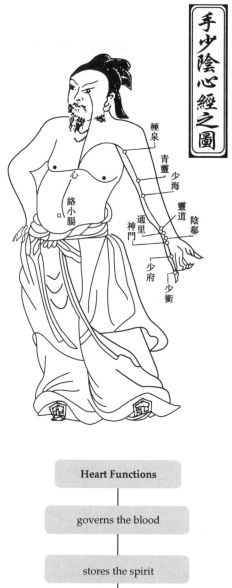

The heart also promotes blood circulation, which is coordinated in two ways. First, heart qi and yang propel, promote and warm the blood. Heart blood and yin are associated with the qualities of nourishing, cooling, moistening, and stabilizing. If this balance is not coordinated, yin or yang will become over-abundant, and this may bring on an illness. When heart qi and heart yang becomes deficient and so fail to promote and warm, the cooling and moistening qualities of heart blood and heart yin will become overactive. As a result, the heartbeat will become affected with impaired blood circulation and obstruction of the vessels. In this case, signs

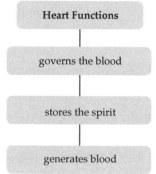

and symptoms include a slow or weak heartbeat with chest oppression or stabbing pain (which in mild cases can be relieved by lying down for a while), and a "choppy" pulse[2]. In severe cases there is excruciating pain with a cyanotic complexion, purple tongue and lips, and profuse sweating. (Similar to myocardial infarction complicated by heart failure.)

---

[1]   This process here can be roughly compared to the biomedical concept of arterial blood formation.

[2]   (sè zhì, 涩滞) unsmooth, stagnant

In contrast, when heart yin is deficient, the cooling and moistening actions will decline where the propulsion, promotion and warmth of heart qi and heart yang will become overactive; this may speed up the flow of blood to the point of damaging the vessels. Signs and symptoms include an accelerated heartbeat with a red complexion, crimson tongue and lips, a rapid pulse with a surging quality, and in extreme cases, hemorrhaging.

Shén (神)

The *shén* is translated as "spirit" and is also the "spirit" most closely associated with the heart[1]. The concept of the spirit, or *shén*, in a narrow sense refers to mental activities that include consciousness, cognitive thinking and emotion. In the broad sense, *shén* refers to the "ruler" or "emperor" of all human physiological and psychological activities as well as the outward manifestations and actions of life. These activities of the heart system include the formation of ideas, consciousness itself, memorization and thought and thinking. Therefore the Chinese theory of the "heart-spirit" includes what other sciences would consider brain functions.[2]

The heart also controls all physiological activities of the organs and tissues within the body.[3] As long as the heart-spirit remains normalized, the activities of the organs and tissues will be well-regulated and healthy. The heart also controls all psychological activities, which in Chinese philosophy include the five spirits (spirit/ *shén*, ethereal soul/*hún*, corporeal soul/*pò*, thought/*yì*, will/*zhì*) and the seven emotions (joy, anger, anxiety, thinking, sorrow, fear, fright). When a person's heart functions normally to govern the spirit, one will be full of energy and consciousness, think and respond appropriately, and have an easygoing mood and sleep well.

The normality of the heart in governing the spirit depends upon the nourishment provided by heart blood, which is considered the foundation of all mental activity. Plentiful blood keeps the spirit sound. If the heart blood becomes deficient or otherwise circulates abnormally, this will affect the equilibrium of the heart-spirit with manifestations including palpitations, anxiety, insomnia, restlessness, and slowed responses. The function of the heart in storing the spirit also affects the function of the heart in governing blood, with symptoms of hemorrhage in various tissues and

---

[1] Each of the 5 *zang*-organs have "spirits" associated with them.

[2] Yanhua Zhang. *Transforming Emotions in Chinese Medicine*. Albany: State University of New York Press; 2007. p. 39.

[3] These include activities such as the heart circulating blood, lung controlling breath, spleen governing transportation and transformation, liver governing the free flow of qi, kidney storing essence, stomach governing reception, small intestine controlling digesting the bile, large intestine conveying the waste, as well as movement, speech, vision, smell, and hearing.

organs. When the heart-spirit is in a good condition, the functions of generating and circulating blood will be well-controlled and regulated. If the heart-spirit declines or becomes disturbed, the generation of blood will be affected. Signs and symptoms include a lusterless complexion with pale lips and nails. The function that heart stores the spirit can be the key for life or death. Therefore, there is a saying in Chinese medicine that "with the spirit one lives, while without it one's life ends".

The Spiritual Pivot, (as translated here by Zhang Yan-hua) gives a more complete picture of the *shén*, mental capacity and consciousness:

"What responds to environment (the outside world) is called *xīn* (heart , 心).

What *xīn* brings out is called *yì* (imagery, 意).

What *yì* stores is called *zhì* (memory, 志); because of *zhì*, knowledge is reorganized.

This is called *sī* (thinking, reflection, 思); because of *sī*, one thinks for the future.

This is called *lǜ* (strategy, planning, 虑); because of *lǜ*, one makes decisions and takes actions.

This is called *zhì* (wisdom, 智)."

Zhang goes further to point out that the above concepts are "not different things, but descriptions of different phases of the same continuous process of heart-spirit, where emotions and mores are not separated from thinking and perceiving".[1]

The heart corresponds to fire

The heart is a yang *zang*-organ that circulates blood that is unimpeded and sustains normal mental activities. [The Chinese characters used for these phrases are *chàng tōng* (畅通), which describes the smoothness of the heart vessels, and *míng* (明), as the clarity and brightness of the heart-spirit.] In terms of yin-yang theory, the heart pertains to "*taiyang* within yang". To emphasize the important actions performed by the yang qi of the heart, it is also referred to as a "yang *zang*-organ" or the "fire *zang*-organ". Yang qi of the heart can drive its rhythm, warmth and smooth the blood and vessels, and stimulate the spirit. (In acupuncture channel theory, the heart channel pathway is referred to as "hand *shaoyin*".[2])

The heart's structure includes the vessels

The heart is structurally connected to the vessels (*mài*, 脉), thus all blood vessels

---

[1] Yanhua Zhang. *Transforming Emotions in Chinese Medicine*. Albany: State University of New York Press; 2007. p. 41.

[2] The discrepancy between the heart as being *taiyang* and *shaoyin* deserves some explanation. As the text explains, the heart is associated with fire and also the ultimate activator of the entire body and spirit. However, the heart as a *zang*- or yin-organ is categorized *shaoyin* or "lesser yin". The heart is located lower in the body than the lung (*taiyin*) organ, so it is lesser in position. On the body, the heart channel is most medial. Students will probably be best served by emphasizing that the heart acupuncture channel is the "hand *shaoyin*" channel.

are controlled by the heart, and this direct connection with the vessels creates a closed-circuit "pipe system". The normal flow of blood within the vessels requires sufficient heart qi, adequate blood and smooth blood vessels. If the heart becomes disordered, this will lead to either overly rapid or slow pulses, with stagnation or breakage within the vessels. The pulse descriptions associated with heart patterns include rapid, racing, forceful, thready, choppy, knotted or regularly intermittent pulses.

Heart qi expresses itself in the face

Because blood and qi are sent upward from the heart to the face and head, these areas contain an especially abundant number of vessels. Changes in the facial complexion can therefore indicate functional changes of the heart. Healthy heart qi and abundant blood provide the face with a pleasing and lustrous hue. When heart qi becomes deficient, this can result in a dim or pale-yellow complexion, and with heart blood deficiency, the complexion becomes lusterless. When the heart vessels become stagnated or obstructed, facial cyanosis (a blue or purple color) may appear. Exuberant heart fire may show as a reddish face.

The heart opens to the tongue

The tongue is rich in vessels that are governed by the heart, which is said to connect to the tongue body through the heart channel. The tongue reflects heart function and the essence-qi of the heart; for this reason, it is also regarded as the outward orifice of the heart. When the heart blood is abundant, the tongue will be rosy, fresh, soft and flexible. The heart can affect taste as well as the voice and speech; clear speech and taste sensitivity rely on sufficient heart qi and blood as well as a sound heart-spirit. When the heart function is disordered, not only will the tongue change in appearance, but there may be speech problems such as stuttering, dysphasia, aphasia or inappropriate and/or incoherent speech.

The flavor of the heart is bitter

Bitter flavors act to drain internal heat from all órgans, but especially from the heart. Bitterness moves downward strongly, and is often used in herbal preparations for purgation and draining of toxins and heat. The representative herb for this flavor is *huáng lián* (Coptidis Rhizoma, 黄连) which strongly drains heart-heat. However, excessive administration of bitter herbs can easily damage the stomach and spleen.

Sweat

Sweat is the secretion associated with heart. Sweat (*hàn*, 汗) is a body fluid (*jīn yè*, 津液) that is carried by the "steam" (*zhēng*, 蒸) of yang qi. Blood (*xuè*, 血) contains aspects of both *ying* qi and the body fluids, and body fluids are considered to also move through the body along with the blood. *Essentials of Chinese Medicine* states, "When infused into a blood vessel, body fluid becomes a component of blood. Some components of blood may also seep out of the vessels and become part of body fluid."[1] The *Basic Questions (Sù Wèn, 素问)* states, "The nutritive/*ying* qi moves through the channels, like a mist. The blood in the channels moves like water in a canal." Also, "The *ying* qi secretes the *jīn yè* fluids that pour into the vessels and transform into blood." With sweating, the *jīn yè* fluids of the vessels leave to nourish the skin; however, excessive sweating can eventually lead to dryness and deficiency within the blood. Fluids can also leave the surface on the body to nourish the deficient blood, but this can create dry skin. Fluids and sweat are thus interrelated and interactive.

The generation and excretion of sweat is also controlled and regulated by the heart-spirit. A clear and bright heart-spirit normalizes perspiration, whereas a lack of sweating can be an indication of heart blood deficiency. Abnormal perspiration may be the result of damage to the heart-spirit due to nervousness, mental irritation, and emotional fluctuation or simply from damage to the heart as in a heart attack. Excessive sweating can itself cause mental agitation or severe physical conditions; excessive sweating can consume the blood, qi and yang and the spirit to such an extent that the damage can be fatal. According to these ideas, Chinese medicine has warned repeatedly against excessive sweating in those who have suffered either blood loss or in those with patterns of blood deficiency.

The digestion of food is the source of both blood and fluids, therefore it is said that "sweat and blood share the same source". This relationship between the heart and sweat may seem strange to the modern reader, but we do in fact know from modern anatomy that there are networks of blood vessels that surround the sweat glands. Perhaps the ancient Chinese doctors knew of this connection as well.

The heart is associated with the emotion of joy

Xǐ (喜) means joy or happiness, which obviously is a desirable state of mind in most cases. With sufficient heart blood and a normal heart-spirit, a person can maintain a positive outlook despite their external environment or circumstances. "Appropriate" joy is the body's reaction to favorable condition and this creates favorable heart functions including governing the blood.

Excessive emotions could also hurt the viscera. Over or endless elation can hurt the qi, blood and the spirit of the heart. Persons may seek over-joy through entertainment, sex, drugs, over-eating and alcohol, which eventually will cause damage if not

---

[1]   Liu Zhan-wen, Liu Liang. *Essentials of Chinese Medicine*. Vol. 1. London: Springer; 2009. p. 122.

moderated.

Simply put, eventually, all excessive emotions can damage the organs. As the heart is the ruler of the spirit, extremes of any of the five emotions can affect the heart-spirit, thus impairing normal function of the heart. On the other hand, when one's heart blood becomes deficient, there is a lack of energy and a propensity for sorrow and grief.

In five-phase theory, fire is held in check by water, which is more stable, constant and "willful" than fire. If the kidney-water is deficient, there may be anxiety, insomnia, agitation or manic behavior caused by rising heat. We see this most extremely in mentally ill people who are constantly or inappropriately laughing.

Summerheat

The heart corresponds to "summer-qi", corresponding with the hottest season of the year. The heart, as an organ, is *taiyang*[①] and thus has the greatest yang qi, much like the summer.[②] Naturally occurring physiological signs in the summer include a stronger heartbeat, a relatively red complexion, a red tongue tip, and a rapid surging pulse, all of which are all activated by the qi of yang-heat.

Many heart yang deficiency conditions can be relieved with the assistance of the yang qi of summer. However, emotional diseases and also patterns of hyperactive yang with yin deficiency can become worse during this season when an individual is intolerant to the summer's predominance of yang-heat qi. Chinese medical theory recommends that physicians "treat winter diseases in summertime, and treat summer diseases in wintertime". For example, it is said that a heart yang deficiency pattern (a winter issue) that is treated in the summertime can get twice the effect with half the effort.

Heart Blood, Heart Qi, Heart Yin, and Heart Yang

Heart blood flows through the heart and circulates within the vessels. The functions of heart blood include nourishing the heart and vessels as well as generating the heart-spirit. A case of heart blood deficiency often manifests with palpitations, insomnia, profuse dreaming, amnesia, dizziness or vertigo, a pale complexion, a pale tongue, and a weak thready pulse[③]. Prescriptions for nourishing heart blood such as *Zhì Gān Cǎo Tāng* (Honey-Fried Licorice Decoction, 炙甘草汤) can be used. With blockage of the heart vessels due to qi constraint, turbid phlegm,

---

① Again, we point out that the heart is *taiyang* and a fire-organ, yet *shaoyin* in terms of its channel affiliation.

② This is an example of "correspondence between humans and nature".

③ In this case, to nourish heart blood, *Zhì Gān Cǎo Tāng* could be prescribed.

and/or cold, a pattern of heart blood stasis may develop. Signs and symptoms include palpitations, chest distress, heart pain, and a dusky or purple tongue. Note that both heart conditions above involve palpitations, thus underscoring the necessity of formulating a correct diagnosis. If one were to nourish heart blood when the issue is a pattern of heart blood stasis, the clinical results could be disastrous.

Herbal Formulas for Deficiencies of Heart Qi, Heart Yin, and Heart Yang

The heart qi is an aspect of the overall qi distributed within the heart and vessels. Heart qi is transformed from heart blood, and this combines with *zong*/pectoral qi which then flows back into the heart and vessels. The functions of heart qi include propelling and regulating the heartbeat, relaxing and contracting the vessels, and regulating mental activities. A case of heart qi deficiency commonly manifests with palpitations, chest distress and shortness of breath that worsens with exertion. Signs and symptoms may include mental fatigue, weak breathing, reluctance to talk, a pale complexion, spontaneous sweating, a pale tongue with a whitish coating, and a weak thready pulse. In this case, the treatment principle is to supplement and boost heart qi with a formula such as *Yǎng Xīn Tāng* (Heart-Nourishing Decoction, 养心汤).

The heart yin is the aspect of heart qi that is cooling, moistening and calming with an inhibitory action. Heart yin deficiency commonly manifests with palpitations (usually with tachycardia/rapid heartbeat), restlessness, insomnia or profuse dreaming, agitation (*xīn fán,* 心烦) with a feverish sensation in the chest, hot palms and soles, afternoon fever, and night sweats. The tongue is often red with little or no coating, and the pulse is weak and thready. A typical formula for nourishing heart yin is *Tiān Wáng Bǔ Xīn Dān* (Celestial Emperor Heart-Supplementing Elixir, 天王补心丹).

The heart yang is the aspect of heart qi that warms, propels, and excites. Heart yang deficiency can lead to palpitations, shortness of breath, chest oppression or heart pain that worsens with exertion. Signs and symptoms include intolerance to cold and cold-feeling limbs with fatigue, weak breathing, reticence, a pale complexion, spontaneous sweating and drowsiness. The tongue is pale and enlarged, and the pulse is slow, weak and intermittent. For this condition, *Guì Zhī Rén Shēn Tāng* (Cinnamon Twig and Ginseng Decoction, 桂枝人参汤) is a suitable treatment formula.

KIDNEY (*SHÈN*, 肾)

Main Physiological Functions of the Kidney

The kidney stores the essence to govern growth, development, reproduction, and organ-qi transformation

Essence is the most indispensable substance in the human body for maintaining life activity. As the origin of life in the body, essence is also the material basis for all functional activities.

Prenatal (innate) essence comes from the essence of the parents (which in modern times we can compare to genetic material), and this innate essence is stored in the kidney. Normal physiological function depends upon the storage of essence which acts in coordination with the propelling action of kidney qi and yang. Before birth, essence is the foundation of fetal development, and after birth, essence promotes growth, development, and reproductive capacity.

Postnatal (acquired) essence originates from food-essence that has been transformed by the spleen and stomach. The acquired essence is then transported by the spleen to the whole body to promote and support the organs and tissues. The surplus parts of various organ-essences are also transported to the kidney to supplement and "nourish"[1] the prenatal essence. Furthermore, the warming and propelling actions of kidney yang provide the spleen and stomach with the ability to produce acquired essence; therefore, the innate essence of the kidney and the acquired essence of the spleen act to support and sustain one another.

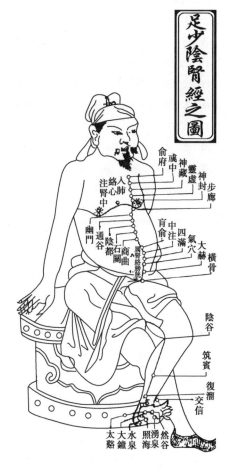

The kidney governs water

One kidney function is to govern and regulate fluid metabolism. This includes the action of kidney qi in promoting the function of organs that are involved in the metabolism of fluids, and also the action of kidney qi in the production and discharge

---

① (*bǔ*, 补) nourish, mend, benefit, supply

of urine.

Kidney qi is vital to the organs associated with fluid metabolism, specifically those associated with the transporting and distributing functions of the lung qi and spleen qi. In the process of metabolism, the fluids in the stomach, small intestine and large intestine are absorbed and transported through the transformation and transportation function of the spleen and sent upward to the lung. Through the lung function of diffusion-dispersion and purification-descent, fluids are transmitted to moisten and nourish the whole body, including the skin surface and body hairs. The metabolized fluids of the organs and tissues are transported to the kidney where, by the evaporating action of kidney qi, the useful fluid is reabsorbed and

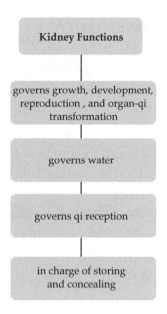

the waste and surplus parts become urine. Water metabolism is performed by the functions of the lung, spleen, kidney, stomach, large intestine, small intestine, *sanjiao*, and bladder. However, it is the kidney qi and its differentiated kidney yin and kidney yang that play the key role in water metabolism. Only under the propelling and promoting actions by the kidney qi, can the qi of the other viscera play their normal functions including the water metabolism of the body.

The kidney governs qi reception

Respiration in the human body is mainly performed by the lung. Nevertheless, the qi from fresh air is transmitted downwards by lung qi to the kidney where it must be "grasped" and stored so as to create an exchange of qi. Therefore, it is said that "the lung dominates qi", while the kidney is the "root of qi". If the kidney qi is weak and thus fails to receive qi from the lung, there will be wheezing, shallow breathing, or difficulty in taking a deep breath. This is called "kidney failing to grasp qi".

The kidney is in charge of storage[1]

A major function of kidney qi is to store essence; it is said that kidney qi "envelops and contains" the essence. When the kidney qi fails to store, the essence will leave the kidney and lead to spontaneous seminal emission, panting, enuresis, incontinence of urine, fecal incontinence; or female leukorrhea, and even frequent miscarriage[2].

---

[1]   (*cáng*, 藏) store, conceal, hide

[2]   (*huá tāi*, 滑胎) slippery fetus

The kidney conceals[1] the ministerial fire

There are two types of fire, the sovereign fire of the heart, and the ministerial fire (associated mainly with the pericardium, liver and kidney). The sovereign fire is the yang qi of the heart, or the physiological fire of the heart. Relative to the heart fire, all the other organs' fires can be seen as ministerial fires. Under normal conditions, they comprise the yang qi of each organ, and are also called the "minor fire". When the fires of the organs are overactive and therefore pathological, they will always be considered as "excess fire". The ministerial fire of the liver is known as "thunder-fire" (*léi huǒ*, 雷火), and the ministerial fire of the kidney is known as "dragon-fire" (*lóng huǒ*, 龙火).

The kidney should conceal the kidney ministerial fire and not let it be "revealed".[2] The ministerial fire of each organ should remain stable and well-contained along with the assistance of the qi of their respective organs. For example, kidney yin qi should be sufficient enough to balance the ministerial fire of the kidney. If not, the ministerial fire of the kidney goes upwards to harass the heart, often manifesting with disturbances of the spirit.

Kidney Structure, Orifice, Emotion, Secretions, and Seasons

The kidney is associated with the bones

The kidney stores the essence, which generates marrow. The marrow includes bone marrow, the spinal marrow, cerebrospinal fluid, and the brain, all of which are created from kidney-essence. The condition of the kidney-essence impacts not only the development of bone, but also the spinal marrow and brain. The spinal marrow communicates with the brain, which is said to be formed by the gathering of marrow. Therefore, the brain is called the "sea of marrow".

When we say that the kidney dominates bone, it also refers to bone growth and development. Only when kidney-essence is abundant can bone marrow be produced. As the bones receive nourishment from the marrow, the bones will be strong and healthy. If the kidney-essence is deficient and fails to generate marrow, the resulting malnourishment leads to conditions such as delayed closure of the fontanel and weak bones in children, and fragile bones that are subject to fracture, especially in the elderly. For many congenital, chronic and deficiency-type diseases, treatment starts with supplementation of the kidney-essence.

Chinese medicine holds that the teeth and the bone both originate and are nourished by kidney-essence. Thus the saying, "The teeth are the extension of the

---

① (*shǒu*, 守) guard, defend
② (*lòu*, 露) show, reveal, betray

bones." Dental problems such as loose teeth or delayed growth in the teeth of children are associated with kidney-essence deficiency.

The kidney's outward appearance is in the hair

Head hair needs the nourishment of blood for growth. It is said in Chinese medicine, "The hair is the extension of the blood." When blood becomes deficient, the hair loses nourishment and become withered, gray and may even fall out. When essence and blood are abundant, the hair will be thick and lustrous. So hair is also the external manifestation of the kidney, as the condition of the hair can directly reflect the abundance of kidney-essence. Clinically, withered and early graying hair, and alopecia can all be signs of kidney-essence deficiency. The treatment principles for these problems are to supplement the kidney, supplement the blood, and nourish essence.

The openings of the kidney are the ears

Hearing is closely related with the abundance of kidney-essence and qi. When the kidney-essence and qi are abundant, the brain receives nourishment and the sense of hearing will be acute. Contrarily, when kidney-essence and qi are in decline, the hearing is affected.

Kidney		
structure	→	bone
outward manifestation	→	head hair
opening (orifice)	→	ears
controls	→	the "two yin"
secretion	→	thick saliva (spittle)
emotion	→	fear
season	→	winter qi

The kidney controls the "two yin"

The two openings of the body in charge of defecation and urination are called the posterior and anterior yin (the "two yin"). The anterior yin excretes urine and is used for reproduction, and the posterior yin is the passage of feces.

The storage and discharge of urine relies on the bladder, and the generation and excretion of urine depends upon the coordination of the evaporating and containing actions of kidney qi. If the evaporating and containing actions of kidney qi become disordered, there may be frequent urination or incontinence.

Defecation depends on the function of the large intestine to convey and transform waste, but it also requires the propelling and containing actions of the kidney qi. When kidney qi is deficient and fails to contain, signs and symptoms of qi deficiency such as constipation, frequent urination, incontinence or prolonged diarrhea may appear.

The anterior yin includes the genitalia for both men and women. When the kidney-essence and qi are abundant, sexuality will be pleasurable, semen is ejaculated normally, and the "intersection of yin and yang will bring new life". When kidney-essence and qi function abnormally, manifestations include impotence (*yăng wěi*, 阳痿), premature ejaculation, spontaneous seminal emission in men, abnormal menstruation in women and weakened libido and infertility in both women and men.

The kidney is associated with spittle

Spittle (*tuò*, 唾) is defined as the stickier and thicker part of saliva. It is secreted in the mouth together with the saliva, and moistens the mouth and food. Spittle is generated from kidney-essence and nourishes kidney-essence when swallowed. Excessive spitting can deplete the kidney-essence; in fact, in many qi gong and tai ji quan practices, practitioners are instructed to conserve and swallow any fluids that accumulate in the mouth during practice.

The kidney is associated with fear

Fear is the emotion associated with the kidney. Fear can cause the kidney qi to go downward or fail to spread upward, thus the sayings, "Fear injures the kidney" and "Fear causes qi to sink". We see this when people with sudden fear have urinary or fecal incontinence. Sudden fear can also turn a person's hair white or cause it to fall out within days. Fear is a result of sudden shock, or it can be associated with an ongoing fearful state.

In *Shen*, Rossi calls fear the "root of all other emotions: the anger of aggressiveness, the sadness of abandonment and loss, the thinking that attempts to control everything, and euphoria that hides the panic of desperation connected to it, and fear embraces them all."[1]

The kidney corresponds to the qi of winter

Winter is the coldest season of the year, and a time when many living things in nature hibernate. The kidney corresponds to water, which is characterized by moistening and downward movement, and it also stores essence, therefore also corresponding with winter-qi. To more effectively store essence in order to meet the growing qi of the spring season, during wintertime one should go to bed earlier and arise later.

---

[1] Elisa Rossi. *Shen: Psycho-emotional Aspects of Chinese Medicine*. London: Churchill-Livingstone; 2007. p. 38.

The taste associated with the kidney is salty

The salty flavor in an herb acts to dissolve masses and drain downward. Modern medicine also tells us that sodium and salt intake can have a dramatic effect on kidney function. As well, and not unrelated, is the fact that sodium influences the retention of fluids in the body.

Kidney-Essence, *Yuan* Qi, Kidney Yin, and Kidney Yang

The terms kidney-essence, kidney qi, kidney yang and yin, and *yuan*/source-qi are a source of frequent debate. Although the idea of kidney-essence is rather clear, kidney qi is often simply described as a combination of kidney yin and kidney yang. As kidney-essence, or *jīng,* comprised mainly of prenatal essence, the qi which results from the transformation of this essence is referred to as *yuan* qi, or source-qi, which can be seen as an "actualization" of the kidney-essence. Outside of reproduction, *jīng/*essence has limited functional ability of its own until it has been transformed into *yuan* qi.

The kidney-essence is the part of general essence stored in the kidney. It comes from the innate essence inherited from the parents and supplemented by parts of foodstuff essence. A part of innate essence stored in the kidney can, under the given conditions, combine with the acquired foodstuff essence to become reproductive essence. This essence is stored in the kidney to serve as the origin of the generation of the embryo. A case of kidney-essence deficiency clinically often presents with delayed development, short physical build, delayed closure of the fontanel, mental retardation, slow movement, and weak bone with no force in children; scanty sperm sterility in men; amenorrhea with sexual hypofunction and acyesis in women; premature senility, loss of hair and loose teeth, tinnitus, deafness, amnesia, trance, flaccid and weak feet, listlessness and apathy.

Clinically, kidney qi deficiency commonly leads to delayed development of the fetus and child, and in adults, premature senility, decreased sexual function, a sore lower back and weak knees, fatigue, dispiritedness, pale tongue with white coating, a forceless pulse or even a predisposition to various illnesses.[1] Kidney-essence deficiency has many of the same signs and symptoms, but often more strongly implies issues associated with aging or reproduction.

Kidney yin and kidney yang are two aspects of kidney qi with distinctly different properties; kidney yin acts to cool, moisten and calm, while kidney yang warms and activates. The harmonious coordination and integration of kidney yin and kidney

---

[1]   Supplement kidney qi with a formula such as *Jīn Guì Shèn Qì Wán* (Golden Cabinet Kidney Qi Pill, 金匮肾气丸).

yang form kidney qi, which acts to activate and regulate the various functions of the kidney. The yin derived from the kidney is seen as the source of all yin qi in the body, and is thus called original yin or true yin; the yang derived from the kidney is the root of all yang qi, called original yang or true yang.

Kidney yin deficiency can manifest with dizziness, tinnitus, insomnia, profuse dreaming, hyper-sexuality, premature ejaculation, scanty menstruation or amenorrhea, tidal fever with a sensation of heat in the bones, flushed cheeks, a red tongue with little or no coating, and a thready and rapid pulse; the teeth can loosen and there can be a hair loss. These signs and symptoms all result from a deficiency of yin and "yin-blood", which over time creates a rising heat within the body. Because kidney yin and liver blood have the same source, kidney yin deficiency can also lead to weakness of the tendons and knee joints due to malnourishment of the liver blood. In serious cases, there can be severe weakness of the muscles of the legs and even atrophy.

If atrophy is present, one can look to *Hǔ Qián Wán* (Hidden Tiger Pill, 虎潜丸) as an herbal prescription. *Formulas and Strategies* discusses this condition, and reveals many of the interlocking terms and concepts studied so far in this book through the use of the herbs *huáng bǎi* (Phellodendri Cortex) and *guī bǎn* (Testundinis Plastrum, 龟板). "*Huáng bǎi* also plays an important role in the treatment of atrophy disorder by drying dampness in the bones and lower *jiao*. Sweet, salty, and cooling *guī bǎn* enriches the yin and anchors the errant yang, augments the marrow, and fills the essence so as to tonify [supplement] the kidney and strengthen the bones. Together, these two substances tonify the insufficiency of both the liver and kidney, while simultaneously draining the ministerial fire that flares out of control."[1]

A standard herbal formula for enriching and nourishing kidney yin is *Liù Wèi Dì Huáng Wán* (Six Ingredients Rehmannia Pill, 六味地黄丸), or when accompanied by signs of deficiency heat, *Zhī Bǎi Dì Huáng Wán* (Anemarrhena, Phellodendron and Rehmannia Pill, 知柏地黄丸). Another condition which comes out of yin deficiency with heat is called yin deficiency with "vigorous fire". In treatment, as the internal fire is drained from the body, yin is nourished at the same time. Often times there will be constant hunger as well, possibly indicating *xiāo kě* (消渴) disease (a condition associated with diabetes).

Kidney yang deficiency usually presents with a sore lower back and weak knees, cold-type pain, and a loss of libido with impotence[2] or infertility. There may also be

---

① Volker Scheid, Dan Bensky, Andrew Ellis, Randal Barolet. *Formulas and Strategies*. 2nd ed. Seattle: Eastland Press; 2009. p. 378.

② (*yáng wěi*, 阳痿) yang atrophy

prolonged diarrhea with undigested food in the stool, a pale or blackish complexion, a fear of cold with cold limbs, listlessness, and clear urine with increased volume or frequent urination at night. The tongue is light red and enlarged with a white glossy coating, and the pulse is deep, slow and forceless or deep and weak. The treatment principle here is to warm and supplement kidney yang with formulas such as *Zhēn Wǔ Tāng* (True Warrior Decoction, 真武汤) and *Sì Shén Wán* (Four-Spirits Pill, 四神丸).

Mìng Mén (命门)

Mìng mén can be translated as life gate, vital gate, or destiny gate and is also known as "the space between the kidneys". *Mìng mén* is also a concept with links to Taoist practices, metaphysics and alchemical processes, where it is referred to as the *dān tián* or "cinnabar field". For some, the *mìng mén* represents another organ altogether, while for others it is simply a functional combining of the left and right kidney. The implicit assumptions are that the *mìng mén* is the source of vitality or yang energy for the entire body, and that the reproductive capacities of both men and women are stored in the *mìng mén*. Ming Dynasty physician Zhao Xian-ke (1567-1644) suggested that *mìng mén* provides the "true fire" of the entire body, and other writings state that the *mìng mén* is in fact the right kidney (corresponding to yang). Others hold that *mìng mén* is the starting point of the breath, so it is sometimes referred to as the "sea of breath".[1] In spite of the interesting historical context, most modern texts state that the *mìng mén* is a fire specifically corresponding with the kidney yang.

◆ *Jueyin* —Liver and Pericardium

The meaning of the term "*jueyin*" is as debatable in the Chinese language as it is in English. *Jueyin*, being the most yin and interior of the six systems, has been variously translated as ultimate yin, terminal yin, reverting yin, and others. The *Treatise on Cold Damage* states that *jueyin* is the deepest level and most critical stage of a disease process; the final stage that occurs after a disease has passed through the other yang and yin channel stages. The corresponding organs are the liver and pericardium, and the substances associated with *jueyin* are blood and wind. At this level, the emotions are also greatly influenced. Wang and Robertson write, "When the body sleeps, blood returns to *jueyin*, where it settles and clarifies. Within *jueyin*, the blood is stored and clarified by the liver while the qi of emotional excess is held, calmed and released by the pericardium."[2]

---

[1]   Isabelle Robinet. *Taoist Meditation: The Mao-shan Tradition of Great Purity*. Albany: State University of New York Press; 1993. p. 80.

[2]   Wang Ju-yi, Jason D. Robertson. *Applied Channel Therapy in Chinese Medicine: Wang Ju-Yi's Lectures on Channel Therapeutics*. Seattle: Eastland Press; 2008. p. 151.

LIVER (*GĀN*, 肝)

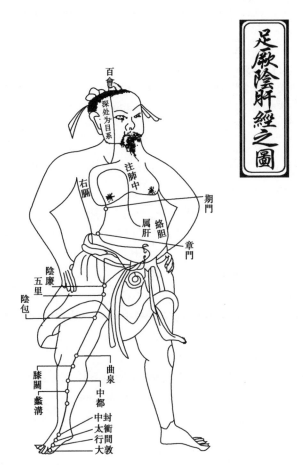

Main Physiological Functions of the Liver

One major function of the liver is to store blood, and the other is to maintain the free flow of qi. In five-phase theory, the liver belongs to wood and is characterized by movement, stubbornness, planning, impatience and irritability (like a military general); thus the liver is called "the general" as well as "the unyielding organ".

The liver governs the free flow of qi

The differences in meaning between the terms "stagnation" and "constraint" are a common source of misunderstanding for students and even translators, and in spite of their differences, the two terms are often used interchangeably. In brief, *zhì* (stagnation, 滞) refers to the qi itself and its lack of movement, often "stuck" in a particular place. *Yù* (郁, constraint) also refers to an impaired or depressed movement of qi, although it can also be in some contexts translated as depression in the psychological sense. Many translate *yù* as "depression", no matter the context. Compared with stagnation, constraint can therefore be understood in a broader sense, and the two conditions are sometimes found used together, as in "liver constraint and qi stagnation". In another context, *yù*-constraint may be found used in combination with the term *jié* (结), which means bound or "knotted".

The TCM statement "the liver governs the free flow of qi" can be more literally rendered as "the liver governs free-coursing" (*gān zhǔ shū xiè*, 肝主疏泄), referring to the liver's ability to free, regulate and soothe the overall movement of qi; the free flow of qi also promotes the circulation and distribution of essence, blood, and fluids, regulate the ascent-descent of the spleen and stomach qi, the secretion and excretion of the bile, adjust the emotional activities, as well as promote the ejaculation, menstruation and ovulation, bile secretion and the ascending and descending of spleen-stomach qi. While the lung governs the overall qi of the body, the liver (as general) ensures that qi flows in an orderly manner. The liver is also associated with the upward and outward movement of qi.

Concerning emotions, the liver failing to maintain the free flow of qi may manifest in two ways; the first involves liver qi stagnation or constraint that manifests with distending pain of the chest, rib-sides and breasts, often associated with frustration, depression or sadness. The second, and more dramatic condition resulting from anger or rage, involves liver impairment (*shāng gān*, 伤肝), which results in a hyperactive ascending of liver qi. Prolonged qi stagnation can also transform into internal fire that rises along with the hyperactive upward movement of liver qi; in this case, signs and symptoms include irritability, insomnia, headaches, red face and eyes, nosebleed, high blood pressure and even stroke.

The liver promotes the flow and distribution of blood and fluids

The circulation of blood and the distribution and metabolism of fluids all depend on the free movement of qi in the organs and channels, which is maintained by the liver. In fact, the circulation of blood and fluids is said to "follow the qi". Liver qi constraint then results in impeded blood flow or blood stasis; this can lead to the formation of internal masses as well as menstrual disorders in women. With resulting fluid distribution disorders, there may be water-dampness or phlegm-fluid retention. In addition, hyperactive liver qi can force blood out of the vessels, leading to profuse menstruation or menstrual flooding and spotting (*bēng lòu*, 崩漏). Therefore, the fundamental treatment principles for patterns of blood stasis, water-dampness or phlegm-fluid retention caused by liver qi constraint are to regulate the liver and correct the movement of qi. For bleeding due to hyperactive ascending of liver qi and internal fire, the main treatment principles are to descend qi and drain internal fire.

The liver promotes spleen-stomach transformation and transportation, and regulates the secretion and excretion of bile

The ascent and descent of spleen-stomach qi should remain interdependent, coordinated and harmonious, while also relying on the "freeing" function of the liver qi. When the liver maintains the free flow of qi, it allows the spleen and stomach to transform and transport substances along with normal secretion and excretion of bile. This promotes normal digestion and the absorption of the refined essences of food and water.

If the liver qi does not flow freely, the ascending and descending of spleen and stomach qi are affected, and digestive function becomes disrupted. Manifestations include a poor appetite, an aversion to fatty and greasy foods, and abdominal distention and pain. With hyperactive ascending of liver qi, bile excretion can become affected, causing a bitter taste in the mouth and jaundice in more severe cases. At the same time, the associated abnormal ascending of stomach qi results in abdominal distention and pain, nausea, vomiting, acid regurgitation and intestinal gurgling.

The liver and emotions

Feelings, affections, moods and sentiments are closely related to the five *zang*-organs. With well-regulated qi movement, a person's outlook is generally positive and balanced, with neither too much excitement nor depression. Often times, liver qi constraint can cause an otherwise happy person to become enraged, and with further constraint, there can be depression and sadness. Abnormal or excessive emotional activities also lead to disorders of qi movement, thus affecting the function of the liver to govern the free flow of qi. Prolonged liver qi constraint can lead to internal fire and hyperactive ascending of liver qi.[1] Unhappiness or frustration at any level, because of the lack of proper qi movement, is most often attributed to liver qi constraint (although the heart-spirit may be involved also).

The liver promotes ejaculation, menstruation and ovulation

Ejaculation in men, and menstruation and ovulation in women are both closely

---

[1] One can turn this around and say that anger is itself the rising of qi and/or fire resulting from liver constraint.

related with the liver function of maintaining the free flow of qi. The storage and emission of the semen requires the freeing actions of the liver qi working in coordination with the closing action of the kidney qi. When the liver qi maintains normal qi flow, semen can be released smoothly and appropriately; when the liver fails to maintain normal qi flow, normal seminal emission can become affected.

The free movement of qi as maintained by the liver is also required for regular and unobstructed menstruation, ovulation, conception and pregnancy. Liver qi stagnation can lead to irregular menstruation, menstrual block, amenorrhea, anovulation and infertility. For these kinds of issues, the general treatment principle is to soothe the liver and regulate qi (*shū gān lǐ qì*, 疏肝理气).

The liver stores the blood

Another function of the liver is to store blood. The liver storing of blood has five aspects: it serves to nourish liver qi, to regulate blood volume, to moisten the sinews and eyes, to serve as the source of menstruation, and to prevent bleeding. This is similar to the liver organ in biomedicine, which also recognizes that the liver contains a large amount of blood as well as multiple clotting factors.

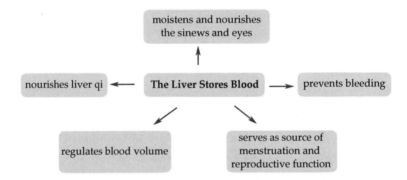

1) Nourishing liver qi

Qi is formless and characterized by motion, whereas blood has form and is characterized by stillness. The qi must attach itself to the blood so as to create a normal and orderly flow of qi and blood. If qi is not carried by the blood, it may circulate in a disordered manner and/or strongly ascend. Therefore, the liver stores enough blood to produce and nourish the liver qi; by maintaining harmony and free movement in this way, the liver qi is prevented from becoming hyperactive. With liver blood deficiency, mental-emotional symptoms such as anxiety or restlessness can also result.

2) Regulating blood volume

The liver stores an appropriate volume of blood for distribution to various parts of the body. Under normal conditions, the amount of blood present in each part of the body is relatively constant; however, the amount of blood in each part can vary according to changes in the body's activity levels, emotions, and changes in the natural climate. When the body is active or the mind becomes agitated, the liver will transport the stored blood into the body's peripheral regions. When a person is asleep or in a quiet state, the demand for blood will decrease, so blood will return from the peripheral regions for storage by the liver. On the emotional level, the spirit of the liver (*hún*) is implicated in many concepts concerning sleep and dreaming.

Modern studies show that blood flow in the liver increases by 25% as one is lying still, and that the whole liver system can store 55% of the body's entire blood volume. In an emergency condition, the liver can provide 1000~2000 mL of blood to guarantee sufficient cardiac output. Chinese medicine states, "When one is exercising, the blood circulates thorough the channels, while resting, the blood returns to the liver."

3) Moistening and nourishing the sinews and eyes

The blood stored by the liver acts to moisten and nourish the liver itself, as well as other organs and tissues. Thus the saying, "When the liver receives blood, one can see. When the feet receive blood, one can walk. When the palms receive blood, one can grasp. When the fingers receive blood, one can hold." If the liver is not well-functioning, this may lead to a shortage of blood with a resulting lack of moistening and nourishing. For example, if the liver blood becomes deficient and fails to nourish the eyes, there will be dryness and discomfort of the eyes with blurred vision or night blindness. If liver blood fails to nourish the sinews, there can be impaired movement or numbness of the limbs.

4) Source of menstruation and reproductive function

The blood stored in the liver also provides the source of menstruation in women. The *chong mai* is an "extraordinary vessel" which is greatly associated with menstruation; the *chong* vessel originates in the lower abdomen, connects with the liver, and is called the "sea of blood". If liver blood is deficient, there will be shortened menstruation or even amenorrhea. For men, both liver qi and blood are often implicated in issues of sexual function in that deficient blood and disordered liver qi are seen as one cause of impotence and/or lack of libido.

5) Preventing bleeding

The liver is in charge of storing blood and one function of qi is to control blood; thus with abundant liver qi, liver blood remains under control. Yin qi is characterized by coagulation, and liver yin acts to restrain liver yang (which can cause bleeding when in excess).

If the liver fails to store blood, various types of bleeding may appear such as in expectoration of blood, nosebleeds, profuse menstruation, or flooding and spotting[1]. There are three main pathomechanisms, the first involving a deficiency of liver qi with failure to astringe; in this condition, bleeding is relatively scant in quantity and light in color. The second involves a shortage of liver yin that leads to hyperactive ascending of liver yang; in this case, bleeding is more profuse and bright red in color, often accompanied by fever, and dry uncomfortable feelings of the eyes. The third pathomechanism involves hyperactive liver fire that scorches the blood vessels and forces blood to extravasate from the vessels; in this condition, the bleeding is profuse with a deep red or purplish-red color.

The liver is yin in form, but yang in function

The structure of the liver enables it to store blood, so its form belongs to yin. The liver governs the free flow of qi, which is a yang function; thus the saying, "The liver is yin in form but yang in function." If the liver blood is deficient and fails to nourish, sinews and eyes can become affected. The liver functions of governing the free flow of qi and storing blood are complementary and interdependent. The freeing function concerns the smoothness of qi movement, and the storing function concerns the storage and regulation of blood; both are required to maintain the harmony of qi and blood. When the liver maintains the free flow of qi, the movement of qi will be smooth and thus blood circulation remains normal, but when the liver fails to maintain the free flow of qi, the resulting stagnation of qi can also lead to patterns of blood stasis. Qi stagnation can also lead to internal fire that causes blood to move frenetically, forcing blood to extravasate from the vessels. With hyperactive liver qi where the blood follows the disordered qi movement, there may be headaches, bleeding, or irregular menstruation. If liver yin becomes deficient, impaired cooling and moistening may lead to hyperactive ascending of liver qi with a stirring of internal wind. *The Yellow Emperor's Inner Classic* states, "When the movement of liver-wood is excessive, this will cause wind, and spleen-earth will be injured."[2] The resulting lack of blood can also cause internal wind. The pattern of deficient blood producing wind is commonly associated with conditions such as Parkinson's disease and other disorders involving tremors.

Physiological Characteristics of the Liver

The liver is the unyielding organ

In five-phase theory, the liver corresponds to wood, which is characterized by qualities of bending and straightening; therefore, the liver qi is said to prefer free

---

[1] "Flooding and spotting", profuse bleeding or menstrual spotting between periods.

[2] Yin Hui-he. *Fundamentals of Traditional Chinese Medicine*. Beijing: China Science and Technology Press; 1992. p. 338.

activity as well as upward movement. However, the liver is also said to be "firm but impatient" [1] in nature, thus called the "unyielding organ". This means that liver qi can grow in a number of directions, but once grown, it becomes difficult to change. We can see this in the imagery of bamboo, which once grown under the eaves of a house, will continue to push upward until the roof itself is lifted[2]. For this reason, liver disharmony often manifests with hyperactive ascending of liver qi or upward flaming of liver fire with signs and symptoms of dizziness, vertigo, a red complexion, irritability, spasm of the sinews, etc.

The liver governs ascent and dispersion

The liver corresponds to the spring season, which is characterized by growth and an ascending movement of qi. Liver qi thus moves upward and diffuses outward, which also acts to prevent qi stagnation. With normal liver qi ascending and diffusion, qi and blood remain harmonious and the five *zang*-organs will function normally. However, it is also said that "liver qi and liver yang are prone to over-activity". Due to this propensity for upward movement and over-activity, liver disharmony is often characterized by hyperactive ascending of qi and yang.

Relationships of the Liver with the Orifices, Emotions, Secretion, and Season

The liver is connected to the sinews

The sinews (*jīn*, 筋) [3] include the tendons and ligaments which adhere to the bones and gather at the joints, the tissues that connect joints and muscles, and the tissues that govern the motion of the joints[4]. The sinews depend upon liver blood for nourishment. If liver blood is sufficient, the sinews receive adequate nourishment, and thus they can move freely and forcefully. Therefore, the liver is called "the basis of resistance to fatigue". When liver blood becomes deficient and the sinews become malnourished, the power of the sinews will decrease. With deficient blood producing wind, signs and symptoms include tremors of the hands and feet, or numbness of the limbs with impaired flexion and extension. If pathogenic heat consumes the liver blood, as sinews lose nourishment there may appear tremors of hands and feet, spasms, and a rigid body. Even slight tremors may reflect a deficiency of liver blood.

The liver's outward appearance is in the nails

The fingernails and toenails are considered as an extension of the sinews and thus

---

① (*gāng qiáng zào jí*, 刚强躁急) firm and impatient
② David Scott, 2010
③ The character itself has the components (radicals) for bamboo, flesh, and strength.
④ Many practitioners state that the sinews encompass the white parts of the muscle and joint system.

are also dependent upon liver blood for nourishment. By inspecting the form, color and luster of the nails, one can determine the condition of liver blood. When liver blood is abundant, the nails will be tough and lustrous. With deficient liver blood, the nails become soft, thin, withered, or even deformed and cracked.

The opening of the liver is the eyes

The vision function of the eyes depends on both the nourishment of liver blood and the freeing action of liver qi. The liver channel ascends to link with eyes where the qi and blood of the liver can reach the eyes through the channel pathway, thus the statement "the liver opens to the eyes". When liver blood is sufficient and the liver qi is harmonious, the eyes can see well and differentiate colors. If liver blood is deficient, there may be eye dryness and discomfort, blurred vision, dizziness and eye pain. If exterior wind-heat invades the liver channel and goes upward, there will be red, painful and/or itching eyes. If liver wind stirs internally, there may be deviation of the eyes. When liver qi stagnates for a long time and subsequently produces internal fire and phlegm, there may be misting and darkness of the eyes with blurred vision.

In addition, the vision function of the eyes also depends upon the nourishment of essence of all the five *zang*-organs and six *fu*-organs. The essence of the five *zang*-organs and six *fu*-organs all go up into the eyes and nourish various parts of the eyes respectively. In "the theory of the five orbiculi" in Chinese medicine, the eye is divided into several parts that correspond respectively to the five *zang*-organs, i.e., "pupil is water orbiculus corresponding to the kidney, the black of the eye is wind orbiculus corresponding to the liver, white of the eye is qi orbiculus corresponding to the lung, canthi are blood orbiculi corresponding to the heart, and eyelids are flesh orbiculi corresponding to the spleen."

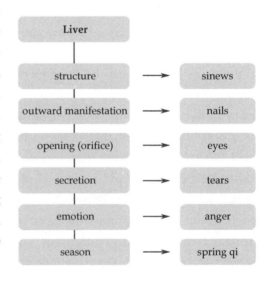

The liver is associated with tears as its secretion

The liver opens to the eyes, and tears act both to moisten and protect the eye; tears are said to be transformed from the essence-blood of the liver. Under normal conditions, the secretions that moisten the eye should not flow freely, but when a foreign body invades the eye, the secretion of tears will increase in order to wash the eyeball and remove the foreign body.

There can also be a pathologically abnormal lacrimation. For example, when liver blood is deficient, the secretion of tears will decrease and there may be dry eyes. If pathogenic damp-heat invades the liver channel or pathogenic wind-fire disturbs the eyes, there may be increased secretions. As well, of course, the emotions of sadness and happiness can cause tears to flow.

The liver is associated with the emotion of anger

From a strictly material viewpoint, anger comes from changes in liver blood and liver qi. Hence, there is the saying that the liver is associated with anger. Generally, everyone experiences anger, which (within a certain range) helps to maintain the physiological equilibrium of the body. However, great or persistent anger will have an extremely negative effect on the body due to liver qi constraint impairing qi flow that affects the normal distribution of essence, blood, qi and fluids. This can result in phlegm and fluid retention, blood stasis, and masses (*zhēng jiǎ*, 癥瘕[1]). Anger can cause hyperactive ascent of liver qi with manifestations of stroke or even coma. For the patient with persistent anger, the treatment principles are to soothe the liver and resolve constraint. For those patients suffering from hyperactive ascent of liver qi caused by great anger, the treatment principles are to soothe the liver and descend qi.

The liver corresponds to the qi of spring

Spring is the beginning of a new year, during which yang qi begins to grow; there is a flourishing in nature with signs of new life. The liver governs the free flow of qi, prefers free activity, and its qi ascends and diffuses upward and outward. These qualities are similar to the nature of the spring season, thus it is said that the liver corresponds with the qi of spring.

The liver's associated taste is sour

The flavor or taste associated with the liver is sour. Sourness pulls inward and prevents qi from moving too aggressively. One of the main herbs associated with the liver is *bái sháo* (Paeoniae Radix Alba, 白芍), which acts to nourish liver blood with its sour flavor and astringent quality. Another herb with which *bái sháo* is often combined is *chái hú* (Bupleuri Radix, 柴胡), which acts to resolve liver qi stagnation. Together, these two herbs reflect the main qualities of the liver: there is a yin function that holds the blood, and a yang function that maintains the free flow of qi.

---

[1] "Concretions and conglomerations", as defined in *The Practical Dictionary of Chinese Medicine* (Nigel Wiseman, Ye Feng. Taos: Paradigm Publications; 1998. p. 92.).

Liver Blood, Liver Qi, Liver Yin, and Liver Yang

The blood stored in the liver is the material basis for the functional activities of the liver, and liver blood is also the origin for the secretion of the bile. The liver blood also has a moistening and nourishing function for the liver, eyes, sinews, and nails. A case of liver blood deficiency may clinically present with dizziness and vertigo, tinnitus, lusterless nails, blurred vision or night blindness, dull pain in the hypochondriac region, or numbness of limbs, joint spasms with impaired movement, tremors of hands and feet, tremble muscles or scanty menstruation with light colored flow, or even amenorrhea, a pale complexion, a light red tongue with a white coating, a wiry and thready pulse. The principle of treatment here is to supplement and nourish liver blood with a formula such as *Sì Wù Tāng* (Four Substances Decoction, 四物汤).

Liver qi is transformed from liver blood. It is a very fine material with powerful actions to activate and regulate the functional activities of the body. Liver qi rises upward (*xiàng shàng*, 向上) and moves outward (*xiàng wài*, 向外) while regulating and freeing the movement of qi (*tiáo chàng qì jī*, 调畅气机). This can promote the flow and distribution of blood and fluids, promote digestion and absorption of food, promote the secretion and excretion of the bile, and make one's mood less irritable and melancholy. The menstruation and ovulation in women and ejaculation in men are closely related with the function of the liver qi.

A case of liver qi deficiency commonly appears as melancholy, timidity, listlessness, lack of energy, dizziness and vertigo, pain in the hypochondria, frequent sighing, and a weak pulse. The treatment principle for this should be to supplement the liver and resolve constraint by using *Xiāo Yáo Sǎn* (Free Wanderer Powder, 逍遥散) plus *rén shēn* (Ginseng Radix et Rhizoma, 人参) and/or *huáng qí* (Astragali Radix, 黄芪).

Liver yin is the aspect of liver qi that cools, moistens, tranquilizes and inhibits. A case of liver yin deficiency presents with dizziness, tinnitus, red eyes, flushed cheeks, burning pain in the rib-sides, vexing heat in the five centers (chest, palms and soles), tidal fever, night sweating, a red tongue with little coating, and a wiry, thready and rapid pulse. To nourish liver yin, one may select the formula *Qīng Gān Yǐn* (Liver-Clearing Beverage, 清肝饮).

Liver yang is the aspect of liver qi that warms, propels and activates. Liver yang deficiency manifestations include chillness, cold limbs, spasm of the scrotum with cold sensations of the perineum, cold pain in the lateral sides of the lower abdomen, abdominal distention like a drum, puffy limbs, loose stools, fatigue, and a thready forceless pulse. *Nuǎn Gān Jiān* (Decoction for Warming the Liver, 暖肝煎) can be used for treatment.

PERICARDIUM (*XĪN BĀO*, 心包)

The pericardium envelops the heart, and in fact the Chinese characters "心包"(*xīn bāo*) literally mean "heart wrapper". Because the heart is the emperor-organ and easily attacked by heat, the pericardium mainly functions to shield the heart from internal heat while also promoting the circulation of qi and blood. Signs and symptoms of an affected pericardium include high fever and mania. The idea of the pericardium shielding the heart is also associated with emotional issues in that when internal heat and phlegm affect the pericardium, the spirit also becomes disturbed. Because of this, many emotional "issues of the heart" are treated through the pericardium. The pericardium is also like the heart, a fire-organ, but the fire associated with the pericardium is considered as a "ministerial fire" as opposed to the heart's "sovereign fire". The pericardium is called an adjunct or associated organ to the other five *zang*-organs.

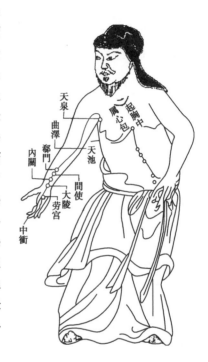

STUDY

	Spleen	Heart	Kidney	Lung	Liver
Structure					
Outward manifestation					
Opening (orifice)					
Secretion					
Emotion					
Season					

	Spleen	Heart	Kidney	Lung	Liver
Taste					
Governs					

CASES

1. Your patient is a 25-year-old woman who complains of headaches located at the top of her head every Sunday evening. She works an office job and goes to school most evenings. She dislikes her job and is involved in a lawsuit involving the job. Her menstrual periods are irregular for the last 3 years, arriving every 20~30 days. Her pulse is wiry, and her tongue is red with a normal thin white coating.

2. Your patient is a 40-year-old man who has a dull pain in his lower back. He is a former athlete who took steroids in high school. He continues to work out for 2 hours a day. He is feeling increasingly tired after his workouts and in response he has begun training with more weight lifting to "build his energy". His tongue is red with no coating, and his pulse is thready and deep.

3. Your patient is a 30-year-old woman with stomach distention after eating. She says that she has a good diet, and that she eats at least one salad each day. Her breakfast consists of a fruit smoothie made from frozen organic fruits. Her tongue is swollen, and her pulse is slippery.

4. Your patient is a 23-year-old woman who had difficult menstruation for several years beginning at her first period at age 14. Her doctors had her take birth control pills for five years, and over the last six years she gained 40 pounds. Her periods now arrive once every 3 months and are of short duration with little menstrual flow. She is beginning to find some hair growth on her face, thus her doctors are testing her for PCOS (polycystic ovarian syndrome). Her tongue is purplish with teeth marks on the edges, and her pulse is thready and deep.

Section 2   Six *Fu*-Organs (*Liù Fǔ*, 六腑)

INTRODUCTION TO THE *FU*-ORGANS

The six *fu*-organs is a collective name for the gallbladder, stomach, small intestine, large intestine, urinary bladder and *sanjiao*. They are viewed as hollow pouches or tubular organs that function as temporary containers and passageways for substances. Their common functions are to receive, transport and transform water and grain

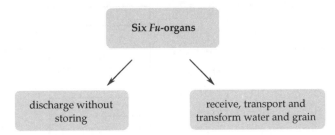

(drinks and food).

In the *Classic of Difficult Issues (Nàn Jīng, 难经)* there is a term called the "seven portals". These are the gates to the outside, or between the *fu*-organs. They include the mouth, larynx, the structures between the stomach and small intestine, between the small and large intestines, and the anus. Food and drink needs to transit through all seven portals in order for it to be digested, absorbed and discharged out of the body. The seven portals help the six *fu*-organs to receive and process food and drink intake, "separate the clear from the turbid", and convey and discharge waste. Therefore, a disorder in any of the seven portals can affect the reception, digestion, absorption and excretion of food and drink.

飞门（唇）flying portal (lips)

户门（齿）house portal (teeth)

吸门（会厌）inhaling portal (epiglottis-entrance to the larynx)

贲门（胃之上口）cardia (upper opening of the stomach)

幽门（胃之下口）pylorus (lower opening of the stomach)

阑门（大、小肠交会）railing portal (conjunction of the large intestine and small intestine or ileocecalcon junction)

魄门（下极）corporeal-soul portal (anus)

Seven Portals

Each of the *fu*-organs has at least one opening that leads to the outside of the body or to another *fu*-organ. Together they are called the 7 portals. Note that each of the Chinese names ends with "door/gate"(门).

"Those that are called the five *zang*-organs (viscera) store essence and qi but don't drain. Thus they are full but are unable to fill up. The six *fu*-organs (bowels) convey and transform things but do not store. Thus they fill up but are unable to stay full."[1]

As *fu*-organs (bowels), with an open-ended tube-like structure, the *fu*-organs can take in substances, process and then later release or discharge them at the appropriate time. Unlike the *zang*-organs, which function best when full with organ-essence, healthy *fu*-organs empty when

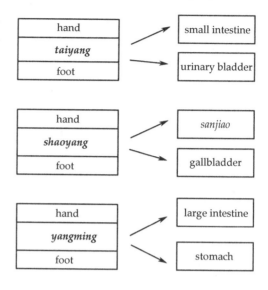

they have completed their transforming and moving actions. The six *fu*-organs therefore function optimally when their qi flows smoothly and freely downward without obstruction.

◆ *Taiyang* — Small Intestine and Bladder

The *taiyang* system opens up to the outside of the body through the channels in two different ways. The foot *taiyang* bladder channel travels from the face to over the head, over the back, and then down the legs. The hand *taiyang* channel also covers a wide area of the upper back. The significance of this is that the *taiyang* channel is the often first to receive outside pathogens which cause an "exterior invasion" type of illness. When in health, these channels will warm the susceptible areas and protect them from exterior pathogens, and will close the pores should an invasion occur. This explains why when we catch a common cold (analogous to one form of an exterior invasion) we first experience a headache, then a stiff neck, and then upper back pain. The *taiyang,* together with the lung, acts to adjust the pores based on the outside environment. Wang and Robertson write, "As the most external of the six channels, the *taiyang* is the first line of defense against external invasion. Defense is achieved by warming and discharging the exterior."[2] The functions of the *taiyang* also explain why urination disturbances are often tied to the onset of colds and flu.

---

① *Basic Questions:* 所谓五脏者，藏精气而不泻也，故满而不能实。六腑者，传化物而不藏，故实而不能满也。
② Wang Ju-yi, Jason D. Robertson. *Applied Channel Therapy in Chinese Medicine: Wang Ju-Yi's Lectures on Channel Therapeutics.* Seattle: Eastland Press; 2008. p. 185.

SMALL INTESTINE (*XIĂO CHÁNG*, 小肠)

The small intestine governs reception and digestion of the chyme (food and drink partially digested by the stomach). After received by the small intestine, the spleen and small intestine then function together to digest the chyme further into essence and waste. If this function of the small intestine is disordered, there will appear abdominal distention, diarrhea, loose stool, and so on.

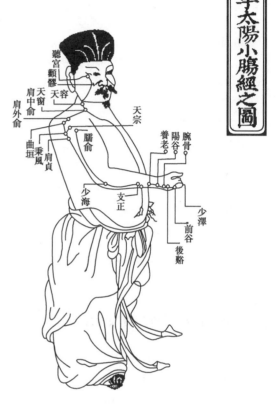

The small intestine is called the official in charge of "separating the clear from the turbid" (*mì bié qīng zhuó*, 泌别清浊). As the small intestine absorbs the essences of food and water, the refined or "clear" fluids are transported by the spleen qi to the other organs and through the body. As the spleen qi transports these essential substances upward, the clear fluids reaching the lung eventually nourish the skin as well.

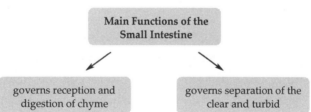

All of these processes involve the exchange of fluids. Some of the turbid materials will be transported from the small intestine down to the large intestine, where they will be further processed and turned into waste. Because the small intestine participates in the fluid metabolism, it is said that "the small intestine governs liquid", and because it separates the clear from the turbid, it is also referred to as "a lower functionary charged with classification".[1]

---

① Wang Ju-yi, Jason D. Robertson. *Applied Channel Therapy in Chinese Medicine: Wang Ju-Yi's Lectures on Channel Therapeutics*. Seattle: Eastland Press; 2008. p.190.

Modern biomedical anatomical study tells us that virtually all food nutrients are absorbed into the blood in the small intestine. These nutrients include electrolytes, sodium, chloride, potassium and the dietary organic molecules of glucose, amino acids and fatty acids. In biomedical terms, *yè-fhid* can be likened to the glandular and lymphatic secretions which are vital to preventing diseases such as diabetes, thyroid disease, celiac disease, and a host of autoimmune conditions. The concept of clear and turbid separation could be involved in the pathology of autoimmune diseases as well.

While it is not always possible to merge the ancient concepts of Chinese medicine with current biomedical knowledge, there are many areas where the insights of biomedicine can confirm ancient thought in order to bring deeper understanding of both.

This function of "classification" is actually more intricate than simply dividing the pure from the impure. The small intestine is connected to the heart-organ through an interior-exterior relationship, and is thus considered a fire-organ as related to the heart through the channels. The clear fluids separated in the small intestine are sent back up to the spleen to be sent through a process of further refinement, and turbid fluids are used to create *yè* (the thicker form of the *jīn/yè* fluids)[1]. *Yè* comprises both cerebrospinal fluid and those fluids which moisten the joints.

BLADDER (*PÁNG GUĀNG*, 膀胱)

The bladder is a hollow organ located in the lower abdomen below the kidney. The bladder, via ureters, connects with the kidney and the urethra at each end, and opens to the external genitalia. The function of the bladder is to store and excrete urine.

The body fluids disperse throughout the whole body to nourish and moisten the lung, spleen, kidney and the other organs. The metabolized fluids enter the kidney where the evaporating action of kidney qi acts to ascend the clear and descend the turbid. The clear parts remain within the body as part of fluid metabolism, and the turbid parts becomes urine.

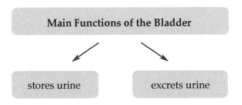

Main Functions of the Bladder

stores urine   excrets urine

① Wang Ju-yi, Jason D. Robertson. *Applied Channel Therapy in Chinese Medicine: Wang Ju-Yi's Lectures on Channel Therapeutics*. Seattle: Eastland Press; 2008. p.190.

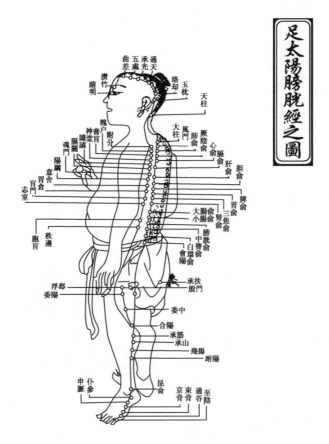

The excretion of urine is regulated through the stimulation and control of kidney qi and bladder qi. With kidney qi acting in harmony with bladder qi, the opening and closing of the bladder will be well-coordinated so that urine is discharged normally.

The bladder function of storing and excreting urine relies upon the coordinated ascending and descending of kidney qi and bladder qi respectively; kidney qi governs ascending, and bladder qi governs descending. The ascent of kidney qi stimulates the production of urine and controls its excretion, while the descent of bladder qi allows the bladder to excrete urine. If the kidney and bladder qi fail to control opening and closing, there can be difficult urination, dribbling urinary blockage, frequent urination, urgent urination, or urinary incontinence.

◆ *Shaoyang* —**Gallbladder and** *Sanjiao*

The *shaoyang* system associated with the *sanjiao* and gallbladder is interesting in both theory and practice. The *shaoyang* is considered to be a "pivot" and is implicated in many mixed cases of exterior and interior disease, issues concerning both deficiency and excess, and chronic problems that develop over many years.

Pathogens are said to be able to "hide" in the *shaoyang*, or to become lodged in between the interior and exterior levels. A classic *shaoyang* disease is malaria, which surfaces periodically with alternating chills and fever. Other conditions associated with *shaoyang* are chronic hepatitis, chronic fatigue, and unresolved colds and flu. Treatment of these diseases can become very difficult because the pathogens are not easily vented nor drained, although they can usually be resolved through "harmonizing" methods of treatment.

GALLBLADDER (*DǍN*, 胆)

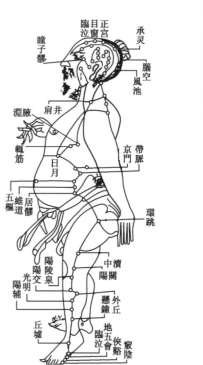

The gallbladder is attached to the short lobe of the liver; it is a hollow structure which contains bile. The bile is a pure, clear, and bitter yellow-green substance called "essential juice" or "clear juice". Because it assists digestion, the gallbladder is known as the "officer of the clear" and "officer of purification".

Proper bile flow depends on the liver function of maintaining the free flow of qi. The bile stored in the gallbladder discharges into the intestine to help with digestion. The longer than normal retention of bile can cause gallstones, jaundice, abdominal pain, diarrhea, and bitter taste in the mouth, among other symptoms. Gallbladder qi functions well when descending as compared to the liver qi, which

functions well when ascending. When bile goes upward or outward to the skin, there can be symptoms of jaundice such as yellow eyes, a bitter taste in the mouth, and a yellowish complexion.

The gallbladder is a *fu*-organ, but is also one of the six extraordinary *fu*-organs. The gallbladder is a hollow organ, similar to the other five *fu*-organs. However, like the five *zang*-organs, the gallbladder also stores an essential fluid. Furthermore, the gallbladder does not directly contact food and water, but only excretes bile into the intestine to promote the digestion and absorption of food and drink. This dual role is the reason the gallbladder is also considered one of the six extraordinary *fu*-organs.

Chinese medicine emphasizes the gallbladder's role in governing judgment and decision-making. These include activities of the spirit, consciousness, thinking, and the process of eliminating negative thoughts. The gallbladder is called the "fair judge" who is said to be "impartial and unbiased". The gallbladder regulates and controls relations between qi and blood, yin and yang, body and spirit, and interior and exterior, therefore serving as a "judge" of the body's state. Consequently, the gallbladder regulates and maintains the optimal state between the body and its external environment, which is a *shaoyang* function. Although this function of decision-making and impartiality may seem rather abstract if not simply esoteric, in clinical practice it is very well-known. Patients who feel "stuck" or unable to make decisions will often make a motion with their hand which unknowingly follows the back and forth path of the gallbladder channel on the side of their head.

SANJIAO (*SĀN JIĀO*, 三焦)

The *sanjiao* is a collective name for the upper *jiao*, middle *jiao* and lower *jiao*. The term *jiao* defies an easy translation, although it contains a suggestion of "fire", and *san* simply means three. For this reason, *sanjiao* is often translated as "triple burner". As one of the six *fu*-organs, the *sanjiao* can be conceptualized in a number of ways. The first is that it has a specific physical form with definite functions. Second, it can also be seen in terms of simple location, referring to the upper, middle and lower parts of the body. Lastly, it can be seen as having specific functions, but with no actual structure; it has therefore been referred to as "an organ without a form". The various ways of looking at the *sanjiao* are not mutually exclusive and can overlap, or they may change given the context of the discussion.

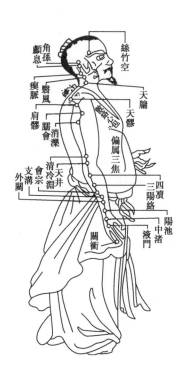
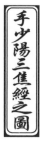

Looking at the *sanjiao* as an organ with a specific shape, structure and function, the *sanjiao* exists in the area between the gastrointestinal tract and the bladder. The physiological function of *sanjiao* is to dredge[1] the water passages and convey water, thus it conducts fluids from the gastrointestinal tract into the bladder. Correlated to modern anatomical studies, the *sanjiao* is associated with the mesentery and peritoneum in the abdominal cavity. These tissues are considered as the passages for gastrointestinal fluids to permeate into the bladder. Because of their hollow structure, all of these qualities correspond to the characteristics of the other five *fu*-organs.

Viewed in terms of location, the *sanjiao* refers to the passages and columns formed by the gaps among the organs and within the organs. The *sanjiao* then can refer to the upper, middle and lower parts of the body, which transmit all kinds of qi and also transport fluids. The heart and lung are in the upper *jiao*, the spleen in the middle *jiao*, and the kidney is in the lower *jiao*; the liver is sometimes considered as being located in the lower *jiao* with the kidney, but it is also viewed as a middle-*jiao* organ in many cases.

There are countless openings in the organs, as the organs communicate with each other through a passageway system which is itself the *sanjiao*. These passageways allow qi to enter and exit the organs and for qi to ascend and descend within the body.

In Chapter 1, we learned how yin and yang can transform into each other. In "qi transformation", yin qi is turned into yang qi and vice versa. For example, food substances are turned into qi which in turn helps activate and nourish the organs. At a basic level, without qi transformation, food would not be digested and the organs would cease to function. This section describes how important the *sanjiao* is to that process.

Because the domain of the *sanjiao* includes the five *zang*-organs and the six *fu*-organs, any sort of general qi transformation can be seen as qi transformation within the organs. Hence, all kinds of qi flow continuously through the *sanjiao*, and all kinds of qi transformation functions occur within the *sanjiao*, especially as related to *yuan* (source/original) qi. The *yuan* qi is said to scatter throughout the whole body through the *sanjiao*. The *sanjiao* is therefore considered a main location for qi transformation.

Transporting fluids

The *sanjiao* serves as the passageway for fluids to ascend, descend and distribute, therefore the *sanjiao* is described as the "officer in charge of drainage, dredging, and the passage of water". The body's fluid metabolism is performed through proper functioning

---

[1]   (shū tōng, 疏通) dredge

of the lung, spleen, kidney, bladder and other organs, but the *sanjiao* is the passageway, and thus the effects of organ function are mainly reflected in the *sanjiao*. In the upper *jiao*, the lung is the upper source of water; in the middle *jiao*, the spleen and stomach transport and distribute water; in the lower *jiao*, the kidney and bladder evaporate water through qi transformation. Viewed in another way, fluid metabolism can be said to mainly take place through the kidney, but this also requires a dynamic and orderly coordination with the other organs. Altogether, this process is called "*sanjiao* qi transformation".

Location

The organs associated with the *sanjiao* are more consistent with their functions than with their physical locations. The upper *jiao* is the chest above the diaphragm, which consists of the upper segment of the body, including the heart, lung, face and head. The upper *jiao* governs the diffusing-dispersing and ascending-dispersing, or diffusing and dispersing of *wei* qi. It scatters the essence of food and fluids to nourish and moisten the whole body. The upper *jiao* functions include those of the heart and lung to diffuse, disperse and distribute essence and qi. The fluids of the upper *jiao* tend to be finer, and are thus compared to a "mist".

The middle *jiao* is the area below the diaphragm and above the navel, including the liver, gallbladder, stomach and spleen. The middle *jiao* digests, absorbs and distributes food and fluid-essence. It includes the functions of the liver, gallbladder, spleen and stomach to digest and absorb food and drink. The middle *jiao* is where food and drink are transformed, and the turbulence created in doing so creates what is compared to a "foam".

The lower *jiao* is the lower segment of the body below the navel, including the kidney, bladder, large and small intestines, and the uterus or essence-chamber (*jīng shì*, 精室). The main function of the lower *jiao* is to excrete waste and urine, so the lower *jiao* is compared to a drainage ditch. One image of the *sanjiao*, particularly in the

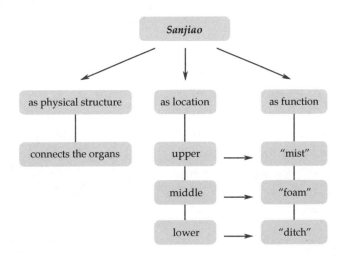

lower *jiao*, is that of a sieve or screen over a drain or at the end of an irrigation pipe.

◆ *Yangming* —Large Intestine and Stomach

The *yangming* system often involves issues of moisture and dryness. Dryness can be the result of heat, and it is thought that many conditions of heat and excess are best treated through the clearing of the *yangming*. When fluids are dry, the stool in the large intestine will not pass downward freely and may clump up, causing constipation; this in turn will cause more heat and dryness. Good bowel movements depend on an exchange of fluids which permeate and then leave the large intestine. Excessive purging of the bowels will eventually cause dryness and other damage to the *yangming*.

The yin-organs that are internal-externally associated with the *yangming* are the *taiyin* organs, the spleen and lung. The lung is the upper source of fluids. The spleen transports fluids upward to the lung and downward to the kidney and bladder. As stated by Yan Shi-lin, "When spleen yin is depleted, fluids are insufficient and therefore cannot enrich the large intestine below." [1]

LARGE INTESTINE (*DÀ CHÁNG*, 大肠)

The large intestine includes the colon and rectum; it is the organ that both absorbs the liquid in the food residue through its drying actions, and changes the residue into stools for discharge. The upper end of the large intestine connects with the small intestine in the "railing" portal (ileocecal conjunction), and the lower end opens to the corporeal-soul portal (rectum). The movement of large intestine qi conveys the stool to the end of the large intestine and discharges it out of the body through the anus, so the large intestine is called the "officer in charge of conveyance". If the conveying function of the large intestine is disordered, a patient may have abdominal pain and/or diarrhea with pus and blood.

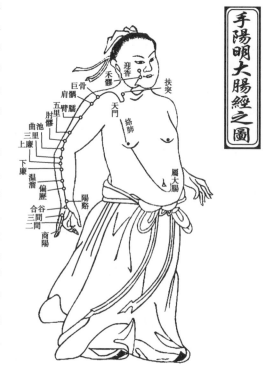

---

[1] Yan Shi-Lin. *Pathomechanisms of the Spleen*. Taos: Paradigm Publications; 2009. p. 193.

The large intestine governs the movement and transformation of waste and liquids. The food residue from the small intestine received by the large intestine includes a large amount of water which the large intestine absorbs as

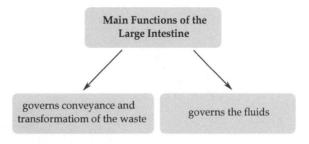

part of fluid metabolism, thus the saying, "The large intestine governs liquid." If there is heat in the large intestine, this can lead to a deficiency of fluids and constipation. On the other hand, if water in the large intestine is not absorbed, but rather goes downward together with the waste, there can be abdominal pain and diarrhea. The clear fluids transformed from the large intestine also nourish the surface of the body, so maintaining a healthy large intestine is very important for treating dermatological issues, especially those involving heat and dryness.

STOMACH (*WÈI*, 胃)

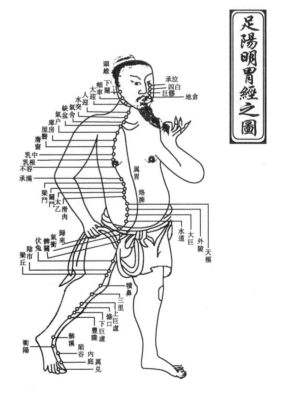

The stomach is located towards the top of the abdominal cavity, and includes the upper, middle and lower parts of the organ. The upper part connects the cardia and esophagus, and the lower connects the pyloric canal with the small intestine. The passageways at the esophagus and the small intestine are considered two of the seven portals. Note that the heart and the stomach share some of the same nerves; often simple stomach issues are confused with heart conditions, and vice versa. Some acupuncture points such as RN 14 (*jù quē*) are associated with issues of the heart. This point's location can be associated anatomically with the upper portion of the stomach.

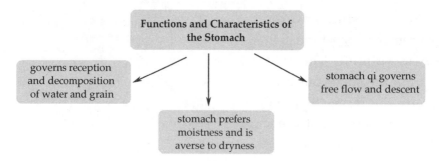

The stomach governs the reception and decomposition of water and grain

The stomach receives and grinds to create the initial digestion of food and drink. Although the decomposition of food and drink into chyme is primarily associated with stomach qi, both reception and digestion are also closely related with the spleen. Because essence, qi, blood and fluids are produced from food and drink, the stomach is called "the sea of water and grain".

The stomach qi governs free flow and descent[①]

The stomach and spleen are both located in the middle *jiao* and are the hub of the ascent and descent of qi movement (*qì jī*, 气机). The descent of stomach qi and the ascent of spleen qi depend on each other. Stomach qi failure to descend not only affects the descending of qi of the six *fu*-organs, but also that of the whole body.

After food is received by the stomach it is "ground up", digested, and then transmitted to the small intestine. It is important that this process has "free flow" and that food is not retained for too long a time. "Descent" refers to free and downward movement of the stomach qi associated with the process of digestion from the beginning of the process through to the elimination and excretion of the waste products.

The stomach is a "yang-earth" organ that is said to dislike dryness and prefer moisture. Diseases easily consume fluids in the stomach, and the stomach requires sufficient fluids to receive and process food and drink. Reception and decomposition in the stomach relies both on stomach qi and the moistening fluids present in the stomach. For stomach qi to descend normally, stomach fluids must be available in sufficient amounts.

The severity of a disease and its prognosis can be determined according to the strength of the stomach qi.[②] The patient may be strong or weak, but if the stomach qi

---

① (*tōng jiàng*, 通降) free flow and descent

② As a specific pulse position for assessing stomach qi, pulses were often taken on the top of the foot at acupuncture point ST 42 (*chōng yáng*), also known as the *fuyang* pulse.

is good, the condition of the illness is relatively mild and the prognosis is good. When there is a severe lack of stomach qi, the prognosis is poor as the condition may be chronic or even fatal. Therefore, when talking with a patient with a chronic disease, questions regarding diet, taste, appetite and elimination are all very important.

The state of the stomach and spleen is easily seen on the tongue. A dry or peeled coating at the very middle of the tongue indicates stomach yin deficiency. In a serious disease, the appearance of a moist coating on a tongue that had been previously dry is a sign of recovery.

CONCLUSION

The *fu*-organs, although often thought of as simply carriers of waste material, are actually very interesting in terms of their functions after digestion. The *jīn/yè* fluids are processed and transported by the *fu*-organs, and both the small intestine and the *sanjiao* have at times been speculated to carry immunological materials. Further biomedical studies may be required to fully appreciate the value of the *fu*-organs as presented in the Chinese medical classics. [1]

STUDY

1. Can you name the *zang*/yin-organ that corresponds with each of the *fu*/yang-organs?

2. Do you know the five phase associated with each *zang* and *fu*-organ?

3. Do you know which of the *zang* and *fu*-organs are *taiyin, taiyang,* etc.?

4. Can you describe three ways to view the *sanjiao*?

Section 3   Extraordinary *Fu*-Organs
(*Qí Héng Zhī Fŭ*, 奇恒之腑)

The 6 extraordinary *fu*-organs are the brain, marrow, bone, vessels, gallbladder and uterus. Because they store essential qi without dramatic discharge of it, their functions are similar to the *zang*-organs. However, in that they are also hollow tubes or containers in shape, the extraordinary *fu*-organs are similar to the *fu*-organs. Therefore, we describe the extraordinary *fu* as having structures similar to the *fu*-organs, but with functions similar to the *zang*.

---

[1]   Readers are encouraged to read more on the topic in *Applied Channel Theory in Chinese Medicine*.

With the exception of the gallbladder, the extraordinary organs have no exterior-interior relationship with the *zang-fu* organs. And while there are no correspondences with the five phases, they are related to the eight extraordinary vessels. Again, except for the gallbladder, the six extraordinary organs have no channels or acupuncture points of their own, but can be accessed through the associated channels of the other organs.

BRAIN (*NǍO*, 脑)

The brain is called the "sea of marrow". The brain is where essence-marrow and the spirit converge, and some texts state that the spirit originates from the brain. Recognition of the brain in Chinese medicine was discussed briefly in *The Yellow Emperor's Inner Classic*, which held that the brain has a close connection with the human spirit, intelligence, vision and hearing. After Western medical science was introduced into China, Chinese doctors increasingly correlated memory, the senses and the voice to the brain.

> Traditionally, the theory of *zàng xiàng* or "organ manifestation" holds that sensory functions are governed by the heart, and then further delegated to the other four *zang*-organs. In the head, there are seven "clear orifices" (openings) of the two ears, two eyes, mouth, tongue and nose (the nose is one opening). All of the upper seven orifices rely on nourishment from the essence-qi of the five *zang*-organs, and upon the moisture of the brain marrow. The organs associated orifices are the liver and eyes, the tongue and heart, the nose and lung, the mouth and spleen, and the ears and kidney. Therefore, disorders of the eye are associated with disharmony of the liver, disorders of taste with the spleen, nose disorders with the lung, and ear disorders with the kidney.

The brain is formed by marrow, which originates from the *jīng*/essence stored by the kidney. Therefore, the brain and the kidney have a close relationship. Kidney-essence consists mainly of prenatal essence, yet it requires the constant supplementation and nourishment of postnatal/acquired essence. When the essence-qi of the five *zang*- and six *fu*-organs are abundant, they nourish the kidney-essence. When the kidney-essence is ample, the brain marrow will be replenished so that the brain can function normally. Larre and Rochat de la Vallee write, "The clear yang rises up to allow the superior function of the brain and the upper orifices, facilitating communication with heaven and the exterior way through the orifices with the eyes, the ears and the nose."[1]

---

[1]　Larre and Rochat de la Vallee. *The Eight Extraordinary Meridians*. London: Monkey Press; 1997. p. 37.

We most clearly see the relationship between the brain and the kidney-essence in conditions of the very young and the elderly. Slow childhood mental development (*wǔ chí*, 五迟) is seen as a lack of essence from the kidney. *Liù Wèi Dì Huáng Wán* (Six-Ingredient Rehmannia Pill, 六味地黄丸) is a spleen and kidney yin-supplementing formula developed to help correct this condition. Alzheimer's disease, senility, and a failing memory in the elderly or late middle age are seen as a pattern of diminished essence.

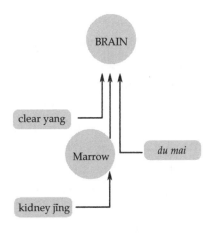

UTERUS (*NǓ ZǏ BĀO*, 女子胞)

The Chinese word for the uterus (*nǔ zǐ bāo*, 女子胞) contains three characters: one for a woman, a child, and a wrapper/container. The uterus governs first onset of menstruation (menarche), subsequent menstruation, and the embryonic gestation, which requires the actions of qi and blood from the organs and channels to produce the reproduction-stimulating essence (*tiān guǐ*, 天癸) in women. (It is also said that *tiān guǐ* in men creates sexual maturity and potency).

The functions of the uterus are intertwined with those of the organs and blood. The heart governs blood, the liver stores blood, and the spleen both controls blood and is the source of qi and blood production. For this reason, restlessness of the heart-spirit can cause menstrual disturbances, a lack of qi and blood due to heart and spleen deficiency which then creates scanty menstruation, delayed menstruation, amenorrhea and infertility. Spleen qi deficiency with failure to control blood can result in "insecurity" of the *chong mai* and *ren mai*[1] which manifests as profuse menstruation or spotting between periods. Liver qi and liver blood functions are also extremely important. Normal menstruation and ovulation require the liver to dispel constrained qi and to store the blood. Infertility treatments in Chinese medicine often require "soothing" of the liver qi as well as the building of liver blood.

When kidney-essence and kidney qi are abundant, *tiān guǐ* supports the development of the reproductive organs to produce menstrual onset and ovulation. *Tiān guǐ* also adjusts different variations of the body with increasing age.

The healthy functioning of the *chong mai* and *ren mai* (*mài*, 脉, vessels) are regulated by *tiān guǐ* and the uterus. The *chong mai* is the "sea of blood", and the *ren mai* controls

---

① The *chong mai* and *ren mai* are "extraordinary vessels", which are discussed fully in the chapter on channels and collaterals.

the development of the embryo and fetus. If the twelve main channels are full of qi and blood, only then can qi and blood pour into the *chong mai* and *ren mai*. Qi and blood will then "infuse" into the uterus, contributing to both regular menstruation and nourishment for the fetus in pregnancy. If the *chong mai* and *ren mai* are disordered, there will be menstrual irregularities such as flooding and spotting, "menstrual block" (amenorrhea), or infertility.

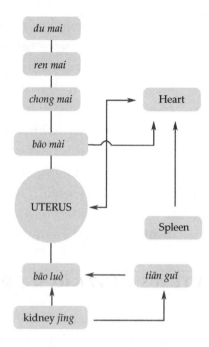

In addition, there is another vessel and collateral system called the *bāo mài* and *bāo luò* (*luò*, 络, channel) that connect the uterus to the kidney and heart, and is also closely related to the actions of fertility. Lyttleton writes, "The heart, kidney and uterus are linked by the *bāo mài* and the *bāo luò*".[1] The *bāo mài* is said to open during ovulation and this action relies on the functions of the heart. The uterus closes by the actions of the kidney. Therefore when kidney qi is weak, it can cause spotting between the menses. The *chong* empties during menstruation, and during the time of ovulation, the *bāo mài* and *bāo luò* bring essence and *tiān guǐ* to the uterus from the kidney, and blood from the heart. The *ren mai* then becomes active again after ovulation.

The stages of fertility are specifically defined in the *Basic Questions* (*Sù Wèn*, 素问), "At the age of fourteen, the *tiān guǐ* arrives, the *ren mai* flows, the *chong mai* fills, the menses come and she can bear children.... at 49, the *ren mai* empties, the *chong mai* weakens, *tiān guǐ* is exhausted, the passages of the earth are cut, and she can no longer bear children." The same text says about males that, "At age 16, his kidney qi becomes even more abundant, his sexual energy arrives, he has semen that he can ejaculate and sex with women will bring children."

The male equivalent to the uterus is called the essence-chamber (*jīng shì*, 精室) and includes the testes, vesicular gland, and prostate; from here, male essence is produced and stored. The essence-chamber is also closely connected with the functions of the kidney, liver, heart, *tiān guǐ*, *chong mai*, and *du mai*.

---

① Jane Lyttleton. *Treatment of Infertility with Chinese Medicine*. London: Churchill Livingstone; 2004. p. 21.

MARROW (*SUǏ*, 髓)

The Chinese medical definition of marrow includes the bone marrow, but it is also broader than that. *The Spiritual Pivot* states that the essence and *yè*-fluids produced from food create a rich paste- or grease-like substance which seeks out and penetrates into the hollows of the bones. The marrow circulates by following the hollows inside the bones to eventually communicate with the brain.

Marrow has three functions related to the kidney. First, marrow nourishes the other extraordinary *fu*-organs as well as the brain. The brain itself is called the "sea of marrow", which communicates this close relationship. Secondly, the marrow supplements the bones. Finally, the marrow produces or "engenders" the blood.

Marrow is vulnerable to heat and dryness, especially in serious diseases. This may come about by heat in the channels, yet the subjective feeling is one of deep cold. In this state, yin and yang are imbalanced and also consume one another. Other pathological states include "bone steaming fever", where the deepest parts of the bones feel painful and hot. This occurs in serious diseases, in old age or as a side effect in modern therapies such as radiation and chemotherapy.[1]

If the sea of marrow is weak, there can be vertigo, tinnitus, fainting, dizziness, blackouts, and mental confusion. Marrow can be seen as related to the Western concept of bone marrow as well as the cerebrospinal fluid. In biomedicine, the bone marrow creates blood cells; dysfunctions are seen in diseases such as sickle cell anemia, aplastic anemia, and leukemia. The functional connection of the kidney with the bones, marrow, and blood illustrate the ancient Chinese medical axiom, "the origin of blood is the kidney".

VESSELS (*MÀI*, 脉)

The *mài* are vessels which act as pathways for blood or qi, variously translated as veins or pulses, depending on context, although they are not exactly the same as either. The *Basic Questions* states, "The vessels are the house of the blood." Therefore we can view the *mài*-vessels as a network of circulation, and the heart as the governor of the vessels. Qi from solid foods enter the stomach and the "clear qi" which is produced goes to the heart. From there, the refined essences enter the vessels as nutrition for the rest of the body. The vessels are then considered as the main route of circulation for essence, qi and blood. Because "the heart governs the blood and vessels", the vessels are also associated with fire.

A more advanced view involves the movement of *ying* qi and *wei* qi within

---

① Bone steaming is also often a feature of withdrawal from opiate drugs, especially methadone.

and outside the vessels; where *ying* qi runs inside the vessels, and *wei* qi runs outside of the vessels. Because *wei* qi is like a mist, and is "lively and quick", it cannot enter the vessels. The *ying* qi is thicker in quality and "embanks" the sides of the vessels. A related idea is that ideally, the "vessels should be large and full of blood, or small and empty of blood". This means that if the vessel is small and the blood "full", this can create "heat in the blood", and if the vessel is large and the blood is deficient (empty), then "wind" can enter. The blood, or more specifically the embanked *ying*, acts to protect against wind inside the vessels. For that reason, to treat internal wind, often the treatment principle is to boost the blood.

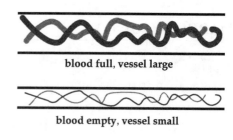

blood full, vessel large

blood empty, vessel small

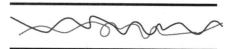

blood empty, vessel large: allows wind

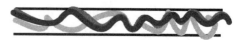

blood full, vessel small: creates heat

BONE (*GǓ*, 骨)

The bones are the outgrowth of the kidney-essence and marrow; bone stores the marrow and the marrow nourishes the bones. The bones also have the obvious functions of supporting the body and protecting the internal organs. Long-term bone problems are therefore treated through nourishing essence and the marrow. Damage to bone is often seen first in the teeth, as the teeth are viewed as "an extension of the bone". Surplus qi and essence unused by the organs and bone is returned to the kidney; in turn, that qi and essence is turned back into blood. Once again, Chinese medicine views the kidney along with marrow as a source of blood.

GALLBLADDER (*DǍN*, 胆)

The gallbladder is considered an extraordinary organ as well as a *fu*-organ because it both stores essence and discharges substances; its tubular structure is also characteristic of the *fu*-organs. The functions of the gallbladder are described in the previous section concerning the *fu*-organs.

Section 4   Relationships among Organs and Substances

This chapter further explores the relationships between the organs and their interconnected physiological processes. Essence, qi, blood, and fluids are the material basis for this system, while the channel and collateral system creates a network between the *zang*-organs, the *fu*-organs, and the extraordinary *fu*-organs.

The relationships among the organs involve the physical and functional ways in which the organs activate, restrict, depend upon and cooperate with each other. Physical functions and dysfunctions of any organ do not act in isolation, but also interact with the other organs as well as the channel system, the fluids, blood, etc. The *zang-fu* organs are the structural and functional centers of storage and activity within the body, whereas the channel and collateral systems are the connecting passageways for the circulation of qi, blood, and fluids throughout the body. Understanding the impact of these interrelationships is extremely important in Chinese medical diagnosis and treatment.

We can look at these relationships from various theoretical perspectives. For example, in the classification of organs, for example, the liver, gallbladder, sinews, eyes, and nails are all associated with the liver system. Another level of relationship is the five-phase system, where organs interact through the generating, restraining, and cosmological sequences. We can also view the interactions between the organs themselves and how they impact the yin and yang actions of qi, essence, and blood. A final consideration is the transformation and movement of qi and its importance to the functioning of all systems. While none of these individual perspectives supersedes another, some perspectives will prove more relevant than others, depending upon the presenting condition of a particular patient. In that there are many correct ways in which to frame a diagnosis and formulate treatment, these different viewpoints are also not mutually exclusive. The art of Chinese medicine involves sorting out which perspectives and approaches are most useful for diagnosis and treatment at any particular moment in time.

This chapter and those that follow begin a review and re-contextualization of many concepts from previous chapters. Students should now begin to create connections and relations between previously learned fundamental principles.

RELATIONSHIPS AMONG THE *ZANG*-ORGANS

Heart and Lung

Both heart and lung are located in the upper *jiao*. The heart is considered the emperor- or monarch-organ of the body, while the lung acts as prime minister. The heart governs blood circulation, while the lung governs respiration and the qi of the entire body. When propelled by heart qi and supported by lung qi, blood is able to circulate constantly. The lung "links with all the vessels", generates *zong*/pectoral qi, and assists the heart in the circulation of blood.

Zong qi promotes respiration and blood circulation because it enters through the heart vessels. When a deficiency of lung qi affects the generation and circulation of *zong* qi, this can lead to dysfunctions of the lung as well as stasis of the heart blood. A disturbance of blood due to heart qi or yang deficiency may also impact the functions of the lung with signs and symptoms of chest tightness, wheezing, and cough.

Heart and Spleen

The heart governs and circulates the blood, while the spleen generates and controls the blood. Their relationship involves a coordinated interaction of blood generation and circulation.

Blood generation

The heart governs the blood of the whole body. The spleen transports the clear food-essence to the lung and heart vessels where it is transformed into "red blood". The spleen governs transportation and transformation and also acts as the source of qi and blood production. A well-functioning spleen guarantees an ample source for the generation of blood, which includes the heart blood. When the spleen becomes weak, the generation of qi and blood is impaired, eventually leading to patterns of heart blood deficiency with signs and symptoms including vertigo, palpitations, insomnia, and profuse dreaming.

Blood circulation

In order to flow smoothly and with proper strength in the vessels, blood must be activated by the heart qi. The blood is also controlled and contained by spleen qi to prevent it from coming out of the vessels. If the movement of blood is impaired because heart qi is deficient to move, this can lead to patterns of heart blood stasis with signs and symptoms of heart pain with cyanotic (purplish-blue) lips and tongue. If spleen qi is deficient and fails to control the blood, blood may extravasate out of the vessels to create bleeding in various parts of the body, or the patient may become bruised easily.

With the proper diagnosis, one can supplement and nourish the heart and spleen with such formulas as *Guī Pí Tāng* (Spleen-Restoring Decoction, 归脾汤). To treat chronic bleeding or bleeding due to deficiency, one can strengthen the spleen and boost the qi to contain the blood with a formula such as *Huáng Tǔ Tāng* (Yellow Earth

Decoction, 黄土汤).

Heart and Liver

The heart circulates blood and stores the spirit, and the liver stores the blood. The liver also governs the free flow of qi, and stores the "ethereal soul" (*hún*).

Functions to move and store blood

The heart, as the hub of blood circulation, also governs the movement of blood. The liver stores and regulates the amount of blood circulating in the vessels. Sufficient heart blood and qi maintain normal blood circulation and provide the liver with blood, which it stores. When the heart fails to generate sufficient blood and the liver fails to store, patterns of blood deficiency may result. If the heart fails to move blood and the liver cannot dispel stagnant qi, various patterns of blood stasis may occur.

Regulation of mental activity

The heart commands mental activity and stores the spirit, so the heart is also in charge of consciousness, thought, and memory. The liver maintains the free flow of qi and regulates qi movement in regards to emotional activity, so the interaction of the liver and heart helps to maintain normal and balanced emotions. Sufficient heart blood nourishes the spirit, thus contributing to a predominantly positive mood with a lack of depression or constraint.[1] If the heart-spirit is restless and the liver qi constrained, there may be depression, sadness, or other negative emotional states. If either heart fire or liver fire becomes overactive, there may be insomnia or excessive anger and agitation.

Chinese medicine holds that abnormal emotional activity impairs the corresponding *zang*-organs according to the specific emotions involved. It is equally important to remember that the seven emotions first affect the heart-spirit, and that several emotions may be involved. Generally speaking, emotional disorders primarily affect the heart and liver, while also impeding the free movement of the qi of the other organs.

Heart and Kidney

Of the five phases, the heart belongs to fire and the kidney to water. The relationships between the heart and kidney involve the interaction between fire and water, the interdependence of spirit and essence, and communication of heart and kidney.

The coordination between water and fire

The heart is located in the upper *jiao* and belongs to yang, while the kidney is

---

① Constraint, 郁 (*yù*), refers to both qi constraint within the body and to mental depression.

located in the lower *jiao* and belongs to yin. In terms of the ascent and descent of yin and yang, that which is in the upper area goes downward, while that which is in the lower area goes upward. Therefore, heart-fire descends to the kidney to prevent the kidney-water from becoming too cold, while kidney-water rises to the heart to prevent heart-fire from being overactive. The descending of heart-fire and the ascending of kidney-water maintain a normal balance between the two organs.

Kidney qi includes both kidney yin and kidney yang, and the ascent of kidney yin (water) depends upon the activation of kidney yang. Heart qi includes heart yin and heart yang, while the descent of heart-fire relies on the cooling function of heart yin. Activated by kidney yang, kidney yin (water) rises up to replenish and cool the heart. Cooled by the yin, heart-fire goes downward to assist the kidney. This balancing process is called the "interaction between water and fire".

The interdependence of essence and spirit

The heart stores the spirit, while the kidney stores essence. The essence, as the source for qi and spirit, can transform into qi and generate spirit, while the spirit dominates and controls essence and qi. An ample supply of essence in the kidney thus creates the conditions for a vigorous heart-spirit. A clear and bright heart-spirit will, in turn, regulate the storage and appropriate release of kidney-essence. This relationship is called the "interdependence of essence and spirit".

Both monarch and minister organs in their proper positions

Heart fire is referred to as sovereign or imperial fire, while the kidney fire is called ministerial fire. Sovereign fire is located in the upper part of the body, and acts to govern the whole body. Ministerial fire is located in the lower part of the body, and is the root of all yang qi in the body, also known as the fire of the gate of vitality (*mìng mén*, 命门)[①]. It is also considered as the root of the spirit. When the *mìng mén* fire is well-stored, heart yang remains abundant and the heart "satisfied". When kidney yin becomes weak, this creates a relative predominance of yang where yin deficiency-type heat then rises to "harass" the heart.

Disorders involving this dynamic balance between fire/water, yang/yin, and spirit/ essence of the heart and kidney are called "non-interaction of heart and kidney" or "heart and kidney not communicating", typically manifesting with patterns of yin deficiency with internal fire. When the relationship between the heart and kidney becomes disturbed, the methods used in treatment will often become more complex. *Formulas and Strategies* states, "A vicious cycle whereby exhausted yin is unable to control the up-flaring fire, while the fire continually scorches and thereby depletes

---

① As stated earlier, ministerial fire is also held in the other *zang*-organs.

the yin, can only be treated by a strategy known as "cultivating the root and clearing the source." Cultivating the root refers to nourishing and enriching the yin-essence; clearing the source refers to draining the internal fire. Both aspects of treatment are essential: if only the root is cultivated, it will be difficult to clear the fire, and if only the source is cleared, the disorder will recur with more intensity".[1]

We also see that heart and kidney yang deficiency can cause water-dampness to overflow; such patterns often include signs of edema. This pattern can be compared to heart or kidney failure as described in modern medicine.

Lung and Spleen

The lung controls respiration, while the spleen governs transportation and transformation. The lung also acts to "free and regulate the waterways", while a major function of the spleen is to transform and transport fluids. Thus both organs are involved in the generation of qi and fluid metabolism.

The generation of qi

The lung governs qi and controls respiration, and the spleen governs the transportation and transformation of food-essence and qi. Merging in the lung, the qi of inhaled air and food-qi comprise *zong* qi. The *zong* qi then merges with the *yuan*/original qi to become the overall qi of the body. *Yuan* qi is derived from prenatal congenital essence, which has a fixed amount in the body, while the lung and spleen supply much of the postnatal acquired essence; the *yuan* qi is then in turn nourished by the postnatal essence.

The food-essence, qi, and fluids transformed by the spleen rely on the diffusing and descending action of lung qi in order to spread throughout whole body. In addition, the necessary food-essence, qi and fluids for the lung all depend upon the spleen qi function of transforming and transporting fluids and food. The production of *zong* qi is made possible only when the lung and the spleen are well-coordinated, thus the saying, "the lung serves as the hub for governing qi, and the spleen is the source of qi production.

Fluid metabolism

Fluid or water metabolism depends on the combined actions of many organs. Taking the lung and spleen as an example, the dispersing and descending action of lung qi acts to free and regulate the waterways, while spleen qi acts to transport and distributes essence and fluids to the lung. Water from the middle *jiao* is transported

---

[1] Volker Scheid, Dan Bensky, Andrew Ellis, Randal Barolet. *Formulas and Strategies*. 2nd ed. Seattle: Eastland Press; 2009. p. 373.

upward by spleen qi to the lung, where it is distributed through the body and sent down into the kidney by the lung. The coordination between lung and spleen in this way creates normal fluid distribution and discharge. If either becomes disordered, fluid metabolism is impaired, leading to abnormal retention of water-dampness or phlegm-fluids. Thus, Chinese medicine holds that although issues of fluid metabolism are apparent in the lung, the root cause is often the spleen. Often these retained fluids will become internal phlegm, thus the saying, "the spleen is the source of phlegm, while the lung contains it." Therefore, when treating edema or cough with phlegm, the primary treatment involves spleen, while treatment of the lung is secondary. In this scenario, the dysfunctional spleen is the "root condition" while the phlegm retained in the lung is the "branch manifestation". The principles of treatment are to strengthen the spleen, dry dampness, transform phlegm, and promote urination.

Lung and Liver

The liver governs ascent and dispersion, while the lung governs purification and descent. Therefore, both organs are involved the ascent and descent of qi movement. *The Yellow Emperor's Inner Classic* states, "right and left are the two ways of yin and yang", which means that the movement of yin qi is ascribed to the left side, while yang qi movement is ascribed to the right. Among the five *zang*-organs, the liver belongs to yin and is located in the lower *jiao*, while the lung belongs to yang and is located in the upper *jiao*. Therefore, the lung qi goes downward while liver qi tends to move upward. It is also said that, "liver qi circulation begins on the left, while lung qi circulation begins on the right." The idea that "the left rises while the right descends" is also consistent with the five-phase cosmological sequence.

The coordination between the ascent of liver qi and the descending of lung qi plays an important role in the smoothness of qi movement within the whole body, which also creates the conditions for harmony between qi and blood. Sufficient lung qi with normal purification and descent contributes to the normal ascent of liver qi and in turn, the free flow of liver qi.

The contrary motions of liver qi and lung qi mutually restrict and also supplement each other. However, there are many cases where liver qi can ascend too quickly or lung qi does not descend normally. Liver qi that is constrained can transform into fire where lung yin will then become consumed by the internal heat. Signs and symptoms of liver fire invading the lung include cough, chest pain, and coughing with blood.

Similarly, when lung qi fails to purify and descend, the resulting dryness and heat will impair liver yin, which then leads to ascendant hyperactivity of liver yang. Signs and symptoms include headache, agitation, and pain in the area beneath the ribs. This helps explain why breathing is also important management of anger.

Lung and Kidney

The lung is the upper source of water, while the kidney governs water. The lung governs qi and controls respiration, and the kidney governs qi reception. Of the five phases, the lung belongs to metal and the kidney to water, so in this case we say that metal and water supplement each other. The lung and kidney relationship is therefore mainly reflected in fluid metabolism, respiration, and the dual supplementation of yin and yang.

Fluid metabolism

The lung is located in the upper *jiao*, frees and regulates the waterways, and is the upper source of water. The kidney is located in the lower *jiao*, governs water, and is the lower source of water. The descending functions of lung qi are dependent on the activation of kidney qi. Lung qi sends fluids downward to the kidney, where the kidney qi then evaporates it and sends it upward again to the lung. The coordination between lung qi and kidney qi affects the normal transportation, distribution, and excretion of fluids within the body. Dysfunctions of the lung and kidney can disturb fluid metabolism and lead to lung edema and other conditions.

To treat fluid metabolism disorders involving the lung and kidney, the treatment principle is to diffuse the lung in order to eliminate dampness. If the predominant pattern is kidney yang deficiency, the principle of treatment is to supplement the kidney in order to drain internal dampness.

Respiration

The lung governs qi and controls respiration while the kidney stores essence and governs qi reception. Though governed by the lung, respiration is assisted by the kidney function of receiving qi. Only when kidney-essence and qi are full and well-stored can the qi from inhaled air reach downward to the kidney, thus maintaining the depth of respiration. The purifying and descending functions of lung qi therefore act to promote the kidney's function of qi reception.

Mutual supplementation of yin and yang

Lung and kidney yin and yang act to supplement one another. The lung belongs to metal and the kidney belongs to water, thus metal is the mother of water. Therefore, lung yin moves downwards to the kidney to support the yin of the kidney. Water is the child of metal, and kidney yin is the root of all yin, so kidney yin moves upward to supplement the yin of the lung. Five-phase theory thus states, "Metal and water supplement each other." Consequently, patterns of lung yin deficiency and kidney yin deficiency can occur simultaneously, or one may lead to the other. The result is internal heat due to yin deficiency of both lung and kidney.

Liver and Spleen

The liver governs the free flow of qi, while the spleen governs transportation and transformation. The liver stores blood, and the spleen generates and controls blood. The liver and spleen relationship is mainly reflected by interaction between the free flow of qi and transportation-transformation, and also through coordination between the respective organ functions of storing and controlling blood.

The interaction of the free flow of qi and transportation and transformation

The liver governs the free flow of qi, which in digestion requires coordinated ascending and descending of the spleen and stomach qi. The liver also makes possible the secretion and excretion of bile into the intestinal tract to assist food-essence absorption and transportation. Spleen qi function replenishes the liver to promote the harmony and free flow of liver qi. When the liver fails to govern the free flow of qi, qi becomes stagnant or constrained, which then causes failure of the spleen to transport. Such patterns of liver and spleen disharmony may include signs and symptoms of poor appetite and digestion, diarrhea, abdominal distention, abdominal gurgling (borborygmus), chest distress with sighing, and depression. When the spleen fails to transport, the free flow of liver qi may be affected where dampness and heat are consequently produced, which in turn further restrains the liver and gallbladder. Bile secretion and excretion are also affected which in severe cases results in jaundice.

The coordination between storing blood and controlling blood

Although governed by the heart, blood circulation is also closely associated to the liver and spleen. The liver stores blood and adjusts the volume of blood, while the spleen generates and controls blood. Healthy and active spleen qi will control the blood and provide the liver with adequate blood for storage. Weak spleen qi can cause blood deficiency due to either a lack of blood generation, or from bleeding due to failure to control blood within the vessels. Blood deficiency manifestations include dry eyes, amenorrhea, insomnia, blurred vision, and tremors of the hands and feet.

Liver and Kidney

It is said, "The liver and kidney are from the same source." The liver stores blood, while the kidney stores essence. The liver governs the free flow of qi, and the kidney governs preserving and storing. In five-phase theory, the liver is the child of water, and the kidney is the mother of wood. The liver and kidney relationship is based on the fact that they share the same source of essence and blood, that they are interdependent in storing and freeing, and that they mutually supplement and restrict yin and yang.

The same source of *jīng*/essence and blood

The liver stores blood, while the kidney stores essence. Both essence and blood come from and are replenished by food-essence. As the kidney receives and stores essence from the organs, the essence can also be transformed into liver blood. However, for the kidney to remain full of essence, it must be regularly replenished and nourished by liver blood. This is why, in the clinic, liver blood deficiency and kidney-essence depletion often appear together. Patterns of essence-blood deficiency include signs and symptoms of dizziness, visual distortion[1], a lack of balance, tinnitus, deafness, and lower back pain with weakness of the knees.

Furthermore, the kidney is associated with bone, where the marrow acts to generate blood; thus the saying "The kidney is the source of blood".

The interdependence of storing and freeing

The liver governs the free flow of qi and the kidney stores essence. The free flow of liver qi allows the kidney to preserve and store, and the kidney's conserving function prevents liver qi from becoming hyperactive. The two organ functions of freeing and storing both oppose and complement each other. This balanced dynamic helps to regulate menstruation and ovulation in women and ejaculation in men. If disordered in women, there may be irregular menstruation, profuse or scanty menstruation, amenorrhea, and ovulation failure. In men, the disorder may result in impotence, seminal emission, and premature or difficult ejaculation.

The mutual supplementation and restriction between yin and yang

Liver qi, which is comprised of both liver yin and yang, is transformed from and nourished by liver blood and essence, where kidney qi is transformed from kidney-essence. So, liver blood and kidney-essence have a close relationship, as do the yin and yang of the liver and the kidney. Kidney yin and yang is the root of the yin and yang of all five *zang*-organs. Kidney yin nourishes and couples with liver yin to prevent liver yang hyperactivity, while kidney yang nourishes and couples with liver yang to warm the liver channel, thus preventing cold stagnation in the liver channel. This yin and yang relationship of mutual supplementation and restriction maintains a coordinated balance between the liver and kidney. Liver and kidney yin deficiency typically involves hyperactive ascending of liver yang with signs and symptoms

---

① (*tóu hūn mù xuàn*, 头昏目眩) visual distortions and/or dizziness with possible lack of balance

including high blood pressure, dizziness, and even stroke. Deficient kidney yang may affect liver yang and lead to a predominance of internal yin-cold. Such patterns of deficiency cold in the lower *jiao* with cold stagnation in the liver channel include signs and symptoms of cold pain in the lateral aspect of the lower abdomen, genital coldness, lack of libido, and impotence or infertility.

Spleen and Kidney

The spleen is the foundation of the postnatal (acquired) constitution and the kidney is the foundation of the prenatal (innate) constitution, thus their relationship involves both the innate and acquired essence. Because the spleen transports water and the kidney governs water, they also have a close relationship with fluid metabolism.

The mutual promotion and assistance between postnatal/acquired and prenatal/innate foundations

The spleen governs the transformation and transportation of food-essence to generate blood, and so is the basis of the postnatal essence. The kidney stores prenatal essence which is the origin of the life of the body. The spleen transforms and transports food-essence, but this requires the assistance of kidney qi. The prenatal essence and the *yuan* qi in the kidney require constant replenishing by the food-essence refined by the spleen. The postnatal/acquired and prenatal/innate essences also interact with each other; the prenatal warms and stimulates the postnatal, while the postnatal replenishes and nurtures the prenatal.

The relationship to fluid metabolism

The spleen and kidney are closely linked through fluid metabolism. The kidney function of governing water metabolism and distributing water relies on the assistance of spleen qi and spleen yang. When spleen qi is deficient and spleen yang has declined, water-dampness will accumulate, although deficiency of kidney qi can also result in stagnant water-dampness, further impacting the function of spleen qi and spleen yang to transport water. Signs and symptoms include edema, abdominal distention, loose stools, fear of cold with cold limbs, and an aching lower back with weak knees.

RELATIONSHIPS AMONG THE *FU*-ORGANS

The six *fu*-organs are in charge of transforming and transporting water and food and distributing body fluids. When food enters the stomach it is decomposed into chyme (partially digested food), and then sent downward to the small intestine.

From there, it is further digested and separated into clear and turbid parts. The clear part, known as food-essence, is transported throughout the body as nourishment, while the remaining fluids filter downward through the *sanjiao* into the bladder to be discharged as urine. The turbid part is transmitted downward, where through the drying and moving actions of the large intestine it is discharged out of the body through the anus. This process also involves the secretion of bile and the functions of the *sanjiao*. It is said that "when there is no obstruction and qi descends smoothly, the six *fu*-organs function well."

Diseases occur when there is stagnation or blockage. For example, excess heat in the stomach will scorch the body fluids, causing failure of the large intestine to transmit and conduct, resulting in constipation. Constipation due to intestinal dryness may cause stomach qi to rise, which may result in belching, nausea, and vomiting. When damp-heat accumulates in the stomach it may "steam" the liver and gallbladder to cause an overflow of bile, manifesting with a bitter taste, jaundice, and other symptoms. Diseases of the six *fu*-organs are usually of the excess type; therefore, herbal treatment for the *fu*-organs often aims to free the movement of qi and to descend qi.

RELATIONSHIPS AMONG THE *ZANG*-ORGANS AND *FU*-ORGANS

The relationship between the *zang*-organs and *fu*-organs refers to the pairing between yin and yang organs, or what is known as the exterior-interior relationship. To review, these pairings are the heart/small intestine, lung/large intestine, spleen/stomach, liver/gallbladder, and kidney/bladder. The *sanjiao* is paired with the affiliated organ of the pericardium.

The exterior-interior relationship has several aspects, the first involving the connections and affiliations of their respective channels. For example, the hand *taiyin* lung channel connects with the hand *yangming* large intestine channel, which means that disease of the large intestine can be treated by accessing the lung channel. Pathogens can also easily transmit between exterior and interior pairs, for example, a case of excessive heart-heat may lead to a dysfunction of the small intestine that creates blood in the urine.

The transportation and transformation of water and food by the six *fu*-organs is normally regulated by the qi of five *zang*-organs. For example, the storage and discharge function of the bladder requires the evaporating action of kidney qi. Conversely, the functions of the five *zang*-organs also require support from the six *fu*-organs.

Heart and Small Intestine

Connected and affiliated by their channels, the heart and small intestine have an exterior-interior relationship, thus interacting with each other physiologically. The functions of the small intestine are influenced by the heart's governance over the blood and vessels, the heart yang warming function, and the moistening and nourishing function of heart blood. In turn, the small intestine is enabled to digest the chyme, separate the clear from the turbid, and to absorb food-essence and water. The component of digested material that is rich in nourishment, the "clear", is conveyed by spleen qi to the heart, where it is transformed into blood.

The heart and small intestine also influence each other pathologically. Excess-heat in the heart channel can move downward to the small intestine creating difficult or burning urination with dark or bloody urine. The method of treatment is to clear heart fire and clear small intestine heat while concurrently promoting urination. On the other hand, heat in the small intestine can also affect the heart to cause agitation, mouth and tongue sores and other symptoms. Furthermore, if the small intestine is affected by deficiency-type cold, food-essence cannot be produced normally; if prolonged, signs and symptoms of heart blood deficiency may appear.

Lung and Large Intestine

Connected and affiliated by their channels, the lung and large intestine have an exterior-interior relationship. The relationship between the lung and large intestine is mainly reflected by the interaction between the purifying and descending functions of lung qi and the conducting and transmitting functions of the large intestine. The lung qi purifies and descends to promote both smooth qi movement and the dispersion of body fluids which also supports the transmission and conduction of waste products by the large intestine. Conversely, when the large intestine functions well, the purifying and descending action of lung qi is also supported.

The lung and large intestine can also impact each other pathologically. When lung qi is congested, impaired purifying and descent can lead to dryness and obstruction of the intestinal qi, resulting in constipation. On the other hand, when excess-heat invades the large intestine, the resulting stagnation of bowel-qi may also impact the diffusion and descending action of lung qi with manifestations including fullness of the chest, cough, and panting.

Spleen and Stomach

The spleen and stomach have an exterior-interior relationship. Both associated with the earth-phase, are located in the middle *jiao*. The spleen and stomach function as a pair, perhaps more than any two organs. Larre and Rochat de la Vallee write, "It is often difficult to distinguish between the functions of the stomach and those of the spleen. Even the traditional texts say that the stomach (and spleen) is the trunk where later heaven is rooted."[1] As the postnatal acquired foundation and source for the generation of qi and blood, the spleen and stomach both play a significant role in the process of absorption, transformation, and transportation of food-essence. Their relationship can be reflected in three aspects, namely, the coordination between transportation and reception, the interdependence between the ascent and descent of qi movement, and the mutual complement between the yin and yang of dryness and moisture.

The stomach governs reception and decomposition of water and food

The spleen acts to govern transportation and transformation, digest food and water, and to transform and transport food-essence. It also supports the stomach while providing other preconditions for further ingestion of food and water. Their close cooperation maintains the normal digestion of food and the transportation and transformation of essence and fluids. Failure of the spleen to transform and transport can harm the reception function of the stomach, while a disharmony of stomach qi can also cause a disorder of the spleen in transformation and transportation. Both scenarios result in a disharmony between the transportation function of the spleen and the reception function of stomach; signs and symptoms include poor appetite, abdominal distention sensation of blockage (*pǐ*, 痞), and diarrhea, among others. Failure of transportation and impaired descent usually happen concurrently.

The failure of the stomach to normally descend creates "food retention", and the treatment method in such cases is to support the stomach to promote digestion and direct qi downward. Herbs are employed in combination to treat the stomach while also boosting qi and fortifying the spleen.

The interdependence between the ascent and descent of qi movement

The spleen and stomach are both located in the middle *jiao*. The rising of spleen qi helps kidney and liver qi to rise, while the descending of stomach qi helps heart qi and lung qi move downwards. In food digestion and absorption, the ascending of spleen qi lifts the food-essence and fluids upward. The normal descending of the stomach qi sends the chyme (partially digested food) downward to the small intestine. The interdependence of spleen qi ascent and stomach qi descent creates a normal condition for the reception and transportation of food. The lifting action of spleen qi also maintains the relatively constant positions of the internal organs.

A case of spleen qi sinking may lead to the failure of stomach qi to normally descend, and thus to counterflow upward. In turn, the ascending and transporting

---

[1]   Larre,Schatz, Rochat de la Valle. *Survey of Traditional Chinese Medicine.* Tai Sophia Press; 1986. p. 199.– later heaven is synonymous with postnatal/acquired essence.

function of spleen qi is affected. Both cases are characterized by sagging and distending sensations in the abdomen, dizziness, diarrhea, vomiting, hiccups, or even prolapsed internal organs. As the hub of qi movement in the body, spleen and stomach functions should be also considered whenever the qi movement of other *zang* or *fu*-organs is disturbed.

A typical example for treatment is the herbal formula *Chái Hú Shū Gān Sǎn* (Bupleurum Liver-Soothing Powder, 柴胡舒肝散), a formula for soothing the liver and resolving qi. In this formula, *chái hú* (Bupleuri Radix) acts to soothe liver qi while also raising spleen qi, while *zhǐ shí* (Aurantii Fructus Immaturus, 枳实) acts to descend stomach qi. This method of pairing one herb with an ascending function with another for descending maintains the hub of qi movement, thus making it possible for the qi of other organs to recover.

Mutual complement between yin and yang of dryness and moistness

The spleen prefers dryness and is averse to dampness, while the stomach prefers moistness and is averse to dryness. Active spleen yang is required for normal transportation and transformation which also prevents the spleen from becoming overwhelmed by excessive dampness. Spleen yin helps the stomach from becoming too dry, but when dampness in the spleen becomes excessive or the dryness in the stomach impairs yin, the spleen will fail to transport and the stomach will fail to receive.

Liver and Gallbladder

The liver and gallbladder act together to control the free flow of qi and also to "govern courage".

Controlling the free flow of qi

The liver governs the free flow of qi which allows for the secretion of bile. The gallbladder is attached to the liver and in charge of storing and discharging the bile. Their cooperation allows bile to be discharged into the small intestine to help the spleen and stomach digest food. The smooth discharge of bile can be greatly affected by constraint or stagnation of liver qi. In cases of gallbladder damp-heat, the free flow of liver qi can also be affected.

Governing courage

The liver is compared to an army general who governs the design of strategy, while the gallbladder is compared to an impartial judge of justice who governs decision-making. The designing of strategy is a process of planning and considering the future, a precondition to decision-making, while a decision is the final judgment to be implemented. Therefore, cooperation between the liver and gallbladder maintains normal emotional and mental activity which provides for appropriate action in one's life. In addition, the governance of decision-making by the gallbladder also concerns bravery. A person with sufficient gallbladder qi is fearless and able to maintain a calm state of mind in the face of stressful situations, and thus able to make accurate judgments and choices. If gallbladder qi is deficient or liver qi constrained, the circulation of gallbladder qi can be affected to result in mental depression, timidity, fear or anxiety. The general treatment principle in such cases is to "regulate the liver and boost the gallbladder". Furthermore, remembering that the heart stores the spirit and governs all activities of the spirit, treatment can also include methods that calm the heart and mind with a formula such as *Ān Shén Dìng Zhì Wán* (Spirit-Mind Calming Pill, 安神定志丸).

Kidney and Bladder

The kidney is the water *zang*-organ, while the bladder is the water *fu*-organ. Their duties include the generation, storage and discharge of urine. The kidney governs water, and has its openings at the "two yin"[①]. The bladder stores and discharges urine, although its function depends on the abundance of kidney qi. When kidney qi is abundant and functions effectively, it both evaporates fluids and controls the urine. In turn, as the bladder appropriately stores and discharges the urine, it can also support the kidney to govern water. If kidney qi is weak, the bladder's function to store and discharge urine will be affected, which can lead to frequent urination, incomplete urination or incontinence. Patterns of damp-heat in the bladder or bladder failing to control can lead to changes in the color and quality of urine.

Problems of urine discharge are divided into either excess- or deficiency-type patterns. Those caused by dysfunction of the kidney are usually deficiency patterns, which should be treated by supplementing the kidney primarily and promoting urination secondarily. Those induced by the dysfunction of the bladder usually belong to a pattern of excess where the treatment principles are to clear heat and promote urination. Because these two treatment strategies are quite different, a careful differential diagnosis is required for all urinary syndromes.

RELATIONSHIPS BETWEEN THE FIVE *ZANG*-ORGANS AND SIX EXTRAORDINARY *FU*-ORGANS

The five *zang*-organs and the extraordinary *fu*-organs both share the characteristic of "storing essence-qi without undue discharge". Except for the gallbladder, none of

---

① Urethra and rectum

the extraordinary *fu*-organs has its own channel; however, the extraordinary *fu*-organs do have many connections with the extraordinary vessels. Thus the extraordinary *fu*-organs and eight extraordinary vessels closely interact and are mutually involved pathologically.

RELATIONSHIPS BETWEEN THE FIVE *ZANG*-ORGANS AND THE UTERUS

Heart and Uterus

The heart stores the spirit, governing all physical and mental activities, while the uterus functions to produce menstruation and gestate the fetus. Both uterine functions are influenced by mental activities, and therefore are regulated by the heart-spirit. Therefore, a stable emotional state with a predominantly positive mood is an important factor for orderly menstruation and timely ovulation. The heart also governs the circulation and generation of blood. Because women have "blood as their basis" (man's basis is said to be qi), the abundance of heart blood, which nourishes heart vessels, and the sufficiency of heart qi, which moves blood, can greatly supplement and activate the uterus in both menstruation and conception. Uterine function may become impaired by a disturbance of the heart-spirit, an insufficiency of heart blood, or by a deficiency or decline of heart qi, which may result in irregular menstrual cycles or amenorrhea.

Liver and Uterus

The liver governs the free flow of qi and stores blood, and is at the center of the regulation of qi and blood and emotional activities. One of the main functions of the uterus lies in storing and discharging blood. The liver is the *zang*-organ that governs the storage of blood and is called the sea of blood. Liver blood, when sufficient, will flow downward into the *chong mai* (also known as the "sea of blood") to keep it full of blood. The liver governs and regulates qi movement. If the liver qi is functioning well, it means that there is a smooth circulation of blood. Under these ideal conditions, the *ren mai* will flow smoothly and the *chong mai* will be abundant with blood.[1]

The free flow of liver qi keeps the movement of qi smooth and creates a happy mood. If the mind is at ease, menstruation is more likely to come at the appropriate time. In women, menstruation and fertility rely on blood for substance and qi for proper functioning. All menstrual issues are associated with qi, blood, and emotional activities, and this explains why the constraint of liver qi and an uneasy mood often

---

[1] The *ren mai* and *chong mai* extraordinary vessels are particularly associated with women's menstruation and conception.

accompanies menstrual disorders. The treatment principles for menstrual disorders often involve soothing the liver and regulating qi, for this, the classic formula *Xiāo Yáo Sǎn* (Free Wanderer Powder, 逍遥散) is frequently selected.

Spleen and Uterus

The spleen governs transportation and transformation, generates and controls blood, and is the source for the generation of qi and blood. Chinese medicine holds that in women, the blood in the upper part of the body becomes milk, while blood in the lower part generates the menses. Vigorous spleen qi provides an adequate source of blood production as well as the power to control the blood in the vessels, but if the spleen qi is weak, then not enough blood will be produced for menstruation. In addition, because spleen qi holds the blood within the vessels, if it is weak there may be bleeding or spotting between the periods. In this state, there is the paradoxical issue of blood deficiency along with that of bleeding outside the normal period. In a classic case, the blood itself would be pale in color, and the pulse would have a "thready" or thin quality.

Kidney and Uterus

The abundance of kidney-essence and qi controls growth, development, and reproduction; the relationship between the kidney and the uterus is mainly reflected in the presence of *tiān guǐ*, menstruation, and gestation. In puberty for women, the arrival of *tiān guǐ* is a result of abundant kidney qi which matures the uterus to create the conditions required for menstruation and ovulation. As a woman ages, she eventually loses the ability to ovulate because of diminished kidney-essence and qi. At this stage, *tiān guǐ* becomes depleted, thus ending menstruation and the capacity for childbearing.

RELATIONSHIPS BETWEEN THE FIVE *ZANG*-ORGANS AND THE BRAIN

The functions and pathological changes of the brain are subordinated to the heart and the affiliated five zang-organs. It is believed that the heart, as the emperor organ, dominates all the organs as well as all activity of the mind and spirit. Therefore, consciousness, thinking, and emotional activities are all subordinated to the heart; thus "the heart stores spirit". Furthermore, the term "spirit" refers to both an overall spirit as well as the *shén* (spirit, 神), *hún* (ethereal soul, 魂), *pò* (corporeal soul, 魄), *yì* (thought, 意) and *zhì* (will, 志). Together, these aspects of the spirit are called the "five-spirit zang-organs" which can only function well when the essence of the five zang-organs is abundant and the qi of the five zang-organs flows freely.

Heart and Brain

The spirit requires nourishment from blood to sustain its normal functions. The heart governs blood, which flows upward to nourish the brain. If heart blood becomes weak, the brain will lack nourishment which leads to listlessness, apathy, dizziness, and headaches.

Lung and Brain

The lung governs qi, links with all the vessels, and assists the heart to maintain blood circulation. Normal lung function supports the fullness of qi and blood which generates and nourishes the *pò* (corporeal soul).

Spleen and Brain

The spleen is the source of qi and blood generation. A strong spleen and stomach generates qi and blood so that the clear yang can move upward to the upper sense orifices and the brain. However, if the spleen and stomach are weak, the orifices will be blocked and the brain will be malnourished. Spleen qi deficiency with yang qi failure to ascend manifests with dizziness and headache. In such cases, the treatment principles are to supplement the spleen and stomach, boost qi, and raise yang.

Liver and Brain

The liver governs the free flow of qi, regulates qi movement, and stores blood. A harmonious state of qi and blood with smooth qi movement acts to maintain the clarity and consciousness of the brain. The *hún* (ethereal soul), which is associated with the liver, also receives nourishment from qi and blood. If the flow of qi is disordered, liver qi becomes constrained or ascends hyperactively, which can lead to disorders of the spirit or emotions, or even stroke. If the liver fails to store blood and leaves the spirit malnourished, the *hún* may become unstable; manifestations include movement disorders, and sleepwalking or sleep-talking.

Kidney and Brain

The kidney stores essence, while essence generates marrow. The marrow replenishes the brain, which is called the "sea of marrow". The marrow is created from essence, with kidney-essence providing abundant marrow for the brain. When kidney-essence is deficient, the sea of marrow will also become insufficient.

RELATIONSHIPS BETWEEN THE FIVE *ZANG*-ORGANS AND THE VESSELS

The vessels are the passageways through which the blood circulates. Their flexibility of dilation and contraction and the free flow circulation of blood are both directly related to the functions of the five *zang*-organs.

Heart and Vessels

The heart governs the blood and vessels. The heart and vessels obviously have a close interdependent system involving blood circulation. The system depends on a regular heartbeat, which is seen as the activation and regulation of heart qi, yin, and yang. The heart qi and heart yin and yang act to propel and regulate not only the heartbeat, but also the contraction and dilation of the vessels. If heart qi is deficient, there may be a lack of strength along with signs of blood stasis. If deficient, the heart yang warming function is impaired, resulting in a slow heartbeat and signs of blood stasis. If heart yin is deficient, its function of cooling and moistening will become weak, resulting in an accelerated heartbeat due to the relative increase in yang heat. The heart blood circulating through the vessels nourishes not only the other organs and areas of the body, but the heart itself as well as the vessels. Additionally, the spirit, which is stored in the heart, commands the movement of qi, thus exerting actions which regulate both the heartbeat and the circulation of blood.

Spleen and Vessels

The spleen governs blood. When spleen qi transports, contains, and controls the blood, the blood will circulate within the vessels and not escape. When spleen qi is deficient and unable to control blood, blood may extravasate from the vessels, which is known as "spleen qi not holding the blood". The spleen is also the source for the generation of qi and blood which nourishes and flows within the vessels.

Lung and Vessels

The lung governs qi and links with all the vessels; therefore, it also assists the heart function of activating and regulating blood circulation. The lung also takes part in the generation of blood, as normal respiration provides fresh air to the blood which nourishes the heart and vessels. This process largely involves the actions of *zong*/pectoral qi.

Liver and Vessels

The liver governs the free flow of qi, which helps to maintain a regular heartbeat while also regulating emotional activity, which also in turn helps maintain a regular heartbeat.

Kidney and Vessels

The yin and yang of the kidney is considered the source of the yin and the yang of the five *zang*-organs. Kidney yang can supplement heart yang, activate the heartbeat and contract the vessels. Kidney yin supplements heart yin, slows the heartbeat, and causes the vessels to dilate. When deficient heart yin fails to inhibit the heart yang, heart yang becomes overactive. The treatment principle is to enrich and nourish the yin of both heart and kidney. On the other hand, weakened vessel dilation or contraction is often created by a relative prominence of heart yin as a consequence of heart yang deficiency failing to inhibit heart yin. The treatment principle here is to warm and supplement the yang of both heart and kidney.

RELATIONSHIPS BETWEEN THE FIVE *ZANG*-ORGANS, BONE AND MARROW

The kidney stores essence, which transforms into marrow to nourish the bones. Abundant essence ensures both abundant marrow and fully-nourished bones. The marrow, as one of the extraordinary *fu*-organs, includes the brain marrow, bone marrow, and spinal marrow. Because the kidney-essence is related to the respective essences of the five *zang*-organs and the six *fu*-organs, the growth of the bone and marrow is also closely related to organ-essence.

Chapter 4

Etiology and Pathogenic Factors

Introduction

Etiology, or the causes of disease, are also called pathogenic factors (*bìng yīn*, 病因). To explain the causes of disease and their pathogenic characteristics, ancient Chinese doctors classified several etiological factors. In *The Yellow Emperor's Inner Classic*, pathogens were first divided into categories of yin and yang. Yang-pathogens are associated with extremes of the climate, usually affecting the body surface. Yin-pathogens affect the internal organs and are associated with improper diet, poor living conditions, irregular lifestyle, sexual overstrain, and extremes of emotion.

Chen Wu-ze in the Song Dynasty (AD 960-1270) theorized three categories of etiology. These included the "six external pathogenic factors", "internal damage by emotional factors", and a third category which includes dietary factors, overstrain, traumatic injuries, incised wounds, and injuries by insects and animals. This third group has been referred to as either "miscellaneous diseases" or those "neither interior nor exterior" (*bù nèi wài yīn*, 不内外因). Currently, a fourth category has also been included which involves dividing the second cause, "internal damage by emotional factors," into two separate categories: "internal causes" and "secondary pathogenic factors". Therefore, we now divide TCM etiologies into four categories.

1) **External contraction** involves pathogenic factors that invade the body from the outside, usually via the surface of the body or the mouth or nose. In general, there are two kinds of external causes: the six pathogenic factors (wind, damp, dryness, heat, cold, summerheat), and those due to epidemic or pestilential qi.

2) **Internal damage** are internally-generated causes including the seven emotional factors, dietary factors, and lifestyle issues of work and rest.

3) **Secondary pathogenic factors/products** include phlegm and fluid-retention, static blood, stones, and others. This category includes all pathological products which result from organ dysfunctions in the course of a disease. During the progression, new symptoms often result from obstruction or stagnation as associated with these pathological materials.

4) **Miscellaneous diseases** are those sustained from falls and accidents, injuries

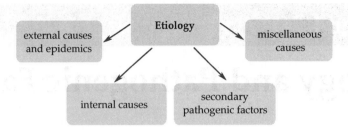

by animals and insects, frostbite, burns and scalding, injuries from metallic objects, parasitic infections, etc. Many Chinese texts also list improper qi gong or meditation as a miscellaneous cause.

Section 1   Six External Pathogenic Factors (*Liù Yín*, 六淫)

The "six pathogenic factors" is a collective term for six different pathogens that can be contracted from the external environment. In Chinese medicine, nature is said to contain the "six qi" of wind, cold, summerheat, dampness, dryness and fire (heat). As these environmental factors change from one to another, a healthy person can easily adapt to them under normal conditions. However, abnormal climate changes may be beyond the capabilities of the body, especially when an individual has lowered resistance to exterior invasion due to insufficient *zheng* qi. One or more of the six qi can then invade the body and create disease; under these circumstances, the six qi are referred to as the six pathogenic factors.[1]

Diseases produced by the six pathogenic factors are called "externally-contracted" or "exogenous" because they always invade the body from the exterior environment. The six pathogenic factors most often invade through the skin, mouth or nose. For example, pathogenic wind, cold and dampness most frequently invades the surface of the body, while warm and heat pathogens usually invade through the mouth and nose.

The six external pathogenic factors are closely connected with seasonal changes, so they are also called "seasonal diseases". Wind-disease often invades in spring, summerheat in summer, dampness in late summer, dryness in autumn, and cold in winter. However, these seasonal correspondences are not absolute, just as seasonal changes are not always consistent; thus a cold-disease may also occur in the summer or a heat disease may occur in the winter.

---

①   From a biomedical perspective, the six pathogenic qi might be comparable to bacteria, viruses, and chemical factors, in addition to the traditional climatic factors.

The six pathogenic factors are also closely associated with the areas and conditions in which people live and work. For example, pathogenic dryness naturally occurs more often where the climate is dry, or pathogenic dampness can often be contracted by a person living in a damp living space. The factor of environment becomes especially complex in modern society due to the proliferation of artificial climates created by heating and air conditioning. People who live in hot climates often have working environments that are filled with cold air, and hot and dry heating units may be overused during a cold winter. This can create a situation where a person may encounter several extremes of temperature or climate within the same day.

Each of the six pathogenic factors may invade the body alone or in combination. For example, a common cold may be caused by wind-heat, diarrhea by damp-heat, or *bi*[①] (obstruction, 痹) by wind-cold-dampness.

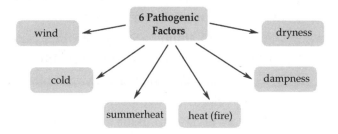

PATHOGENIC WIND

A pathogen that causes a disease that moves and disperses quickly is called a wind-pathogen. Wind is common in spring, but may occur throughout the year. Whenever wind becomes excessive enough to cause disease, it will become a pathogen. Wind pathogens usually invade the human body via the skin or into the muscles to lead to external wind disease. Chinese medicine believes that the wind-pathogen is an important factor in externally contracted disease, so it is called "the first and foremost factor of the various diseases". Wind easily combines with other factors, causing wind-cold, wind-heat, wind-dryness, etc. The wind-pathogen was regarded from the beginning of Chinese medicine as the general term for external pathogenic factors and the main cause of illnesses.

The wind-pathogen is considered yang in nature and tends to attack the upper yang parts of the body such as the head, neck, and back. A wind-pathogen is characterized by movement, lightness, opening, and dispersing. Dispersing-opening means that the wind-pathogen is apt to invade the upper portion (the head and face), yang channels, body surface, and make the striae and interstices (*còu lǐ*,

---

① *Bi* is more or less pronounced like bee, the insect.

腠理-compared to the surface, the "grain of the skin" and the areas immediately underneath) open when it invades the body. It can create headaches, sweating, and an aversion to wind.

A disease caused by a wind-pathogen is characterized by sudden onset, constant movement, and rapid change in the process of the disease. This means that wind is apt to come on quickly, move quickly, and then perhaps move unpredictably around the body. For example, a *bi* (obstruction) syndrome that changes locations indicates a wind-pathogen and is called "migratory *bi*" or "wind *bi*". Another example of wind is a rash on the surface of the skin that may come and go quickly and change locations.

If a wind-pathogen invades the body, the patient may have facial spasms, or dizziness, tremors, convulsion, or stiffness of the neck. Facial spasms or deviation of the eye and mouth (such as in Bell's palsy) can be the result of wind pathogens attacking the channels and collaterals. Invasion by wind pathogens following traumatic injury may lead to symptoms such as convulsions.

Wind often invades the body in combination with other pathogens. Because the wind-pathogen has a dispersing and opening nature, other pathogens (cold, dampness, heat, dryness, and fire) often invade the body in conjunction. The result is the external contraction of wind-cold, wind-dampness, wind-heat, and wind-dryness. The wind-pathogen can attack any organ and tissue externally or internally or invade the body through any of the upper orifices.

Today we can categorize many symptoms and diseases as wind. Signs and symptoms of wind include fainting, dizziness, tremors, convulsions, and facial spasms. Diseases may include (with the appropriate symptoms) colds and flu, dermatological conditions, stroke, Bell's palsy, Parkinson's disease, Tourette's syndrome, and epilepsy.[1]

PATHOGENIC COLD

An external pathogen with the characteristics of cold and congealing is called a cold-pathogen. Cold-pathogens are often seen in winter, but diseases caused by cold can happen in any season. A sharp drop in temperature, being caught in the rain, swimming, exposure to wind while sweating, or exposure to cold air-conditioning can all contribute to an external invasion of a cold-pathogen. If the cold-pathogen attacks the body surface and constrains the *wei* (defensive) yang qi, the case is called "cold-attack". When the cold-pathogen invades the interior directly and damages the

---

[1] Some modern practitioners have extended a wind diagnosis to auto accidents (especially being "rear-ended") because they often have the characteristics of wind; being sudden, affecting the upper body first (neck "whiplash") and lingering with moving pain. This then is a combination of traumatic injury with wind.

organ's yang qi, it is called "cold-strike".

Cold is created from an excess of yin qi, so it is called a yin pathogen and therefore easily damages the yang qi. When a cold-pathogen invades the body, the yang qi of the body will rise to resist it. But if the cold-pathogen is too excessive, not only will the yang qi fail to dispel the pathogen, but the yang will be damaged by the cold. The damage to yang qi by a cold-pathogen may lead to an excess cold pattern due to constraint of *wei*-yang[①] by the cold, or a deficiency-cold pattern due to the decline of yang qi. If a cold-pathogen invades the body surface and the *wei*-yang is constrained, it can cause aversion to cold, fever, lack of sweating, stuffy nose, and a thin or watery nasal discharge. If a cold-pathogen invades the spleen and stomach directly and damages the spleen yang, there will be cold pain in the abdomen, vomiting, and diarrhea. If a cold-pathogen invades the *shaoyin* channel in a patient with heart and kidney yang deficiency there can be symptoms of intolerance of cold, lying with the body huddled-up, cold extremities, watery diarrhea with undigested food, fatigue, and a faint and thready pulse.

Cold is characterized by contraction, condensation, and obstruction. This means that cold-pathogens can easily slow the flow of qi and blood and fluids and obstruct the channels. Once a yin cold-pathogen invades the body, yang qi will be damaged and lose its warming action. This will cause blood stasis and qi stagnation. A common saying is that "obstruction comes before pain", so pain is an important clinical symptom in diseases caused by cold-pathogens.

When a cold-pathogen invades the body, it leads to a constrained flow of qi, constricted skin surfaces, and contracted channels, sinews, and vessels. If a cold-pathogen attacks the body surface, it will make the surface of the skin closed and create aversion to cold, fever, and a lack of sweating. If a cold-pathogen attacks the blood vessels, it will lead to constriction and spasms of the blood vessels, causing general pain, headache, and a "tight" pulse. If a cold-pathogen invades the channels and joints, a patient may have contractions and spasms of the channels with symptoms of spasmodic pain, impaired joint movement, or coldness and numbness of the limbs.

Cold in the Clinic

There are many characteristics of diseases caused by cold-pathogens. The first is the sensation of cold in the body or the pronounced desire to avoid cold ("aversion to cold"). The invasion of external wind-cold will often lead to a headache or pain in the body. Because cold congeals, cold-pathogens can make the blood and qi in the body slow and fail to flow smoothly, which results in pain. Joint pain in Chinese medicine is often a manifestation of a *bi*-obstruction syndrome. *The Yellow Emperor's Inner Classic*

---

① *Wei* qi is often referred to as *wei*-yang because wei qi is yang in nature.

states, "invasion of wind, cold, and dampness together will cause *bi* disease" and "invasion of predominant cold will cause painful-*bi*". For wind, dampness, or cold-*bi* conditions, the treatment principles are to dispel wind, eliminate dampness, warm the channels to expel cold, and activate blood to stop pain.

PATHOGENIC DAMPNESS

Pathogenic dampness is characterized by qualities of heaviness, turbidity, stagnation, density, and downward movement. The nature of dampness is sticky, stagnant, and creates diseases that are slow to develop and are difficult to resolve. Although it can happen at any time of the year, dampness is said to be most common in summer and especially at the turn of summer to autumn. Dampness is often contracted in damp climates, when exposed to rain or when swimming, or when living and working in damp environments.

Dampness is a yin-pathogen and easily damages yang qi and slows the flow of qi. When a yin-pathogen invades the body, the yang qi of the body will fight against it. The invasion of external dampness often affects the spleen and spleen-yang. The resulting failure of the spleen to transport and transform then leads to retained water-dampness. Consequently, the patient may have loose stools, diarrhea, scanty urine, and edema. Because of its heavy, turbid, and substantial properties, when dampness invades the body, the dampness will most likely be retained in the organs and channels. This leads to disturbance of the ascending and descending qi flow as well as obstruction in the channels. Signs and symptoms include chest distress, an oppressive feeling in the stomach cavity (*pǐ*, 痞), scanty urine with unsmooth urination, and incomplete defecation.

Dampness can be heavy, turbid, thick, sticky, or greasy and tends to linger. Heaviness here often manifests as a heavy feeling of the body and head, and sore and heavy sensations of the limbs. Dampness is similar to water, which tends to go downward and as such is apt to attack the yin (lower) portions of the body. Turbidity means that diseases caused by dampness pathogen have thick, foul discharges or secretions, dysentery with pus and blood in the stool, turbid urine, leukorrhea in women, or a dirty complexion and "dampness-type" eczema.

The diseases caused by pathogenic dampness are often chronic, relapse repeatedly, and are difficult to cure. For example, damp-warm diseases such as eczema and dampness and fixed *bi* can repeatedly return. Even for an experienced practitioner, diseases of dampness are notoriously stubborn and difficult to treat.

The Differences and Similarities between Pathogenic Cold and Pathogenic Dampness

Of all six pathogens, only pathogenic cold and dampness are associated with yin, so they both can damage the yang qi. Cold-pathogens primarily constrain the *wei* yang (protective yang qi) and therefore inhibit its spread outward. Cold-pathogens can also damage the yang qi of the organs, which leads to deficiency and shortage of yang qi in the organs. Dampness "surrounds" the yang qi, thus preventing the yang qi from dispersing. The internal dampness also inhibits the spleen yang which in turn creates even more water-dampness. Cold congeals, while dampness creates thick fluids, and thus they both can obstruct qi transformation and movement. Diseases caused by cold often manifest as pain because of the contracting nature of pathogenic cold. However, diseases caused by dampness usually manifest with edema and a local and fixed pain with a sensation of heaviness due to the sticky and lingering qualities of dampness.

Cold is invisible because its main manifestation is discomfort as felt by the patient, while dampness always has substance, even if concealed deep within the body. Of all six external pathogens, only the dampness pathogen is tangible; however, tangible pathogens often serve as a home for the other invisible or intangible-type pathogens. Cold often combines with dampness, such as in cases of cold-dampness diarrhea, cold-dampness dysentery, and cold-dampness headache.

Dampness in the Clinic

Because diseases involving dampness usually are chronic and difficult to cure, the symptoms often change. Dampness pathogens impairing the functioning of the spleen and stomach can include chest and stomach distress, vomiting, difficult urination, incomplete defecation, diarrhea and edema.

Other symptoms caused by the heavy and turbid dampness yin include a heavy sensation of the head like being bound by bandages, depression, a heavy feeling of the body, aching and heaviness of the limbs, a dirty complexion with excessive secretions of the eyes, turbid urine, leukorrhagia in women, dysentery with pus and blood in the stool, etc. Dampness obstruction (*bi*) causes aching, heaviness, and pain of the joints. There can also be symptoms of difficult defecation with sticky stools, a greasy tongue coating, dysentery, leucorrhagia, edema of the lower limbs, and urinary difficulties with turbid urine. Dampness can also transform into phlegm, which can create conditions that are often even more difficult to treat.

PATHOGENIC DRYNESS

Pathogenic dryness invades the body mostly through the mouth and nose and first injures the lung. Diseases caused by dryness are divided as warm-dryness and cold-dryness. Dryness is most apparent in the autumn when the heat of the late summer is still present. Dryness and heat together attack the body, which creates warm-dryness disease. In late autumn, closer to winter, dryness and cold together attack the body to create cold-dryness.

Dryness is apt to consume yin-fluids, leading to dryness of the mouth, lips, hair, nose, as well as chapped and rough skin, scanty urination, and constipation. The lung is a "fragile" organ that desires moisture and has an aversion to dryness, so dryness tends to impair the lung. The lung governs qi, controls respiration, directly communicates with the air, is associated with the skin and hair, and its opening (orifice) is the nose. Pathogenic dryness tends to consume lung fluids which leads to lung qi's failure to disperse and descend. This can result in a dry cough with little sputum, or sticky sputum which is hard to expectorate, or expectoration with blood, difficult breathing, and chest pain. The lung and large intestine have an exterior-interior relationship, so as the dryness pathogen consumes the lung-fluids, the large intestine will fail to be moistened. This creates dry stools and difficult defecation.

Dryness in the Clinic

Some of the diseases caused by dryness pathogen are cough with little sputum or dry cough, dry throat, dry and uncomfortable eyes, dry nose, dry skin, dry stools, vaginal dryness and irritation, infrequent menstruation or amenorrhea with dryness of the blood, emaciated muscles, and dry hair.

PATHOGENIC HEAT AND FIRE

Fire and heat can be seen as one pathogen "fire-heat" or as two different pathogens "fire and heat", depending on the severity and presenting symptoms. Therefore, fire and heat are in the same category but are called by different names. The main difference is that heat-pathogens cause a fever in the whole body, while fire-pathogens are mostly isolated in one part of the body. Examples of fire are redness, swelling, local pain, sores on the mouth and tongue, or red eyes with swelling and pain.

Fire-heat belongs to yang because of their nature to burn, scorch and move upward. Excessive yang-pathogens will lead to pathological hyperactivity of yang qi, and when a yang-pathogen invades the body, the yin qi of the body will fight against it. Excess-heat pattern manifestations include a high fever, aversion to heat, agitation, thirst, sweating, and a full rapid pulse. Fire tends to go upward, so fire and heat often attack the upper portions of the body, especially the face and head. Signs and symptoms include red eyes with swelling and pain, swelling pain of the throat, red skin sores, sores of the mouth and tongue, swelling pain of the gums, and swelling pain in the ear with pus.

Fire and heat are associated with the heart, and fire-pathogens tend to irritate the heart-spirit (*xīn shén*, 心神). When fire and heat invade the *ying-* and blood-levels, they have a strong tendency to affect the skin as well as the heart-spirit. In a relatively mild case, these pathogens disturb the heart-spirit to cause agitation and insomnia, while serious cases may present with mania, delirium or even coma.

Pathogenic fire and heat consume qi and fluids. A fire-heat pathogen typically creates two scenarios; the first being where heat forces the fluids out of the vessels and the body so that qi is consumed along with the loss of fluids. The second situation is when heat directly consumes and scorches fluids, thus causing damaging the yin qi of the body; this is called "impairment of yin by exuberant heat". So, in addition to signs of extreme heat, fire and heat symptoms are usually accompanied by impairment to fluids with yin deficiency. Manifestations include thirst with a desire for cold fluids, dry throat and tongue, scanty urine and constipation. When fire and heat becomes so excessive that it consumes qi, there may also be qi deficiency symptoms such as fatigue, shortness of breath and a reluctance to talk.

Fire and heat also tend to stir up liver wind, and cause bleeding. Fire-heat invasion may scorch the liver channel and exhaust fluids where the sinews and channels are then deprived of nourishment; this can lead to the pattern of "liver-wind stirring internally". Because the liver-wind is caused by extreme heat, this is also called "extreme heat producing wind". Manifestations include high fever, convulsions of the limbs, upward staring of eyes, and other severe symptoms. "To cause bleeding" signifies that when the fire-heat invades the blood vessels, it speeds the circulation of blood and forces it to move outside of the vessels or "run recklessly" with frenetic movement. When it invades the blood-level, a fire-pathogen can accumulate locally and cause infections on the skin; the sores and carbuncles caused by fire are usually red, swollen, hot and painful. A common but mild example of this is teenage acne, while more serious cases of fire-heat can manifest with bleeding disorders such as hematemesis, epistaxis, hematuria, purpurae, hypermenorrhea, and spotting and bleeding between periods.

PATHOGENIC SUMMERHEAT

Summerheat is an external yang-pathogen pathogen originally defined as occurring between the summer solstice and the beginning of autumn. It appears following the fire-heat of midsummer, with fire-heat and summerheat both belonging to yang. Therefore, invasion of summerheat may cause yang-heat signs and symptoms such as high fever, agitation, flushed face, a large pulse, etc. It tends to move quickly upward and disperse, often combining with dampness. Summerheat is a transformation from fire-heat. The diseases caused by summerheat can be divided into categories of summerheat damage and summerheat strike. Summerheat damage occurs more slowly and is a milder condition, whereas summerheat strike occurs more rapidly and with greater severity, commonly known as "heatstroke".

The upward dispersion of summerheat rises can easily disturb the spirit and attack the head while also consuming qi and fluids. Manifestations include chest distress, dizziness, giddiness, a flushed face and other symptoms. Dispersion implies that summerheat invasion causes the striae and interstices to open which results in heavy sweating that depletes fluids and qi. So, in addition to fluid consumption, thirst, and scanty dark urine, summerheat may also give rise to shortness of breath, diminished energy, fatigue, or even sudden collapse and coma with unconsciousness. Bensky and Barolet write, "When summerheat penetrates to the interior there is fever, irritability, dark scanty urine, and a rapid pulse. The heat 'steaming' internally forces to open the interstices and pores and causes profuse sweating. Summerheat, a yang pathogenic influence, is very apt to injure the fluids, which is compounded by profuse sweating."[1]

Summerheat often combines with dampness. In summer, a hot and humid climate prevails with rain. Dampness and heat thus intermingle to create summerheat signs and symptoms of fever and thirst along with manifestations of dampness obstruction such as a lingering fever, fatigue with a heavy sensation of the limbs, chest distress, vomiting and nausea, and diarrhea.

Similarities and Difference between Summerheat and Fire-heat

The similarities between summerheat and fire-heat are that both are external yang pathogens characterized by extreme heat that rises and disperses. Both can invade the head and eyes, disturb the heart-spirit, and consume qi and fluids. Summerheat only occurs in summer, where fire-heat pathogens, although most commonly seen in summer, can also occur in other seasons. Summerheat is externally-contracted and cannot be produced internally; however, the fire-pathogen is often produced interiorly, also resulting in disharmonies of the organs, qi and blood, and yin and yang through the flaring up of heart fire and liver fire. Summerheat often combines with dampness to cause a pattern of mixed summerheat and dampness. The fire-pathogen tends to stir up liver-wind, and can also cause bleeding, sores and carbuncles.

Section 2   Epidemic Qi (*Lì Qì*, 疠气)

Epidemic qi (*lì qì*) are external pathogenic factors that generally appear when the environment changes sharply. They are capable of producing intense infections, often

---

[1]   Dan Bensky, Randall Barolet. *Formulas and Strategies*. Seattle: Eastland Press; 1990. p. 107.

leading to epidemics. Epidemic qi has been referred to in various sources as "epidemic toxin", "malignant infectious qi", "morbid qi", "unusual pathogens", "noxious qi", and "perverse qi". In the Ming Dynasty, Wu You-ke posited that because of their highly infectious nature, epidemic qi were different from the normal six pathogenic factors.

The character lì (疠) suggests an illness that is extreme and sudden. The recognition and understanding of epidemic qi became especially prevalent after 1600 AD during a time of devastating plagues. From this era developed new theories of "warm disease". Epidemic qi theory allows for a disease cause that is not strictly environmental nor generated internally; i.e. diseases passed from person to person. In modern Chinese medicine, this often describes diseases that have biomedical correlations such as mumps, scarlet fever, dysentery, diphtheria, small pox, abdominal typhus, cholera, plague, acute infectious hepatitis and epidemic hemorrhagic fever. In even more recent times, acquired immune deficiency syndrome (HIV/AIDS), hepatitis B and C, and severe acute respiratory syndrome (SARS) have been called epidemic qi patterns even though they do not always strictly conform with the original definition. Biomedical testing can now detect HIV and hepatitis long before any major symptoms appear; regardless, such diseases can be associated with the category of epidemic qi as well as with other specialized theories including "lurking pathogens" and "toxic qi".

There are many factors which create an epidemic, the primary factors including climate as well as other environmental and social factors. Prevention and control should be a special priority in social policies and personal responsibility in that epidemic qi may either cause sporadic attacks in a local area, or in modern times, attack globally as with HIV/AIDS, hepatitis, or SARS. Abnormal changes of climate such as in prolonged drought, heat, floods, and earthquakes all may lead to epidemic qi. For example, an epidemic of cholera often follows natural disasters. Environmental factors such as polluted water, air, and food may also produce and spread epidemic qi such as in acute infectious hepatitis (HAV) and dysentery which enter the body through food.

Social factors such as extreme poverty and poor sanitation or working conditions have a definite effect on the onset and proliferation of epidemic disease. With accessible and widespread public health risk-reduction measures, epidemic diseases can be better controlled.

Comparing Epidemic Qi and the Six Pathogenic Factors

Common pathogenic characteristics

1) **External:** The six pathogenic factors come from the external environment and invade the body via the body surface, mouth and nose.

2) Seasonal: The six pathogenic factors are closely associated with the seasons.

3) Epidemic: The six pathogenic factors are related to living and working conditions as well as the environment.

4) Mixture: The six pathogenic factors can also cause disease either alone or in combination.

5) Transformations: The pathological nature of a disease caused by the six pathogenic factors can under certain conditions transform into another pathogenic factor.

Pathogenic characteristics of epidemic qi

1) Highly infectious: Epidemic qi is distinguished by its intense infectivity and epidemic nature.

2) Specific and similar symptoms: Epidemic qi is specific, in that one strain of epidemic qi causes only one specific epidemic disease. Most epidemic qi will have special affinity to a defined part of the body. Therefore, the clinical symptoms are often the same for a specific epidemic qi.

3) Epidemic qi is classically defined as a toxic yang-pathogen with abrupt onset and a virulent nature. Clinical manifestations include excessive heat, consumption of fluids, disturbed spirit, bleeding and the stirring of internal wind. Many kinds of epidemic disease have a high death rate; in some cases patients can contract such a disease and die within the day.

The similarities and differences between the six pathogenic qi and epidemic qi

1) Epidemic qi can infect many people sporadically in a local area or epidemically in a large area.

2) The onset of disease caused by epidemic qi is more sudden and severe than those caused by six pathogenic factors.

3) Epidemic qi causes a specific disease with the same symptoms, whereas manifestations of the six pathogenic factors will generally show more variation.

4) Epidemic qi and the six pathogenic factors are both connected with abnormal climate change, where epidemic qi is also closely associated with environmental pollution, food, social factors, and lack of prevention.

Section 3   Damage from the Seven Emotions
(*Qī Qíng Nèi Shāng*, 七情内伤)

The seven emotions are joy, anger, grief, thinking, sorrow, fear, and fright. The "seven emotional injuries"[①] involve excesses or changes of emotion that cause disease. Historically, emotions have been considered as main factors in the cause of internal damage. They are said to often attack the internal organs directly where existing diseases are exacerbated or caused to deteriorate more rapidly. Chinese writings tend to stress the detrimental effects of excess emotion and over-stimulation of the spirit.

RELATIONSHIP BETWEEN THE SEVEN EMOTIONS AND ORGANS' ESSENCE-QI

In most cases, emotions are normal reactions to various objects and phenomena outside of the body, and therefore do not cause problems. However, when emotional stimulation is sudden or intense or prolonged, normal physiological or psychological adaptation can be exceeded. At this time, any one of the seven emotions can result in damage to the essence and qi of the organs.[②]

The seven emotions involve complex reactions in the body to the changes of internal and external environments based on the organs' essence-qi. Therefore, the essence-qi of the organs is also the physiological basis for emotional activity. The five organs store essence, which can transform into qi, and the reactions of qi to environmental factors cause emotional activities. In this way, the essence-qi of the five organs will produce corresponding emotional activities. As is stated in *The Yellow Emperor's Inner Classic*, the liver governs anger, the heart governs joy, the spleen governs thinking, the lung governs grief, and the kidney governs fear. Emotions are rooted in the strength of essence-qi of the five organs, as well as the smooth flow of qi and blood. If there is an excess or deficiency of essence-qi, the yin and yang of the five organs, or when the flow of qi and blood is disturbed, abnormalities of the emotions can also result.

The heart and liver play an especially important role in emotional activity. The heart stores the spirit and is the emperor of the five *zang* and six *fu*, governing and controlling both physical and the emotional activities. All emotion can be seen as a product of the harmony of essence-qi or the yin and yang of all the organs as dominated by the heart-spirit. Because the heart governs the spirit, any attack by any of the seven emotions will inevitably disturb the heart-spirit. An injury to the heart-spirit may then also affect the other organs and impair the free flow of qi, thus giving rise to disease.

---

① (*qī qíng nèi shāng*, 七情内伤) seven emotional injuries

② Astute readers may notice that the seven emotions often times number six or five. Zhang explains: "In order to correspond to the functions of the five *zang*-organs, seven emotions are sometimes reduced to the five emotions by consolidating *yōu* (worry) with *sī* (thinking) and *kǒng* (fear) with *jīng* (fright)." Yanhua Zhang. *Transforming Emotions with Chinese Medicine*. New York: SUNY Press; 2007. p. 66.

Normal emotional activities depend upon abundant essence-qi from the five *zang*-organs as well as the smooth flow of qi and blood. The liver governs the free flow of qi while promoting and regulating the circulation of qi and blood. The liver thus plays an important role in adjusting emotional activities and maintaining a stable positive mood.

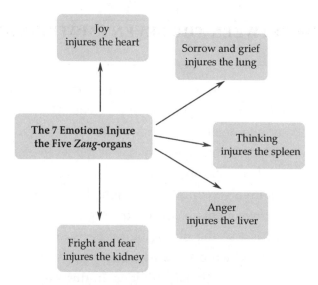

PATHOGENIC CHARACTERISTICS OF THE SEVEN EMOTIONS

Injuring the *Zang-Fu* Organs

The heart governs blood and stores the spirit, while the liver stores blood and maintains the free flow of qi. The spleen is considered the hub of qi movement in terms of ascending and descending, and is also the source for the generation of qi and blood. Because of these functions, the seven emotional injuries greatly affect the heart, liver, and spleen. Too much joy or fright may injure the heart and cause disturbances of the heart-spirit, leading to palpitations, insomnia, amnesia, and mental illness. Intense melancholy and anger can lead to liver qi stagnation and injury to the liver with rib-side pain, chest distress with sighing, or a feeling of obstruction of the throat by a foreign body ("plum pit" sensation). In women there may be menstrual disorders or concretions and conglomerations (*zhēng jiǎ*, 癥瘕) (comparable to uterine fibroids or endometriosis). Pensiveness injures the spleen and leads to poor appetite, loose stools, and epigastric distention and fullness among other symptoms. Sadness causes the qi to contract, leading to depression and fatigue.

Influencing Motion of Qi in *Zang-Fu* Organs

The motion and changes of organ-qi play an important role in the activities of the seven emotions. Because the factors that stimulate the emotions are different, the movement of the different organs' qi is also different. There are special changes of qi movement that correspond to the changes in specific emotions. Note that emotions need not be so extreme to have dramatic effects on the body; even subtle emotional tendencies can cause the qi to flow in less than healthy ways.

"Anger makes qi rise" implies that when the liver qi rises too strongly, blood will rise also. This results in anger with headaches, a flushed face with red eyes, nose bleeding, fainting, or even stroke. "Transverse invasion of the liver qi" (liver qi moving sideways) to the spleen and stomach can create abdominal pain, lack of appetite and diarrhea.

"Joy makes qi slack" implies that over-joy injures the heart where the heart qi becomes sluggish. More severe cases lead to acute depletion of heart qi or an "escape" of the spirit from the heart. Manifestations include absent-mindedness, mental confusion, mania, heavy sweating, weak breathing, and a faint pulse which is nearly undetectable.

"Sorrow and grief consume qi" implies excessive sadness/sorrow or grief which injures the lung. This causes failure of the lung qi to disperse and descend or a lessening and consumption of the lung qi. Manifestations include depression, shortness of breath, chest distress, fatigue, or a reluctance to talk with others. We often see this in chronically depressed people.

"Fear makes qi sink" implies that fear injures the kidney and makes the kidney qi unconsolidated (unable to store), leading to the downward sinking of qi. Manifestations include urinary and fecal incontinence. Fear tends to be a condition of the "personality" that is internally generated while the next emotion, fright, is the response to a real but unexpected external trigger.

"Fright makes qi disturbed" implies that sudden fright injures the heart and kidney and causes a restlessness of the heart-spirit, disorder of qi movement, and an un-consolidation of kidney qi. The Chinese character for "disturbed" here is *luàn* (乱) and suggests chaos, confusion, disorder and/or something messy. Manifestations include palpitations, panic attacks, mental confusion, or sudden urinary and fecal incontinence.

"Thinking makes qi stagnate" means that over-thinking often injures the heart and spleen, leading to a stagnation of the qi movement of the heart and spleen. The resulting dysfunction of transformation and transportation can lead to fatigue, slow reactions, lethargy, poor appetite, epigastric fullness, abdominal distention and loose stools. Too much thinking can cause "student syndrome" or "burn-out" that can lead to a deficiency of heart qi with palpitations.

Damage by the seven emotions can lead to disordered organ-qi which disturbs the course of qi transformation as well as abnormal metabolism of essence, qi, blood, and fluids. Prolonged stagnation of qi may produce heat and fire and an adverse rising of qi. The overactivity can also produce internal heat and fire. The circulation and distribution of essence, blood, and fluids may become obstructed due to qi stagnation, also causing essence stagnation, blood stasis and phlegm-fluid retention. The combining of static blood and retained phlegm-fluids may create an abdominal mass or a tumor. The pathological changes of diseases caused by the seven emotional injuries are often complex with many associated types of disease.

Being Apt to Lead to Mental Diseases

The term of mental disease first appeared in *The Classified Classic (Lèi Jīng*, 类经) by Zhang Jie-bin in the Ming Dynasty. This has the implications of the kind of diseases whose occurrence is connected with emotional stimulation and abnormal emotional activities. Mental diseases include the following:

1) Diseases that are caused by emotional stimulation, such as depression and mania.

2) Diseases that are induced by emotional stimulation, such as chest *bì*, chest pain (angina pectoris), dizziness.

3) Diseases that are caused by other factors but with additional symptoms of abnormal emotional changes, such as *xiāo kě* (wasting-thirst, 消渴), malignant tumors, chronic hepatic and biliary diseases. These diseases can present abnormal emotional symptoms, and their conditions usually change in accordance with the emotional changes. For the treatment of these mental diseases, psychological counseling and emotional adjustments are essential.

Affecting the Condition of Illness

The seven emotions can affect the condition of illness in two respects. First, the seven emotions can facilitate a recovery from illness. In a person with repressed anger, appropriate expression or acknowledgment of that anger may lead to recovery from disease. The same is true with sadness, however not so much as to become more depressed. On the other hand, inappropriate emotions such as depression and pessimism can aggravate an illness. As another example, if a person with a history of dizziness becomes enraged, an extreme rising of liver yang may cause severe dizziness or even stroke. In this case, an excessive emotion aggravates the condition very rapidly.[1]

---

[1] Readers are directed to the writings of Elisabeth Rochat and Claude Larre for in depth discussions of the emotions in Chinese medicine.

Section 4　Improper Diet
(*Yǐn Shí Shī Yí*, 饮食失宜)

An improper diet may lead to organ disharmony or damage to *zheng* qi that can result in disease. Improper diets can be divided in two categories; the first is over- or under-eating, and the second involves inappropriate or unhygenic diets.

Food is primarily digested and absorbed by the transformation and transportation of the spleen and stomach, so an improper diet will primarily injure the spleen and stomach, and thus is called "internal injuries by dietary factors". In the course of a disease, dietary factors may also cause retention of food, accumulation of dampness, heat, phlegm production, and a shortage of qi and blood. Therefore, improper diet is one of the major pathogenic factors of internal damage.

Good eating habits should be moderate. Protracted under-eating will lead to malnutrition with decreased generation of qi and blood. A malnourished person may have general weakness due to deficiency of qi and blood which also leads to a shortage of nourishment for the organs and tissues. External pathogens can also more easily invade a body with insufficient *zheng* qi. Under-eating may also injure the stomach qi, resulting in stomach discomfort and pain. When a person purposely restricts and over-controls their food intake for a long period of time, anorexia may develop. When a person eats excessively and then purposely vomits to remove the food from their system over a period of time, the disease has developed into bulimia. This also leads to malnutrition as well as tooth decay resulting from the repetitive exposure to stomach acid in the throat and mouth.[1] Others may use pergatives to excess and damage their stomach and intestines.

A person who overeats may overwhelm the spleen and stomach. In a mild case, there may be internal stagnation or "food accumulation" as a pathological product. Manifestations include abdominal distention, fullness and pain, belching with fetid odor, acid regurgitation, vomiting, diarrhea, aversion to food, and a loss of appetite. More serious cases may lead to diabetes, obesity, hemorrhoids, and heart-vessel obstruction. If the pathological products of food accumulation stagnate internally for

---

[1] Additionally, in modern times there exists a form of disordered eating where the person will often overeat or "binge" and then instead of throwing up the food, will exercise for an excessive amount of time to burn off the added calories they have eaten. This is known as "exercise bulimia", a subset of bulimia. This diagnosis may also apply to those individuals who exercise excessively with a fear of gaining weight and do not rest adequately between exercise, leading to a state of malnutrition or damage to muscles, sinews, and bones, as the person continues to exercise (often with injuries).

a long period of time, the spleen and stomach may be further damaged leading to other diseases associated with internal dampness, heat, or phlegm.

An unhygenic diet refers to the consumption stale decayed food, parasite-contaminated food or those containing epidemic toxins. Obviously this type of eating is involuntary in most cases, or occurs when a person is particularly careless. The diseases caused by an unhygenic diet mainly involve the stomach and intestines. For instance, intake of rotten food can disturb gastrointestinal function and give rise to abdominal pain, nausea and vomiting, borborygmus, and diarrhea or dysentery. Intake of food polluted by epidemic toxins can cause some kinds of communicable diseases. Intake of poisonous foods can lead to abdominal pain, vomiting, and diarrhea in mild cases, or even death when toxic-qi attacks the heart. Hepatitis A often results from an unhygenic diet where food has become contaminated by the hands of a food-handler of fruits and vegetables. Hepatitis A is a very strong pathogen that can cause illness for several weeks, and can be fatal for those already weakened through age or another condition.

A "peculiar diet" refers to an addiction to foods with specific properties or flavors, or addiction to some kind of food which may cause disease. For example, addiction over a long period of time to alcohol, cold or hot foods, or one of the five flavors will cause an imbalance of yin and yang. Many "fad" diets can be considered as a peculiar diet which may actually mask an underlying eating disorder. A person who eats only salads or raw foods causes the spleen to become overworked and thus create internal dampness. Cool- and cold-natured foods can consume the yang qi of the spleen and stomach, while spicy hot and dry foods may cause an accumulation of heat in the stomach and intestines causing constipation or hemorrhoids; generally speaking, all foods should be moderate in temperature. Heavy alcohol consumption leads to an accumulation of internal dampness, phlegm, and the generation of internal heat. Addiction to alcohol can, of course, be fatal. Some individuals may only have access to or choose to eat only processed foods or "fast foods", and often times the body will become overwhelmed by excessive fats, oils, and non-naturally occurring chemicals.

The Five Flavors

The five flavors include sour, bitter, sweet, spicy, and salty, and there is a one-to-one relationship between each of the five flavors and the five *zang*-organs. Any predilection for or addiction to foods of one flavor over a long period of time may cause a relative overabundance of qi with dysfunction of the corresponding organ. Addiction to one flavor can also affect the other organs by way of their five-phase relationships.

Section 5   Imbalanced Periods of Work and Rest (*Láo Yì Shī Dù*, 劳逸失度)

An appropriate balance between work and rest is essential for good health, where over-working or over-resting for extended periods of time is not beneficial. Overstrain or overwork (*guò láo*, 过劳) includes physical overwork, mental overwork, and sexual overstrain. [1]

Diseases caused by overwork have two pathogenic characteristics. First, overwork consumes qi and the essence-qi of the organs, causing subsequent weakness and dysfunction. Because the lung is the "dominator of qi", and the spleen is the source of qi production, overwork consumes the qi of the spleen and lung. Typical manifestations include fatigue, abnormal sweating, shortness of breath and a reluctance to talk.

PHYSICAL OVERWORK (*LÁO LÌ GUÒ DÙ*, 劳力过度)

Physical overwork usually refers to physical laboring that damages the body. Manual labor can help to maintain good physical condition, but too much work can damage qi and blood. Repetitive work can injure the tendons, joints and muscles and bones, and working while ill or deficient in qi and blood puts further strain on the body systems and will aggravate any existing injury. Often, those with office jobs which otherwise are physically undemanding, may suffer from back strain or carpal tunnel issues through repetitive use or inappropriate posture. Similarly, a factory worker or a housecleaner may perform repetitive tasks which eventually damage the tendons. Overwork can also refer to over-exercising, where someone continues to run or lift weights even though their muscles and tendons have been damaged.

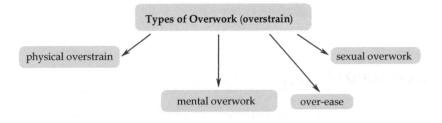

---

[1]   Some text will list nervous overstrain (*yòng nǎo guò dù*, 用脑过度) in the overstrain category.

MENTAL OVERWORK (*LÁO SHÉN GUÒ DÙ*, 劳神过度)

Mental overwork is also called "spirit overstrain" which refers to over-thinking and excessive mental activity over a long period of time that damages the spirit. The heart stores the spirit, and the spleen is responsible for thought (*yì*, 意). The blood is an important substance for balanced emotional activity, so ideation (*sī*, 思) and prolonged thinking and pensiveness (*jiǔ lǜ*, 久虑) may injure both heart-blood and spleen qi. This can create malnourishment of the heart-spirit with manifestations of palpitations, forgetfulness, insomnia, and excessive dreaming, whereas spleen deficiency leads to poor appetite, bloating (distention), and loose stools. Contemporary practitioners often talk of "student syndrome" where long hours of over-studying and schoolwork lead to deficiency of both heart and spleen. This pattern is often treated with the formula *Guī Pí Tāng* (Spleen-Restoring Decoction, 归脾汤).

SEXUAL OVERSTRAIN (*FÁNG LÁO GUÒ DÙ*, 房劳过度)

Sexual overstrain is also called "kidney overstrain". This includes over-indulgence in any kind of sexual activity, including masturbation. Sexual overstrain also involves women who become pregnant at too early an age or those who have had multiple and frequent pregnancies. All the above consume the essence and qi of the kidney with manifestations including soreness and weakness in the loins and knees, dizziness, tinnitus, fatigue, sexual hypo-functioning and sexual disinterest.

Chinese medicine also holds that essence and blood depletion can cause premature senility. Many doctors throughout Chinese history have had the opportunity to treat gynecological issues while considering the effects of sexuality on human health. A great deal could be said about cultural, religious and psychological concerns regarding sexuality, but in any case, over-indulgence for one person may be under-indulgence for another. Regardless it is often simply said that one's essence should be conserved and not "wantonly discharged". Many taoist practitioners emphasize the retention or non-expenditure of essence, while others may emphasize that healthy sexuality in a loving relationship can also actually build the essence for both parties involved.

OVER-EASE (*GUÒ YÌ*, 过逸)

Over-ease can mean either physical or mental over-rest and leisure. Humans need daily physical activity to maintain the free flow of qi and blood and active yang qi. Not working or exercising, staying in bed, or not using the mind for long periods of time can affect the organs, channels and collaterals, and essence-qi-blood-spirit.

The pathogenic characteristics of over-ease has three aspects. First, infrequent physical activities cause qi to stagnate; a lack of exercise over a long period will cause a roughness to the movement and qualities of qi. Second, if yang qi is not regularly activated, the *zheng* qi also weakens. Over-ease for long periods of time can reduce yang qi and subsequently weaken organ function. There may be heart palpitations following slight exertion, difficult breathing, abnormal sweating, or susceptibility to invasion by external pathogens. Third, not under-utilizing one's mental abilities together with stagnant yang qi can give rise to debilitation and depression of the spirit.

Section 6   Pathological Products

Pathological products are formed from existing internal pathologies (many of which are described before). Because they are formed in the process of other pathological changes, they are called "secondary pathogenic factors" or "substantial internal pathogens."

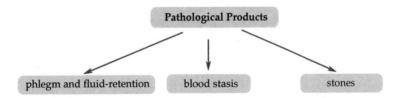

PHLEGM AND FLUID RETENTION (*TÁN YǏN*, 痰饮)

Retention of phlegm and fluids are usually caused by dysfunctions of the spleen, lung, and heart which lead to the retained fluids that later coagulate into phlegm. Phlegm may stay in the *zang-fu* organs and cause pathological problems, as well as move along with the flow of qi to affect the channels and collaterals.

Phlegm and fluid retention can be understood as pathological products resulting from a disturbance of water metabolism in the body. Once formed, the functional activities of the organs, qi and blood are further affected, creating greater dysfunctions in fluid metabolism.

Formation of Phlegm and Fluid Retention

Fluid retention (rheum) implies that as water stagnates in a part of the body, it moves with more fluidity than does internal phlegm. It can remain within the interstices between the organs or tissues, or in the relatively hollow areas of the body; symptoms may vary, depending on the affected area. There are also different forms of fluid retention including "gastrointestinal fluid retention", "pleural fluid retention", "subcutaneous fluid retention" and "thoracic fluid retention".

The formation of phlegm-fluid retention is mostly caused by the six pathogenic factors, injury by the seven emotions, or by irregular eating which leads to organ dysfunction, qi transformation disorders, and disturbances of water metabolism with an accumulation of retained phlegm and fluids. Associated organ dysfunctions mainly involve the lung, spleen, kidney, liver and *sanjiao*.

When the lung fails to disperse and descend, the water passages become obstructed causing impaired distribution of fluids which in turn gives rise to water accumulation and retained phlegm-fluids. If the spleen function of transformation and transportation is impaired, water will not be distributed normally which can also lead to the production of phlegm. If kidney yang becomes deficient and fails to steam or vaporize water, this may cause phlegm-fluid retention. If the liver fails to maintain the free flow of qi, the stagnated qi will fail to distribute fluids normally, also giving rise to the formation of phlegm-fluids. If the water passages of the *sanjiao* become obstructed, water distribution becomes disturbed which can also lead to the formation of retained phlegm-fluids.

There are many causes of phlegm-fluid retention, both external and internal. Externally-contracted dampness can invade and then remain in the body. Fire-pathogens can invade the body and burn body fluids, causing "phlegm-fire". Overindulgence in fatty or sweet foods can lead to the formation of turbid dampness. Damage by the seven emotional factors can cause qi stagnation with water accumulation. All of these conditions may lead to the formation of phlegm-fluid retention. Once formed, retained phlegm-fluids can spread throughout the whole body along with the movement of qi, both exteriorly to the channels and collaterals, skin, sinews and bones, and interiorly to the organs.

Retained phlegm-fluids are pathogens which can flow along with qi, stay in the channels, or stagnate in the organs, thus blocking the qi movement and disturbing the circulation of blood. If retained phlegm-fluids stagnate the channels, the qi movement will be obstructed and the circulation of blood disturbed. In this situation, there may appear numbness and impaired movement of the limbs, phlegmatic nodules or scrofula. If phlegm-fluids stay in the organs, the organ-qi may be disturbed, often resulting in abnormal ascending and descending of qi. For example, if phlegm-fluids are retained in the lung, the lung qi fails to disperse and descend; local symptoms include chest distress, difficult breathing, and coughing with phlegm. Because the lung is "the upper source of fluids", retained phlegm-fluids lead to abnormal distribution of water throughout the body. If phlegm-fluids stagnate in the stomach, the stomach qi will fail to descend normally with symptoms of nausea and vomiting. Phlegm-dampness encumbering the spleen also disturb water circulation. Signs of phlegm-fluids blocking the heart-vessels include palpitations, an irregular pulse, chest distress, and heart pain. Retained phlegm-fluids in the lower *jiao* affect the steaming and transforming functions of the kidney and bladder, thus giving rise to water accumulation.

Compared with the heart-spirit, which is considered to be clear and pure, phlegm is a turbid substance. Turbid internal phlegm can move upward together with qi to cloud the clear orifices and disturb the heart-spirit, manifesting as dizziness, anxiety, and depression. Turbid phlegm can also invade the upper portion of the body in combination with internal wind and fire to disturb the heart and confuse the spirit; in this case, more serious mental issues such as depressive psychosis, mania, delirium, and coma can result. Epilepsy can also be considered part of this pattern. Although these conditions are rather severe, turbid phlegm may also cause less serious symptoms in otherwise well-functioning people, such as simple periodic dizziness and what is colloquially referred to as "brain fog".

Retained phlegm-fluids can move along with the qi to affect any part of the body; they may move inward to the organs as well as outward to the extremities, bones, muscles, and the skin surface, also often combining with other pathogens to cause any variety of complex conditions. So it is said that "the hundred diseases can be attributed to phlegm" and "strange diseases are often caused by phlegm". Retained phlegm-fluids can injure yang so as to produce internal cold, or stagnate the movement of yang qi so as to generate fire. They can combine with wind and heat to invade the head above, the knee and foot below, or they may even transform into dryness and damage yin. Qi constraint can transform into fire and fire constraint can create phlegm. Diseases caused by phlegm and fluid retention are very often both complicated and chronic.

Although the distinction may be considered somewhat academic, many texts will divide phlegm into two large categories of tangible (visible) and intangible (invisible) phlegm. Clavey describes "narrowly defined" phlegm as the tangible phlegm to that which comes out the lung and sometimes by way of the stomach.[1] In other texts, "tangible phlegm" would include formed masses that can be palpated through the skin.

Intangible phlegm may lodge in the organs or the channels and collaterals, sometimes leading to wide range of often inexplicable manifestations including dizziness and mental aberrations. Internal phlegm may form into phlegmatic nodules, large internal masses, and scrofula. Whether termed tangible or intangible, it must be

---

[1] Clavey defines tangible phlegm as "narrowly defined" while others translate it as "visible" phlegm. He uses the definition of intangible phlegm as "widely defined phlegm" which others translate as "invisible phlegm".

stressed that the signs of phlegm are not all so apparent as the phlegm expectorated from the lung, and also that there are forms of phlegm that can transform into one another over time.[1]

Phlegm Patterns

Because phlegm may travel through the body along with qi, the diseases caused by it are both various and changeable. Clavey writes, "Because phlegm follows the flow of qi around the body, and can potentially reach any place where the qi can flow—every organ, every tissue, inside or out, high or low—phlegm theory therefore influences every department of traditional Chinese medicine."[1] Common signs and symptoms include dizziness, headache and heaviness of the head (as phlegm blocks the "clear yang"), chest distress, oppression, or even sharp chest and abdominal pain with an inability to turn the body. Phlegm blocks the chest causing nausea and vomiting. Other symptoms are a sticky feeling in mouth with no desire for drink and loose stools as phlegm blocks the proper functioning of the intestines and stomach, or coughing with phlegm expectoration as it stays in the lung, and numbness of the limbs as it blocks the collaterals. Dry phlegm may cause a persistent non-productive cough.

Phlegm patterns often affect the *shén*/spirit of a patient and can be a source of anxiety, depression, confusion, psychosis, clouded thinking, and lethargy. Phlegm can "mist" the orifices of the heart and head to cause mental illness of various degrees. When the misting is severe, the patient will be disconnected from reality through their inability to hear words clearly (either in volume or concepts), nor can they form coherent speech and may sense non-existent sounds or smells. When combined with fire, there is the example of the mentally ill person pacing on the street corner and raging at the sky; this is a severe case of phlegm misting the heart orifice. Without fire, less serious manifestation include a dull expression, darkness and gloominess around the eyes, obesity, sleepiness, an enlarged tongue body with a moist glossy whitish coating and teeth marks, and wiry, slippery, deep or slow pulses.

Types of phlegm

The disease patterns caused by phlegm often vary due to the fact that phlegm often invades the body in combination with different pathogens. Some common patterns are as follows:

Wind-phlegm is a pattern that has abundant phlegm and symptoms of stirring of internal wind. For example, dizziness and fainting, rales in the throat, a stiff tongue

---

①   Steven Clavey. *Fluid Physiology and Pathology in Traditional Chinese Medicine*. London: Churchill Livingstone; 2008. p. 267.

with slow speech, hemiplegia, deviation of the eye and mouth, fainting, saliva coming out of the mouth, etc. all belong to the wind-phlegm pattern. While the symptoms of wind-phlegm can be tragically dramatic, lesser symptoms can be "simple" dizziness. When other factors such as blood or qi deficiency are ruled out then the cause of dizziness can often be traced to wind-phlegm caused by liver constraint, creating dampness and phlegm, which then turns into wind-phlegm. The herbal formula *Bàn Xià Bái Zhú Tiān Má Tāng* (Pinellia, White Atractylodes and Gastrodia Decoction, 半夏白术天麻汤) is often useful for wind-phlegm.

Cold-phlegm is contraction by external cold, due to intake of cold drinks, or generation of yin-cold internally due to the lack of yang qi which causes the fluid to stagnate. Manifestations include chillness with cold limbs, chest distress and cough, white and thin sputum, a pale tongue with a whitish glossy coating, and a deep and wiry pulse. Cold-phlegm can create a lack of willpower, hopelessness, apathy, and depression.

Phlegm-heat is caused by phlegm and heat. Manifestations include warmness of the limbs, cough, yellow and thick sputum, a red tongue with a yellowish coating, and a rolling and rapid pulse. Mentally, phlegm-heat can cause uncontrolled frustration and anger and both can cause phlegm-heat. Phlegm can easily turn into fire, and then into wind.

Dry-phlegm is caused by a dry-heat pathogen injuring the lung or the lack of lung yin. (The lung is a metal-organ and frequently afflicted with dryness disorders.) Manifestations include a dry cough with little sputum, which may be sticky and difficult to expectorate, a dry mouth and nose, and a red tongue with little moisture. The treatment principles here are to transform the remaining phlegm while also nourishing lung yin. Dry-phlegm often happens after a cold which involved a lot of coughing or when fire has damaged yin. A person who needs to talk a lot during work, such as teachers, often show signs of dry-phlegm. Overuse of herbs that dry dampness can also damage the lung.

Phlegm-dampness is an accumulation of internal dampness with blockage and stagnation of fluids. Manifestations include chest distress, nausea, cough with profuse and easily-expectorated sputum, no appetite, feeling of a heavy body, a thick greasy tongue coating and a slippery pulse. Phlegm-dampness is often the underlying pattern in many cases of clinical depression.

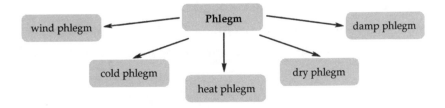

Fluid-Retention Patterns

Fluid-retention[①] (rheum) patterns are of special interest in that they often show as secondary symptoms associated with stubborn problems such as asthma as well as with more serious diseases such as heart and kidney failure. Practitioners may become confused with such ongoing serious biomedical diagnoses, yet an understanding and effective treatment of fluid-retention patterns can go a long way in relieving patients' discomfort while also addressing the underlying disease pattern.

Tán yǐn (fluid-retention in the stomach and intestines, 痰饮)

Water-retention in the intestines and stomach is also called gastrointestinal fluid-retention. Manifestations include abdominal gurgling, vertigo, lassitude, nausea, and vomiting of clear liquid. Because the fluids can rush upwards to disturb the heart, there can also be dizziness and anxiety, palpitations, and shortness of breath. *Tán yǐn* is usually attributed to an inability of spleen and kidney yang to warm fluids with resulting fluid accumulation.

Xuán yǐn (rib-side fluid retention, 悬饮)

Water retention in the rib-sides or hypochondrium is also called pleural fluid retention. The fluids flow freely under the ribs, constricting movement; lying on one side may change the location of discomfort or pain. Fluids can also flow up to the lung area and create shortness of breath and coughing. For these reasons, *xuán yǐn* is often translated as "suspended rheum" because the fluids are not attached to any one particular area. Manifestations include pain in one or both sides of the hypochondrial regions changeable by turning about, shortness of breath, costal pain, etc.

Yì yǐn (subcutaneous fluid-retention in the limbs, 溢饮)

In *yì yǐn*, the fluids flow into the extremities and under the skin. These fluids obstruct the *wei* qi so there is no sweating. The treatment principle is to promote sweating as promoting urination will not help in such cases. *Yì yǐn* can be the cause of many forms of edema. Manifestations include heaviness and pain of the body, edema of the limbs, difficult urination, and aversion to cold with no sweating.

Zhī yǐn (thoracic fluid-retention above the diaphragm, 支饮)

Water-retention in the thorax and diaphragm is called thoracic fluid-retention. The fluids are lodged up against the lung and impede the lung qi. Manifestations include

---

①   Fluid retention is defined as "rheum" in the *Practical Dictionary of Chinese Medicine* (Wiseman).

cough, asthma, difficult breathing, chest distress and shortness of breath, wheezing with inability to lie flat, and a puffy face and limbs.

In addition, there are other types of pathogenic fluid retention such as *liú yǐn* (lingering fluids, 留饮) and *fú yǐn* (lurking fluids, 伏饮). [1]

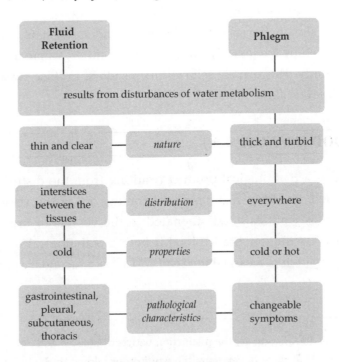

Similarities and Differences between Fluid Retention and Phlegm

Disorders of the Relationships Among Fluids, Qi and Blood

Fluids, qi and blood depend on and supplement one another. When their functions are coordinated, the physiological activities of the human body are regulated. When their functions are not coordinated, there can be water retention with qi obstruction, qi desertion following massive fluid loss, blood dryness with fluid exhaustion, blood stasis with fluid deficiency, and blood stasis with water retention.

1) Water retention with qi obstruction

Water retention with qi obstruction is a pathological state of stagnation of qi movement resulting from stagnation of water-dampness and phlegm-fluids caused by a disturbance in fluid metabolism. For example, when retained water-dampness blocks the lung, manifestations include a sensation of fullness in the chest, cough, dyspnea, and an inability to lie flat. Water retention affecting the heart may cause

---

① Many of the concepts in this section are indebted to *Fluid Physiology and Pathology in Traditional Chinese Medicine*.

palpitations and heart pain. When water retention stagnates in the middle *jiao*, manifestations include dizziness, sleepiness, distention and sensations of fullness in the epigastrium. Water retention in the limbs may cause edema as well as sensations of heaviness and distention in the limbs.

2) Qi desertion following massive fluid loss

Qi desertion following massive fluid loss is a pathological state of acute desertion and loss of qi caused by the loss of great quantities of fluids, where qi leaves the body along with the fluids. This usually follows an episode of profuse sweating, vomiting or diarrhea with severe fluid damage.

STATIC BLOOD (*YŪ XUÈ*, 瘀血)

Static blood is a pathological product resulting from the disturbance of blood circulation in the body. This includes blood coming out of the vessels yet staying within the body as well as blood stagnated in the vessels or organs because of obstructed blood circulation. Static blood is both a pathological product resulting from a faulty circulation process, while it can also act as a secondary pathogenic factor as in "dead blood" (*sǐ xuè*, 死血).

> In Chinese medical language, the distinction between "static blood" (*yū xuè*, 瘀血) and "blood stasis" (*xuè yū*, 血瘀) depends on the word order (although the individual Chinese characters are the same). Blood stasis can be seen as a "generalized" etiological condition, while static blood (also translated as "stagnant blood") is a pathological and specific product (pathology) as most obviously (but not always) seen in clots and bruising.

Static blood is a pathological product which at times, although not always, can be the result of blood stasis. Using the above example, when blood stasis creates clots in the menses, we have signs of static blood. When static blood lodges in an organ or tissue, it usually remains persistent for some time before it resolves, generally remaining in a fixed position and manifesting with a sharp localized pain, or with a palpable mass. If static blood blocks the heart, there can be chest distress and heart pain. If it blocks the lung, there may be chest pain, breathlessness, and the coughing-up of blood. If it blocks the liver, the free flow of qi and blood is impaired causing rib-side pain or a substantial abdominal mass. If it blocks the uterus, there can be amenorrhea, or dark purplish menstrual flow with clots. If it blocks the limbs and skin, there may be cyanotic swelling with pain. If static blood blocks the brain, the obstruction of the brain collaterals may result in sudden fainting and unconsciousness. In addition, prolonged static blood can produce internal heat that can lead to other conditions.

The before-mentioned distinctions not withstanding, the border between blood stasis and static blood is not always clear and blood is often described (like "phlegm") as both a cause and result of disease ("thief and victim"). In addition, English texts, especially older ones, will translate static blood and blood stasis as "blood stagnation" which is actually a distinct and less common condition (*xuè zhì*, 血滞) .

Symptoms Caused by Static Blood

Static blood patterns can display a variety of signs and symptoms, but there are some common features. There may be masses under the skin or within the body, which are usually fixed and immovable; often there is swelling and hardness with a purple color. Sometimes static blood leads to bleeding of dark-purplish blood accompanied by clots. In some cases, there may appear a purplish facial complexion, cyanotic lips and nails, and the tongue may be dark and purplish. With static blood there may be stabbing pains in a fixed area that are aggravated by pressure and become more severe at night. The quality of pain associated with static blood is usually sharp and stabbing, while pain of qi stagnation only type has a more dull quality. Therefore, the general diagnosis of "qi and blood stagnation" is often applied in many pain conditions. Static blood can also create dry skin and abnormal pulse conditions such as a choppy or "knotted" pulse, or a regularly intermittent pulse.

Causes of Static Blood

Various traumatic injuries, falls and surgical wounds can damage the vessels and cause bleeding outside of the vessels within in the body. Bleeding inside the body may also result from failure of the spleen to control blood, or failure of the liver to store blood. When blood which leaves the vessels is not released to the outside of the body, it forms static blood internally, as in cases of endometriosis. Menstruation with clotting can be a mild or a severe form of static blood depending on the quantity.

Blood circulates when qi circulates, and stagnates when qi stagnates. Therefore, if the emotions become constrained, the movement of qi will also become obstructed. When phlegm-fluid retention impedes and blocks the vessels, the unsmooth flow of blood will result in further stagnation and static blood. For this reason, chronic diseases associated with qi deficiency and accumulation will often lead to patterns of static blood.

Qi, as the "commander of the blood" acts to promote and control blood flow, which is also influenced by the amount of qi and fluids within the body. When qi becomes deficient, it cannot promote the flow of blood. When yang qi is deficient, the resulting loss of warmth will affect smooth movement in the vessel system. When yin qi is deficient, the vessel system becomes more rigid due to a loss of the softening and moistening actions of yin qi. Fluids and blood share the same source, and transform into each other; therefore, any shortage of qi and fluids can also affect the blood and its normal circulation.

Temperature also has a great influence on the blood. Blood moves more freely when warm, and becomes more stagnant when cold. When external cold invades the blood vessels, or if excess yin-cold is present in the body, blood stasis may also result. With an invasion of a fire-heat pathogen, or if exuberant yang creates internal fire that invades the blood vessels, the blood and heat will intermingle. As a result, the fluids of the blood become scorched, causing the blood to become sticky, thick, and thus fail to circulate normally. Heat and fire can also force blood to leave the vessels, which also results in static blood.

STONES (*JIÉ SHÍ*, 结石)

Common calculi or stones are sand-like, round or irregularly-shaped and variable in size. Generally speaking, smaller stones are easily discharged, whereas larger stones will often remain lodged within the body. The free flow of liver qi has a major effect on the formation and excretion of bile, and the steaming and transforming actions of kidney qi affect the formation and excretion of urine. Therefore, dysfunctions of the liver and kidney can potentially create stones. Furthermore, the liver and kidney have passages to communicate with the gallbladder and bladder respectively; for this reason, stones are usually found in the gallbladder, kidney and urinary bladder.

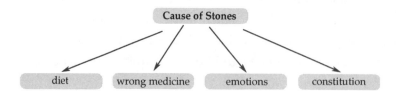

Stones can result from stagnant damp-heat in the body, and so the formation of stones often becomes a chronic condition. Stones are called a "substantial pathogen", with clinical manifestations varying greatly according to the size and position of the stone. Generally speaking, if the stone is smaller, the illness will be mild or asymptomatic. If they stay in the body, they can block the flow of qi and disturb the circulation of qi and blood. There can be intense local pain and distention, and retention of water. If a stone is trapped in a narrow passage such as the biliary tract, the flow of qi and blood can become almost completely blocked. If a stone damages the vessels, there may be bleeding into the urine.

There are complex reasons for the development of stones, and the mechanisms are not always clear. Dietary factors may be a major cause in that overconsumption of sweet or fatty foods can affect the function of the spleen and stomach to cause the formation of damp-heat. Prolonged accumulation of damp-heat in the gallbladder can produce gallstones, and if damp-heat descends and accumulates in the lower *jiao*, it can cause kidney or bladder stones. In addition, water high in minerals and impurities may also contribute to the development of stones.

Emotional disorders can cause liver qi stagnation. If the liver fails to maintain the free flow of qi, obstructed gallbladder qi may lead to impaired bile excretion. Over time, this condition may lead to the formation of gallstones.

Section 7   Miscellaneous Pathogenic Factors

Pathogenic factors not discussed above are called miscellaneous pathogenic factors. They include traumatic injury, parasites, medicinal agents, iatrogenic agents, and congenital factors.

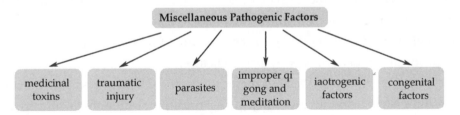

MEDICINAL TOXINS

A medicinal can be used to treat disease, but they can become a pathogenic factor due to improper processing and/or usage. Both medicinal herbs and Western drugs can cause a disorder when they are not prepared or prescribed correctly, if they are out of date, or if the patient fails to follow the instructions.

Many Chinese texts discuss Chinese medicinal toxins at length, as well as common herbal mistakes made by practitioners. However, the modern practitioner is now invariably faced with patients who are using pharmaceutical medications. In addition, many patients will also be seeing other "alternative medical" practitioners. As a result, we often treat patients who are recovering from surgeries or those taking a number of Western drugs, supplements and herbs, as well as receiving aromatherapy, cranial sacral therapy, or chiropractic care, etc. This fact creates several issues for Chinese medicine practitioners and patients. All practitioners should try to be as knowledgeable as possible about any medication that their patients are taking. In most cases, at least outside of Asia, Chinese medicine practitioners are often not licensed nor adequately trained in biomedicine to prescribe Western drugs. In short, such a practitioner should never advise a patient to stop taking prescribed Western medications nor change the dosage. A referral to licensed biomedical practitioners is necessary in many cases.

This does not mean that the Chinese medicine practitioner should simply ignore the Western medications that their patients are taking, as many patients rely on the judgment of their healthcare practitioners to guide them regarding possible side effects and interactions. Strategies for dealing with patients who are taking pharmaceutical medications vary greatly. Some Chinese medicine practitioners are very cautious about giving herbs or even acupuncture to patients who are on certain medications, and others feel that Chinese medicine can only enhance Western therapies. Depending on the circumstances, both viewpoints are valid; the practitioner should consider their level of knowledge and treat each individual case accordingly.

Resolving the interactions of Chinese medicine with other modalities is beyond the scope of this book. Chinese medicine texts that focus on a specialty such as cancer or diabetes often have sections on the combined application of Chinese herbs with Western drugs. Other texts focus on possible or perceived herbal interactions (although modern practitioners rarely create severe or toxic reactions in their patients). Such books can give insight into both the Western nature of herbal medicine as well as the Chinese medical perspective on Western medicines.

When a patient is taking Western medications, the Chinese medicine practitioner faces an interesting conundrum when using traditional diagnostic and treatment techniques. A very common issue is that of high blood pressure which is being controlled with Western medications. Should the practitioner apply herb combinations that will also lower the blood pressure, or should they take the now normalized blood pressure as the new standard? Signs and symptoms such as pulses also change with medication; for example, anti-depressants are notorious for making pulses "deep". In this case, the practitioner must decide whether to see the deep pulse as a side effect, or as a pathological sign that needs to be addressed. These are just a few simple examples of the many issues of the co-existence of biomedicine and Chinese medicine.

TRAUMATIC INJURY

Injuries are usually caused by external force, but can also include burns and scalds, frostbite, and injuries by insects and animals. In a broad sense, they also include injury from lightning, drowning, knocks and falls, and knife or gunshot wounds. A small injury may only cause mild bleeding and contusions, but a serious trauma may also involve broken bones or damage to the internal organs. In a case of extensive burns or scalds, the organs are invaded by fire-pathogens which consume fluids where the resulting depletion of yin and yang may lead to loss of consciousness or even death.

Frostbite is caused by low temperatures for an extended period of time. Local frostbite happens mostly in the hands, feet, ear, nose and cheeks. At the beginning, the local skin is pale, numb and painful resulting from the contraction of cold. Then the skin becomes swollen, dark and purplish, and there is pain with itching or the skin bubbles up. If this continues without treatment, the necrotic tissue may require amputation. General frostbite is caused by excessive yin-cold, and as the body temperature continuously decreases, the patient may have a pale complexion, dark and purplish lips, tongue and nails, numbness which may lead to coma, and death due to the depletion of yang.

"Injuries by insects and animals" can be caused by animals, poisonous snakes, spiders, bees, or ants. In mild injuries caused by wild animals, there may be flesh wounds, bleeding, swelling, and pain. However, in severe cases the injury can damage the internal organs and cause excessive bleeding or even death. Injury by a rabid animal can lead to restlessness, panic, fear of water and wind or even convulsions and death. The stings or bites of bees, scorpions, ants, or centipedes generally cause localized swelling and pain, sometimes with dizziness, palpitations, nausea and vomiting, or coma; this is especially true when the person is allergic to the insect-toxins. Poisonous snakebites can be rapidly fatal. Although there are Chinese medical treatments for such conditions, most are better served with immediate primary biomedical treatment.

PARASITES

The common parasites in the human body are roundworm, threadworm, tapeworm, hookworm and the blood fluke. These parasites not only consume the nutrition of the body but also lead to disease. Different parasites have different pathogenic characteristics.

Intestinal roundworms are the most common parasite in the human body. The rate of infection is higher in the countryside than in the city, and higher in children than in adults. It is primarily caused by intake of unsanitary food that has been polluted by the eggs of roundworm, which then live in the intestinal tract. If the roundworm goes upward and into the biliary tract, it can cause sharp rib-side pain, nausea and vomiting, clammy limbs, or spitting worms. A greater number of intestinal worms can cause intestinal obstructions.

Pinworms are caused by polluted water and food, and the worms live in the intestines. Symptoms include fidgetiness, insomnia, poor appetite, bruxism and emaciation. Diseased babies may weep throughout the night and cannot sleep deeply. Prolonged and repeated infection may influence the physical and psychological health of children.

Tapeworms are primarily caused by the consumption of raw or uncooked pork or beef. The common symptom is pain in the upper abdomen, sometimes very sharp. Taking food can give relief as the parasite has something to feed on. Some infected children will have nausea, diarrhea, or binding pain. At the beginning, there may be vomiting with poor appetite, weight loss, fatigue, and dizziness occurring later.

Hookworms (ancylostomum) is also called "latent worms". Among the worms living in the alimentary canal, the hookworm does the most severe damage. The infestation of hookworm can cause chronic blood loss of the body, causing anemia, as well as symptoms connected with anemia. They live in the small intestine, seriously affecting the functions of the spleen and stomach while also consuming qi and blood. There may appear a dull pain in the abdomen, poor appetite, weight loss with a sallow complexion, general lassitude, palpitations, and shortness of breath. Some infected persons may have allotriophagy, which is a desire for eating unnatural things as food such as uncooked rice, beans, or even clay, cinder, and rags.

Blood flukes (schistosoma) cause a condition called in the ancient literature "*gǔ*"(蛊), or "*shuǐ gǔ*"(water distention, 水蛊). The infection occurs when the skin is exposed to water polluted by the grubs of the blood fluke. In the beginning there are fever, chills, coughing and chest pain, and sometimes abdominal pain, diarrhea, and pus and blood in the stool. Over time, there may also appear an enlarged liver or spleen, ascites or abdominal masses.

It should be pointed out that the above descriptions involve invasions of parasites and worms that can be viewed with the naked eye when exposed. Many current alternative medical practitioners will diagnose "parasites" that may or may not be related to fungal infections. In Chinese medicine, such a condition would possibly be seen as more related to patterns of spleen qi deficiency, cold-dampness, damp-heat, or phlegm. To complicate the discussion further, in contemporary Chinese medicine, there has been a revival of what is called a "*gǔ* syndrome", a unique condition that tends to become deep and chronic in nature.[1]

IMPROPER QI GONG AND MEDITATION

There are a number of self-cultivation methods that people engage in to live longer and more healthy lives, including qi gong, tai ji quan, yoga, and meditation practices. However, all of these methods involve powerful exercises which may in fact cause

---

[1]   The contemporary scholar and practitioner, Heiner Fruehauf, has written several articles concerning "*gǔ* syndrome". Interested readers are directed to the May, 1998 issue of *The Journal of Chinese Medicine* and articles and interviews available.

harm when practiced improperly or under the wrong circumstances.

The physicality of yoga, tai ji quan and even meditation postures can cause damage to the body. Less common but not unknown are "*shén* disturbances", or mental problems caused by these practices. All physical and "mental" practices should be done with the guidance of a teacher. For someone who already has a disturbed *shén*/spirit, unsupervised practices such as qi gong or kundalini yoga that have strong energy-moving capabilities can worsen the condition. Meditation practices for young adults and children may be too intense, and should be carefully monitored. Because young people and those who are *shén*-disturbed are impressionable and/or adventurous, they may attempt practices that are harmful to them in their present condition. In an unstable state, a *shén*-disturbed patient may try to use qi gong or meditation to bring themselves back to normal. The practitioner treating such a patient may be in the uncomfortable position of pointing out the harm of otherwise healthy practices under these circumstances.

IATROGENIC FACTORS

An iatrogenic disease or symptom is one brought on by the unintentional actions or words of the doctor. Iatrogenic problems are not limited to patients of inexperienced or undereducated practitioners, but unfortunately may be the result of unforeseen circumstances. Obviously, practitioners should always try to limit the amount of harm that they may inadvertently cause.

Most modern practitioners will be seeing patients who have access to an array of Western and alternative treatments. For example, the modern Chinese medicine practitioner is often asked to treat patients after they have gone through surgeries. Back and knee surgeries can often cause severe pain to the patient after a seemingly successful procedure. Whether this is considered as iatrogenic or simply a side effect is a matter for discussion.

Each encounter between the doctor and the patient sets the stage for a healing opportunity. Kind words, appropriate behaviors and a compassionate attitude from the doctor can only help to resolve and/or relieve the condition of the patient. If the doctor's words and attitude are uncaring or otherwise inappropriate, it can have negative effects. This type of attitude can worsen the disease or lead to the patient refusing treatment.

In Chinese medicine, there is a saying that "diagnosis is everything". Some inexperienced or poorly educated practitioners will give herbs or acupuncture treatment based on symptoms alone, without forming a proper diagnosis. Others may try to treat based solely on a Western medical diagnosis, which often leads to confusion and an improper treatment. Yet, even the best educated and most experienced doctor can make an error. The worsening of cases induced by previous doctors that are extensively described in the *Treatise on Cold Damage* are examples of "iatrogenic factors".

Although acupuncture is extremely safe with proper training, it is possible to puncture a lung or another organ, especially if a patient has an anatomical abnormality. Some points are inherently difficult to needle, such as those around the eye. Additionally, although extremely rare and through no fault of the practitioner, acupuncture needles can break off within the body. Sometimes needles, *gua sha* or cupping therapy can cause bruising, but such discoloration generally only lasts for a few days. Moxibustion and cupping often involve the use of fire, which can create minor burns. Modern treatment room accidents more typically involve unsteady heat lamps or faulty electro-stimulation machines. For all of these reasons, doctors should always "do no harm" by practicing within their range of education, experience, and scope of practice. The best policy is to remain humble and honest when an iatrogenic issue is created; denying an iatrogenic problem not only damages trust in the practitioner and the profession as a whole, but can also cause the patient further harm.

CONGENITAL FACTORS

Congenital factors refer to pathogenic factors that exist within the individual before birth. (Congenital factors come under the category of constitution.) They include the parents' genetic etiology, those developed during the process of embryonic and fetal development, as well as those due to the process of childbirth. Congenital factors are divided into "fetal feebleness" (inadequate natural endowment) and "fetal toxins". Fetal feebleness means that the fetus received deficient or abnormal essence and blood from its parent, causing so-called birth defects or malnutrition. There are two kinds of issues caused by fetal feebleness. The first involves hereditary diseases derived from issues of the parents' essence. The second is inadequate natural endowment, mostly due to physical weakness or diseases of the parents during pregnancy. Inadequate nutrition may be caused by the parent's irregular or inappropriate diet, injuries by the seven emotional injuries, and overstrain or over-leisure.

Fetal toxins are infections passed on to the child by the mother (such as in HIV and hepatitis B). Fetal toxins also occur in pregnancy (usually early) when the mother is invaded by pathogens or misuses alcohol, medications, drugs, or foods which are harmful to the fetus. Chinese medicine believes that serious emotional issues in pregnancy and various accidents in childbirth will lead to various abnormalities in the newborn after birth. These abnormalities include congenital heart disease, deafness, extra fingers or toes (hyperdactylia) and epilepsy. In modern times, we are more apt to see environmental pollutants, alcohol, drugs, cigarettes and improperly prescribed medicines as being the cause of many problems. Additionally, we now understand that the genetic status of a parent can also be passed on to the offspring. In any case, such children may develop special problems or increased susceptibility to disease. What healthy *jīng* exists must be especially nurtured throughout their lives.

ISSUES OF HERBAL ADMINISTRATION

The improper and/or over-usage of some herbs (especially those toxic) can cause further health problems. Herbs have strict rules of dosage that are learned at the very beginning of any herbal study. As well, there are special requirements and contraindications with many herbs. Some herbs should be decocted first to reduce their toxicity, and strict rules regarding dosage must be observed for others; there are also restrictions and contraindications for pregnant women. Improper usage or disobeying the relevant contraindication can cause toxic reactions, vomiting, or other problems. That being said, properly prescribed herbs and related medicinal substances are normally very safe, and their contraindications are easily remembered; in fact, most toxic or otherwise unfavorable reactions occur as a result of an incorrect diagnosis. Currently, some manufacturers will create Western-oriented herbal drugs using chemical constituents that in no way reflect Chinese methodologies. Drugs made in this way are devoid of the rich chemical constituents of the original herb, and when used outside the context of pattern differentiation they can create side effects that would never appear with traditional prescriptions.

CASES

1. Your patient was caught out in the rain during the springtime. When she got to her air-conditioned office she didn't have a chance to dry her clothes. Over the next week she started to feel increasingly dizzy and often wanted to lie down. She had no cough or headache, her tongue was normal, and her pulse was wiry.

2. Your patient is a 28-year-old male with cystic acne on the back. He works long hours and often goes out drinking after work. The acne is red, large and with yellow pus inside. His tongue is red, and the pulse is rapid and slippery.

3. Your patient is a 22-year-old woman with back pain due to curvature of the spine. She suffers from frequent colds, insomnia, and anxiety. Her pulse is deep and thready, and her tongue is red with no coating.

4. Your patient is a 78-year-old man who had a heart attack 2 months ago. Now he has stuffiness of the chest and swelling in his legs. He has a lack of energy, shortness of breath, a slight cough, and feels that he is unable to take a deep breath. His tongue is purple, large and wet, and his pulse is deep, choppy and weak.

Chapter 5

The Onset and Transmission of Disease

The onset of disease (*fā bìng*, 发病) is a special term referring to the categories, mechanisms, and laws of how diseases occur, as well as the factors which influence their onset. The study of transmission looks at disease processes and progression in relation to the healthy upright/*zheng* qi (正气) and its struggle with the pathogenic/*xie* qi (邪气). If the internal or external environments change beyond the capabilities of the body to adapt, pathological changes result. One scenario might involve drastic changes in climate which create pathogenic factors that invade the body, while another might be long-term emotional stimulation that impairs defensive adaptability, which also results in disease.

The onset of disease has two general aspects which influence each other during the course of disease. The first involves functional disorders of the body itself, and the second is the influence of damage caused by pathogenic factors that invade the body. Disharmony within the body can allow external pathogens to invade, and in return, the invasion of external pathogens can lead to or worsen any existing dysfunction that is already present within the body. In the best case scenario, the *zheng* qi will resist and overcome the invading pathogens while internally adjusting the body and assisting recovery. If the pathogens are overcome, then "*zheng* qi conquers the pathogen" and "yin is calm and yang is sound", so there will be no manifestations of disease. However, if the pathogens cannot be eliminated quickly enough, the pathogens may dominate, *zheng* qi will decline, the balanced coordination of the body will be impaired and the body will become afflicted by disease.

Section 1   Attack of Disease

MAIN FACTORS

There are many factors that influence the attack of disease, but they can be divided into the three large categories of environmental factors, constitutional factors and emotional factors. Environment refers to natural and social environments as related to climatic changes, geographic factors, and living and working conditions. Abnormal changes of seasonal weather provide a condition for pathogenic qi to cause disease. For example, Chinese medicine states that wind diseases are more likely to strike in springtime, heatstroke in summer, dry disease in autumn, and cold diseases in winter. Abnormal weather, such as prolonged wind and rain or extreme hot or cold not only injure *zheng* qi, but also cause the spreading of epidemic pathogens. In addition, the growth or decline of yin and yang qi within the body also varies along with normal seasonal changes. As a result, in different seasons, different pathogens are more likely to attack.

In different geographical regions, the weather, the nature of water and soil as well as the customs of the people are different. All of these are factors affect the physiological characteristics of the local people and the occurrence of disease, thus there are many common local diseases. Naturally, cold diseases are more prevalent in cold climates, and diseases of heat and dampness in hot and humid climates. In some areas, due to deficiencies in the mineral content of the water, people are prone to goiters. Other pollutants from industry, coal mining, and nuclear plants can all be disease factors among groups of people. In addition, when people visit or move to other regions, their defenses may not well-adapt to their new surroundings.

Diseases are often common among people who do the same type of work or are part of the same grouping otherwise, generally involving living and working conditions. Office workers who use computers are often afflicted with carpal tunnel syndrome and shoulder issues, Whereas people who clean houses for a living may develop knee and arm problems. Pollution, environmental toxins, and noise can also be pathogenic factors that cause disease. Various social and educational factors can affect the emotions and cause illness as well as a person's political, financial, family, and interpersonal situations. People with little financial means may not have access to fresh healthy foods, while their constant struggle to survive can lead to a myriad of stress-related health conditions. However, even those with greater financial ability can be more prone to obesity or diabetes, also have many unfulfilled needs and desires or become similarly afflicted with work-related stress or unhealthy lifestyle choices.

ZHENG QI AND CONSTITUTION

The individual constitution is a manifestation of the strength of the *zheng* qi, and so it also determines the progression of a disease. In general, a person with a strong constitution will have strong *zheng* qi, so the body is not easily invaded or influenced by pathogens. Furthermore, when the body of such a person is disturbed by pathogenic qi, the resulting pattern of disharmony will be tend to be excess (*shí*, 实) in nature. This can be understood as there being an abundance of *zheng* qi which can put up a strong fight, with the "by-products" of the battleground (heat, damp, phlegm, etc.) being the excesses. On the other hand, a weak constitution will predispose the body to disease, and those illnesses will typically present as patterns of deficiency, or as mixed deficiency and excess. Weakened *zheng* qi then allows the pathogens to take over and further afflict the body systems.

People with different constitutions have different amounts and balances of essence-qi and yin and yang, so they also will present with different susceptibilities. Someone with a yang deficiency-type constitution can more easily contract cold pathogens, and someone with constitutional yin deficiency may more easily contract heat pathogens. An obese person with excessive phlegm-dampness within the body may be predisposed to pathogenic cold-dampness. A thin person with a yin deficiency-type constitution is more likely to be affected by dry-heat pathogens.

Because of different individual constitutions, affection by the same pathogen may result in different types of disease patterns. For example, being struck by wind-cold may lead to an exterior excess pattern in someone with strong *wei* qi (defensive qi, 卫气), but the same factor will cause an exterior deficiency (or deficiency with excess) pattern in someone with weak *wei* qi. Pathogenic dampness can lead to damp-heat patterns in people with excess yang, but to a cold-dampness pattern in people with weak yang. Furthermore, people of the same constitution may present with the same pattern type even when affected by different pathogens. For instance, a person with a yang-heat constitution may manifest a heat pattern no matter whether they have been invaded by a heat or a cold pathogen.

Emotional states can change the body's balanced internal environment and thus influence the attack of disease. If the mental state is balanced and positive, qi movement is smooth and qi and blood are harmonious, and when organ functions are strong, the *zheng* qi is vigorous. Consequently, pathogens find it more difficult to attack the body and they can easily be driven out. When the emotions are extreme, the flow of qi is disturbed, creating a disharmony of the qi and blood and the organs. Sudden strong emotions or prolonged emotional disturbances will impair qi movement and can even injure the internal organs, such as with chest pain and stroke that follow strong emotional stimulation. Prolonged states of grief, worry, or frustration may block qi movement or result in qi counterflow which over time will affect the body constitution to cause chronic health problems.

We now know that genetic factors also have an effect on the onset of disease, that they influence the constitution, and that they are of course associated with inherited diseases and congenital conditions. Having unfortunate genetic markers does not guarantee that a person will be affected by an inherited disease, but such individuals should consider preventative measures and practices of health maintenance.

TYPES OF ATTACK

Sudden Attack

An immediate or sudden attack[①] occurs immediately after a pathogenic invasion. In terms of the struggle between *zheng* and pathogenic qi, as the *zheng* qi fights strongly against the pathogen, an immediate imbalance of yin and yang then results in obvious clinical symptoms. An immediate attack is most common when newly-acquired external pathogens are strong. Sudden attacks typically involve wind-cold, wind-heat, warm-heat, summerheat, or heat-toxins. Sudden changes of emotion such as rage or severe grief may also lead to an adverse uprising of qi, imbalances of qi and blood, and organ dysfunctions.

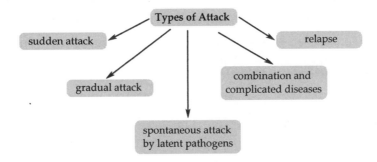

Gradual Attack

A gradual or slow attack occurs slowly after the occurrence of a pathogenic invasion. Gradual attacks are characterized by progressive pathological changes, and are more common in conditions associated with internal pathogens, emotions, unhealthy lifestyles and addictions. External pathogenic dampness, with characteristics of stagnation, heaviness and turbidity, also cause diseases that develop slowly. When a person with weak *zheng* qi is attacked by a mild pathogen, the *zheng* qi resists the pathogen slowly, which also results in a gradual-type attack.

Latent Onset

A latent onset is created after a pathogen first invades the body and does not immediately cause disease, but instead the pathogen lodges and incubates within the body for a period of time; health issues will only appear when induced by some other

① (*gǎn xié jí fā*, 感邪即发) an immediate attack

factor. This kind of type of attack is mostly seen in externally-contracted diseases and with some external injuries. Externally-contracted diseases mainly caused by warm-heat pathogens form what is called "latent-qi warm disease".

Practitioners over time have adapted the theory of latent-qi. The mechanism for the development of a latent onset often involves a relatively mild pathogen that invades and remains in a superficial region, thus the *zheng* qi does not contend with the pathogen; this allows the evil qi to lurk internally, hiding within the body. However, once the insidious pathogen causes a disease, it is often quite serious and also relatively changeable in nature.

Many modern practitioners consider some viral or autoimmune conditions such as HIV/AIDS, chronic hepatitis B and C, Lyme disease and Epstein Barr to be associated with latent pathogenic factors. Here we see that the patient may have contracted the original pathogen decades earlier, also remaining asymptomatic or with only mild flu-like symptoms. As long as the disease is "latent", or held in check by the *zheng* qi, then the patient remains relatively healthy. Many of these diseases only become problematic as the patient ages or when their *zheng* qi diminishes for other reasons, and in these cases, the latent disease may surface quite dramatically.

Secondary Attack

A secondary attack refers to a new disease that occurs because of a primary disease to which it has a close pathological relationship. For example, a deficiency of lung essence-qi may create a secondary onset of heart blood stasis obstruction. Other examples would be a stroke due to ascendant hyperactivity of liver yang, infantile malnutrition with accumulation because of indigestion with food retention, deficiency of lung essence-qi and heart blood stasis obstruction in asthma. All belong to secondary attack.

Combined Attack

The concept of combined attack and complicated attack is a major aspect of the *Treatise on Cold Damage*. A combined attack refers to a disorder that is seen in two or more channels simultaneously. It mostly occurs when the invading pathogen is more excessive while the *zheng* qi is relatively deficient, so that pathogenic qi may attack two or more channels or parts simultaneously. Such examples are a combined disease of the *taiyang* (greater yang) and *shaoyang* (lesser yang) channels, or the *taiyang* and *yangming* (yang-brightness) channels. The symptoms may include a cough that appears concurrently with spleen-stomach symptoms such as diarrhea and abdominal pain. A combined attack therefore causes simultaneous injury to different areas of the body, with multiple disease patterns also present. Line 142 of the *Treatise on Cold*

Damage states, "with *taiyang* and *shaoyang* combined illnesses, the head and neck are very stiff and painful, or there is dizziness with vertigo."

Complicated Attack

A complicated attack refers to a scenario where a pattern associated with one part of the body or system does not completely disappear, and at the same time another part of the body becomes affected. A complicated attack is characterized by pathogenic transference to another part of the body, while the primary diseased site still exists.

Relapse

Relapse means that during the recovery from a disease, it happens again or repeatedly. The mechanism for relapse is that the original pathogen has not been driven out completely, and *zheng* qi has not fully recovered yet. Often there is yet another pathogenic factor such as improper diet or improper medication that can cause the original pathogen to grow again. As a consequence, the *zheng* qi becomes weaker and there is a relapse of the original disease.

Several points concerning relapse are pertinent. Relapse can't help but mean that the body did not fully recover during the healing process of the main disease. The clinical manifestations of a relapse are similar but not exactly the same to those of the original disease. However, because there is not always an exact replay of the original struggle between the pathogen and the *zheng* qi, a relapsing episode is often more complex, extensive and serious than the first. The more episodes of relapse there are, the more incomplete the recovery will be. As well, of course, the prognosis will worsen with the addition of more severe after-effects.

Relapse may be generally divided as relapse with minimal recovery, relapse alternating in intervals, and acute episodes alternating with chronic remissions.

A relapse with minimal recovery is mostly seen during the convalescence time of another disease. When the pathogen has not been driven out completely and the *zheng* qi is weak already and there are factors such as improper diet, improper medication or overstrain, the residual pathogens may develop and make the *zheng* qi weaker. Although the symptoms and signs of the first attack have disappeared through treatment, the root of the disease may still exist in the body. In terms of *zheng* qi, the disease reoccurs because the *zheng* qi is too deficient to get rid of the original pathogen completely. The pathogenic qi may be heavy and turbid that cannot be easily driven out. As examples, epilepsy and various diseases caused by stones are asymptomatic in the remission stage, but can be reactivated with a pathogenic factor.

An acute episode can alternate causing chronic remissions. This actually is an alternation between remission with mild symptoms and an acute attack with more serious symptoms. Once again, it is determined by the state of the struggle between the *zheng* qi and the pathogenic qi. As examples, asthma, chest distress, heart pain and chronic kidney diseases can have mild symptoms for a long period of time, but then become more acute through the influence of excessive emotion, improper diet, overstrain, or exogenous pathogens.

Therefore, to get rid of residual pathogens completely, the pathogens should be driven out while the *zheng* qi is simultaneously strengthened, or soon afterwards. With this, the incidence of relapse can be reduced. Clinically, relapse due to exogenous contraction is common. For example, the *Revised Popular Guide to 'Treatise on Cold Damage' (Chóng Dìng Tōng Sú Shāng Hán Lùn, 重订通俗伤寒论)* says, "Usually relapse occurs when a patient again contracts pathogens before the latent heat has been thoroughly driven out."

If a disease reoccurs after being just cured because of improper diet, it is called relapse due to improper diet. Different diseases and different constitutions have corresponding proper diets. For instance, improper diet can cause the diseases of the spleen and the stomach to reoccur. Shrimps and fish and seafood can cause urticaria and asthma to reoccur. Too much alcohol or spicy food can cause hemorrhoids and urination disturbance to reoccur. Therefore, for the patients with the diseases in the spleen and the stomach or special constitutions, in the course of the disease, proper diet is very important.

Overstrain of the body and mind or sexual activity can cause relapse of a disease and can happen in both exogenous diseases and endogenous diseases. Such endogenous diseases as chronic edema, asthma, hernia, falling of the womb, apoplexy, obstruction of qi in the chest and heart pain can reoccur due to overstrain. The more times it reoccurs, the worse the injury is and the worse the prognosis is.

A disease may reoccur due to improper use of an herbal prescription or medicine. When a disease has just been cured, methods may be used to replenish essence and qi. However, one must be careful to strengthen the *zheng* qi without promoting the strength of the internal pathogen. One common example involves a heat-fire disease that has resolved and yet left the

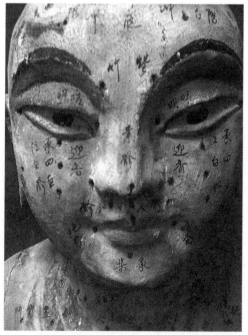

(Photograph of acupuncture face by Douglas Eisenstark, courtesy of Emperors College, Santa Monica, CA.)

patient fatigued; in this case, the overuse of supplementing herbs such as *rén shēn* (Ginseng Radix et Rhizoma) can reactivate a condition of internal heat. A disease may also relapse due to emotional factors that destabilize the balance of yin and yang, affect the circulation of qi and blood, or injure the internal organs directly. Climatic, vocational, social and environmental factors can also lead to relapse and recurrence.

Section 2   Disease Transmission

A disease is in a constant state of movement and change. Every disease has its own unique process of frequency, development and outcome. Many factors, such as pathogenic factors, the patients' constitution and environmental conditions all influence the direction of development and transformation of a disease. The course of a disease is both complex and changeable, thus the concept of disease transmission and change was developed. This unique feature of Chinese medicine was first elaborated in *The Yellow Emperor's Inner Classic*, which over time evolved into several specialized theoretical systems.

We can generalize about the two types of disease transmission and change. The first concerns the location of the disease that we observe according to layers of depth. Pathological changes in one part of the body often transfer or spread to other parts through the channel-collateral system and so leads to new pathological changes. This is transmission of the disease location, where the second kind of change involves the nature of the disease itself.

What are being described below are different "schools" or methods of diagnosis and treatment. Most notably are the cold disease school based on the *Treatise on Cold Damage*, the warm disease school of the *Wēn Bìng*, and the *sanjiao* method. The school of cold disease is the pillar of the latter two. Reading the chapter on history will give a fuller understanding of the context to which these different approaches belong.

TRANSMISSION OF EXTERIORLY-CONTRACTED DISEASE

Generally speaking, the fundamental form of transmission of diseases caused by external pathogenic factors involves transmission between the exterior and interior, while disease originating in the interior is generally transmitted between the *zang-fu* organs. Exteriorly-contracted diseases pass from the exterior to the interior or from superficial levels to deeper levels. However, as an exteriorly-contracted disease moves interiorly, there may also appear transmission among the *zang-fu* organs. Chinese medicine has over the years identified several main forms of transmission. These include transmission involving the six channels, transmission among *wei*-qi-*ying*-blood levels, and transmission through the three divisions of the *sanjiao*.

TRANSMISSION TO THE EXTERIOR OR INTERIOR

The exterior and interior levels are not an absolute pair, but are relative to one another. As a whole, diseases on the skin, orifices, sinews, channels and collaterals belong to the exterior, while diseases in the *zang-fu* organs and bone marrow belong to the interior. Comparing the skin with the channels and collaterals, a disease located in the skin belongs to the exterior, while a disease in the channels belongs to the interior. Viewing from the three yin and three yang channels, the three yang channels belong to the exterior, while the three yin channels belong to the interior[1]. When speaking of the *zang*-organs as compared to the *fu*-organs, a disease in the *fu*-organs belongs to the exterior, while a disease in the *zang*-organs belongs to the interior. Generally speaking, a progression from exterior to interior will exacerbate the condition, while outward movement to the exterior level will be accompanied by clinical improvement.

The passage or transmission of pathogens from the exterior into the interior commonly appears in the beginning or middle stage of an exteriorly-contracted disease. The transmission can be caused by a deficiency of *zheng* qi which allows the pathogens to move more deeply into the body. There can also be a rapid passage of the exterior pathogens into the interior because of especially strong pathogens, or because of improper treatment. For example, in a wind-cold pattern, if the exterior pathogen cannot be eliminated, they will go deep into the interior to affect the lung and stomach. This may transform an exterior cold pattern into one of interior heat.

Under some special conditions, when the *zheng* qi fails to resist the pathogens, they can quickly invade the interior of body, and manifest as a "direct attack". For example, a cold pathogen can invade the exterior and then further invade the *zang-fu* organs directly where the spleen and stomach become impaired. In this process, there is no presenting exterior pattern because the condition first appears with the manifestations of an interior pattern.

Transmission from interior to the exterior is a process in which internal pathogens are released to exterior levels as the *zheng* qi successfully contends with the pathogenic qi. For example, in a "warm disease", because the heat pathogen is rampant internally,

---

[1]   The three yin channels are the foot and hand *taiyin*, *shaoyin* and *jueyin* while the three yang channels are the foot and hand *taiyang*, *yangming* and *shaoyang*. These represent the channels that are used in acupuncture, massage, moxa among the others.

the first symptoms are a high fever, thirst, agitation, chest distress, cough, and difficult breathing. Through the actions of *zheng* qi or with the proper medical treatment, the pathogenic heat may be dispelled through sweating, which also results in alleviation of the main symptoms.

Whether or not the internal pathogens move outwardly mainly depends upon the ability of *zheng* qi to drive out the pathogens. If the *zheng* qi is strong enough, the condition would improve as the pathogens are moved outwardly. On the contrary, with a progressive deficiency of *zheng* qi, the pathogens will move more deeply inward to cause an unfavorable progression of the disease.

In the process of the transmission between exterior and interior, there is an in-between stage referred to as half-exterior/half-interior. Both the cold damage *shaoyang* pathomechanism and the warm disease pathomechanism of latent pathogens belong to a half-exterior/half-interior type pattern. Although in some cases there will be a tendency of inward or outward movement, the pathogens may also remain lodged in the *shaoyang* level, which often leads to a low-level yet chronic disease with frequent periods of relapse.

TRANSMISSION OF INTERNAL DISEASE

Nearly 2000 years ago, the *Treatise on Cold Damage* marked a turning point in Chinese medicine which in fact represents "modern" Chinese medicine. Rather than the result of random "winds" and "spirits" attacking the body, illnesses could now be categorized and followed according to their transmission. Without explicitly using cold disease theory, the following section on transmission is greatly indebted to it.

The organic whole of the human body contains *zang-fu* organs as the center with the channels and collaterals as functional pathways. Physiologically, the *zang-fu* organs are closely related in both disease and health, and the transmission of internal disease largely involves transmission among the *zang-fu* organs.

TRANSMISSION AND TRANSFORMATION BETWEEN ORGANS

Via the channels and collaterals, the five *zang*-organs communicate closely with each other where a pathological change in one organ often affects the others. The heart governs the blood and vessels, and the lung governs qi. If deficient *zong*/pectoral qi fails to move the heart qi, blood stasis may appear elsewhere. Wiseman writes "…when blood becomes stagnant in the lung, lung qi is inhibited… "[1] The lung's dispersion and

---

[1] The heart and lung relationship is also expressed as "The lung faces the hundred vessels". Nigel Wiseman, Ye Feng. *A Practical Dictionary of Chinese Medicine*. Taos: Pradigm Publiations; 1998. p. 273.

descent will become disordered, and there might be symptoms such as cough, shortness of breath, and an inability to lie flat. On the other hand, a prolonged lung disease can cause dysfunctions of qi that affect the normal intake of clear qi and exhalation of the turbid; this in turn may create heart blood stasis. In this case, signs and symptoms would include palpitations, chest distress and bluish-purple lips and nails.

Transmission between *zang*-organs and *fu*-organs involves the passage of pathogens between organs that are interiorly-exteriorly related. For example, the large intestine can conduct and transmit stool as it benefits from the actions of the lung qi. If the lung qi stagnates in the upper *jiao* and fails to purify and descend, this may lead to constipation because of a resulting obstruction of large intestine qi. On the other hand, excessive heat in the large intestine can also influence the purification and descent of lung qi to cause shortness of breath, cough and asthma. Therefore, a lung disorder may affect the large intestine, and vice versa.

Each of the six *fu*-organs also has processes of reception, digestion, conduction and transmission, excretion of food, as well as distribution and excretion of water. If the large intestine fails to conduct and transmit downward, the resulting obstruction of the lower *jiao* may result in ascending counterflow of stomach qi with manifestations of belching and nausea.

TRANSMISSION BETWEEN BODY STRUCTURES AND ORGANS

Pathogens can transmit from the body structures and orifices to their related *zang*-organs, or from the *zang*-organs to the structures and orifices. Pathogens invade the body surface and then spread through channels to the *zang-fu* organs. For example, excessive intake of cold food may damage the yang qi of the spleen and stomach. Because the hand *taiyin* lung channel originates in the middle *jiao*, stomach cold with yang deficiency may through the channels affect the lung, resulting in a failure of lung to diffuse and disperse. If externally-contracted wind-cold invades the body, the lung will be affected as its function of defending the body surface declines. Manifestations might include cough and shortness of breath.

On the other hand, pathological changes also may be transmitted from the *zang-fu* organs to the channels or to the body surface. For example, disorders of the heart or lung may spread to their affiliated channels, with manifestations appearing along the running course of the channels on the body surface. This could include pain in the chest or in the medial aspect of the arms. This principle may also be applied for proper diagnosis.

TRANSFORMATION OF THE NATURE OF THE DISEASE

In the disease process, transmission involves a changing location of disease or a changing nature of the disease pattern. Transmission of the nature of disease mainly includes transformations between cold and heat, and transformations between deficiency and excess.

Transformation between Cold and Heat

Cold patterns can involve excess-type cold or deficiency-type cold, and heat patterns can involve excess-type heat or deficiency-type heat. There are two types of transformation from cold to heat. One is excess cold changing to excess heat. For example, in a *taiyang* exterior cold pattern there is first a severe aversion to cold, mild fever, and a tight floating pulse. This can develop into a *yangming* interior heat pattern with a high fever, aversion to heat, agitation, thirst, and a rapid pulse. Secondly, a pattern of deficiency cold can also change to one of deficiency heat. These changes in pattern are based on the theory of yang impairment affecting yin, as well as the mutual impairment of yin and yang.

The transformation of a heat pattern into a cold pattern can happen in three ways. The first involves the transformation of an excess heat pattern into a deficiency cold pattern due to damage of the yang qi. For example, a patient with high fever due to an external pathogen may have yang desertion caused by profuse sweating. As a result of yang collapse, excess heat may become deficiency cold with manifestations of profuse cold sweat, a sudden lowering of body temperature, cold clammy limbs, a pale complexion, and a faint thready pulse.

The second involves transformation of an excess heat pattern into excess cold pattern. Obstruction in the channels due to internal heat (heat *bi*) can result from stagnation and blockage of wind-dampness and heat pathogens in the joints. With improper treatment or constitutional yang deficiency, this may transform into a cold *bi* pattern with wind-cold-dampness obstruction.

The third involves transformation of a deficiency heat pattern into a deficiency cold pattern which results from yin impairment affecting yang. For more detail, refer to the discussion on mutual impairment of yin and yang.

To sum up, the general laws of disease transformations involving cold and heat are as follows. The condition of a patient with a constitution of yang overabundance with yin deficiency is apt to transform into a pattern of heat and dryness, while the condition of a patient with a constitution of yin exuberance with yang deficiency is apt to transform into a pattern of cold and dampness. A condition of a patient whose *zang-fu* organs and channels and collaterals are invaded by yang pathogens often transforms into a pattern of heat and dryness, while a condition of a patient whose *zang-fu* organs and channels and collaterals are invaded by a yin-pathogen often transforms into a pattern of cold and dampness. With improper treatment damaging yang, the condition will transform into cold, whereas if improper treatment damages yin, the condition will transform into heat. Generally speaking, the transformation of the nature of an externally-contracted disease is more rapid, while transformations of miscellaneous diseases due to internal injury are slower.

Transformation of Deficiency and Excess

Transformations of the deficiency or excess natures of a disease depend on the relative strengths of the *zheng* qi and the pathogenic qi, both of which change during the progression of disease. As should be well-known by now to the reader, an excess pattern is defined as a condition in which pathogens are present and being resisted by the *zheng* qi. However, as the *zheng* qi of the body weakens over time, an excess pattern may transform into a pattern of deficiency.

For example, a summerheat pattern is characterized by heavy sweating that forces fluids out of the body, which may result in "qi desertion following profuse loss of fluids". The disease then rapidly transforms from an excess summerheat pattern into a complex pattern of excess heat with a deficiency of yin. This can lead to further yin deficiency, or even to yin collapse. Typical yin deficiency signs include a thready pulse, a red tongue with no coating, and night sweating with a feeling of heat. Signs of yin collapse include heat on the skin, agitation (or a "clouded" spirit), profuse sweating, heat in the palms and soles, thirst, a dry red tongue, and a thready and rapid and/or weak pulse.[1]

Excess Developing from Deficiency

Excess develops from a deficiency pattern when there is an initial deficiency of *zheng* qi where the disease pattern transforms into a condition in which pathogenic qi becomes relatively predominant, causing an excess condition. Excess developing from deficiency begins with hypo-functioning of the organs with disturbances of qi, blood and fluids. For example, palpitations and breathlessness due to yang deficiency of the heart and kidney may suddenly manifest with retained water overflowing to affect the heart and lung. This results in a blockage of lung qi, thus there appears a critical pattern manifesting with severe palpations and a suffocating sensation in the chest. The *zheng* qi deficiency remains present, yet the pathomechanism of excess becomes predominant.

FACTORS INFLUENCING DISEASE TRANSMISSION

Constitutional Factors

A person's constitution influences the transmission of disease in two aspects. The first is that the constitution affects the strength of the *zheng* qi, and thus influences

---

[1] Nigel Wiseman, Ye Feng. *A Practical Dictionary of Chinese Medicine*. Taos: Pradigm Publications; 1998. p. 709.

the speed of onset and the transmission of the disease. For example, a person with a sound constitution is usually not predisposed to invasion by external pathogens, but if afflicted, the disease will often be acute and with a short course. Most importantly, the disease will not easily transmit to other parts of the body. However, a person with a weak constitution is predisposed to invasion by pathogens that are apt to go deeper into the body. The disease will generally have a longer course, transform into other patterns, and can more easily become chronic.

The second aspect is that constitution plays an important role in the transformation of pathogens. Generally speaking, in those with constitutional yang abundance, the disease tends to become an excess pattern of yang-heat where a pathogen is more likely to produce internal fire. However, in those with constitutional yin abundance, the disease tends to become a pattern of excess cold or deficiency cold patterns where a pathogen often produces internal cold. For example, pathogenic dampness is apt to lead to a damp-heat pattern when it invades a body with yang-heat qualities, but to a cold-dampness pattern when invading a body with yin-cold qualities.

Pathogenic Factors

The speeds of transmission and transformations of a disease are closely related to the quantities and qualities of the pathogen. The speed of transmission is directly related to the nature of the pathogenic qi; for example, the six pathogenic factors, yang, fire (heat), wind, and summerheat pathogens all tend to transmit rapidly. The transmission of yin pathogens is slower. This is especially true of the dampness pathogen due to its properties of thickness and stagnation. Transmissions of dampness, phlegm, water retention and blood stasis are slower than that of other interior pathogens, while the transmission of epidemic qi is most rapid. In addition, obviously if the pathogen is strong, the transmission will be more rapid whereas if the pathogen is weak, the transmission will be relatively slow. The nature of pathogenic wind is characterized by rapid movement as well as in its tendency to combine with other pathogenic factors.

Geographic and Climactic Factors

Geographical factors also contribute to differences in the disease process. In dry areas, acquired pathogens are apt to produce heat and dryness which result in damage to the yin-fluids. In damp locations, acquired pathogens tend to produce dampness resulting in damage to the yang qi.

Lifestyle Factors

The lifestyle of each patient includes emotions, diet, work, and rest. Lifestyle affects the transmission of disease by influencing *zheng* qi. In general, normal emotions, proper diet, and appropriate work and rest will promote recovery. On the other hand, excessive emotion, improper diet, and unbalanced periods of work and rest will aggravate a disease. Many work conditions can contribute to the prolonging of disease, for example when overwork causes undue stress that negatively affects the body and mind. A person with a frail constitution may not be well-suited for heavy manual labor, or because of economic circumstances, a person may work when they are aged or ill.

TRANSMISSION BETWEEN THE SIX CHANNELS

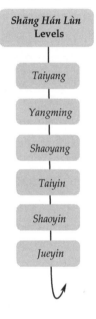

Shāng Hán Lùn Levels

Taiyang

Yangming

Shaoyang

Taiyin

Shaoyin

Jueyin

Zhang Zhong-jing's book, *Treatise on Cold Damage* provides a specific, if not always easily understood guidebook on the transmission of diseases and their appropriate treatment. Although originally written as one book, two separate works were subsequently published as the *Treatise on Cold Damage* and the *Essentials from the Golden Cabinet* (*Jīn Guì Yào Lüè*, 金匮要略).

The basic form of transmission from exterior to interior among the six channels is a transmission from yang into yin, where there are six levels of transmission from *taiyang* to *yangming*, to *shaoyang*, and then to *taiyin*, to *shaoyin* and to *jueyin*. This shows a developing process in which yang qi goes from strong to weak, and a disease goes from being mild to severe. On the contrary, transmission from yin to yang involving the *zheng* qi demonstrates a process of deficiency changing to exuberance, and of a disease changing from severe to mild. When *zheng* qi is deficient, excess pathogens may also directly invade the yin channels; this process is called "direct attack to the three yin".

Treatments with methods from the *Treatise on Cold Damage* are explicitly tied to the stage at which the disease is found. Specific herbs and formulas, often times at specific dosages, are assigned to the levels depending on the history of the disease. Pulse examination and diagnosis is also extremely important in this system.

Modern herbal formula books draw heavily upon the concepts and herbal formulas from the *Treatise on Cold Damage*. One basic precept is that there are levels (phases, warps or stages) through which contracted pathogens progress. An external pathogen will begin at the *taiyang* level, and then move more deeply into the body. Treatment in the initial phase often involves the sweating method, whereas when the deeper levels are affected, methods that promote urination or purgation through the stool are employed. Improper treatment can damage qi movement, cause pathogens to move more deeply into the body, or damage fluids.

Another major concept in the *Shāng Hán Lùn* involves the *shaoyang* disease pathomechanism as described previously in this chapter.

The following excerpt from *Chinese Herbal Formulas* by Yang Yi-fan describes the way in which the herbs in the formula *Xiǎo Chái Hú Tāng* (Minor Bupleurum Decoction) act on the various levels when treating *shaoyang* disease: "*Chái hú* is one of the two chief herbs. It is pungent and neutral, and enters the gallbladder and liver meridians (channels). *Chái hú* has ascending and dispersing properties and can disperse and expel pathogenic cold from the *shaoyang* level. At the same time, it also disperses and spreads the qi. *Huáng qín* is the other chief herb in this formula. It is bitter and cold, and enters the gallbladder meridian. *Huáng qín* can clear heat from the *shaoyang* level and reduce the heat generated by the stagnation of qi. When these two herbs are used together, they open up the obstruction of qi, heat and cold, allowing the qi to move freely in the *shaoyang* meridians." [1]

The *Essentials from the Golden Cabinet* has been called the more "practical" of the two books, primarily because it addresses specific disease categories. In addition to gynecology, the book also provides herbal treatments for malaria, jaundice, worms, and cough, as well as a number of Chinese diseases categories including "running piglet" and "wilting diseases".[2]

WĒN BÌNG THEORY-WARM DISEASE

Wei-qi-ying-xue Transmission

Wei-qi-*ying*-*xue*[3] (defensive qi, qi, *ying* and blood) is another system for viewing the course of a warm-heat disease, as solidified by Wu You-xing after an epidemic in 1642. The differences between "warm disease" theory and "cold damage" theory were first described by Wu. Contemporary author Liu Guo-hui discusses Wu's writings and writes that epidemic diseases "are caused by pestilential qi" that "can be transmitted from one person to another, unlike wind, cold or dampness". They act "as a toxin once invading the body". Epidemic qi (*lì qì*) is contagious and "attacks through the mouth and nose rather than through the skin and muscles, as cold damage is said to do." Finally, this special pathogenic factor "does not manifest symptoms soon after the exposure to the pathogen".[4]

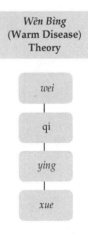

Relatively soon after Wu You-xing first developed the four-stage *wei*-qi-*ying*-*xue* concept, Ye Tian-shi fully developed this into the "warm disease" theory of treatment. The "warm disease" theory of *wei*, qi, *ying* and *xue* has special relevance for many contemporary practitioners treating conditions such as

① Yifan Yang. *Chinese Herbal Formulas*. London: Churchill Livingstone; 2010. p. 370.
② Sung Yuk-ming. *Understanding the Jin Gui Yao Lue*. Beijing: People's Medical Publishing House; 2009.
③ *Xuè* (血) is pronounced more or less like "shway".
④ Guohui Liu. *Warm Pathogen Diseases: A Clinical Guide*. Seattle:Eastland Press; 2005. p. 14.

HIV/AIDS, hepatitis and other conditions thought to be viral in nature.

Transmission through the *wei-qi-ying-xue* stages commonly begins at the *wei*-level, then moves to the qi-level, the *ying*-level, and finally the blood level. This describes the process of pathogenic movement from superficial to deep levels, and the tendency of disease to change from mild to severe. When pathogens, after entering the *wei*-level, invade the *ying*-level or blood-level without first going through the qi-level, this is called "contrary transmission".[①]

The *wei*-level is involved at the beginning stage of a warm-heat disease, concentrating on the lung or *wei* qi. This is basically approximate to an attack of external wind in other systems. The qi-level is at the middle stage of a warm-heat disease, involving the stomach, intestine, spleen, lung, and gallbladder. The *ying*-level is a more severe stage of warm-heat disease that affects the pericardium and heart and as such may cause emotional agitation. The *ying*-level often also has signs of heat in the blood, such as spots of red on the skin. The *xue*- or blood-level is at the final stage of warm-heat disease, involving the liver, kidney and heart.

Transmission from the *wei*- and qi-levels to the *ying*- and blood-levels reflects a deteriorating condition, whereas transmission from the *ying*- and blood-levels to the

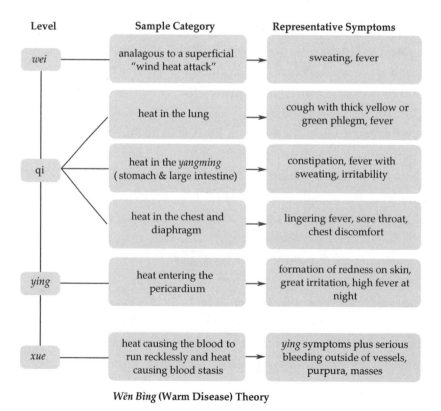

Wēn Bìng (Warm Disease) Theory

---

① (*nì chuán*, 逆传) contrary transmission

qi- and *wei*-levels shows improvement or recovery.

Wēn bìng (warm disease) theory is often useful in the modern clinic. For example, when a patient with a serious disease such as HIV begins to exhibit great irritability and signs of rashes, we can determine that the pattern may have progressed to the *ying* stage. Herbs and acupuncture techniques that cool the blood and protect yin may be selected. The *ying* and *xue* stages of a heat disease represent the point at which hospitalization is often needed.[1]

SANJIAO THEORY

The theory of the transmission through the *sanjiao* was established by Wu Jutong (1758-1836) in *Systematic Differentiation of Warm Diseases (Wēn Bìng Tiáo Biàn,* 温病条辨). This system describes the movement of heat-pathogens that enter the nose and lung which then descend to the lower *jiao* to eventually affect the liver and kidney. *Sanjiao* theory is often combined with the four-stage warm-disease theory as described above.

Transmission through the *sanjiao* involves transmission and changes of the disease location through the divisions of the upper, middle and lower regions of the body. The three *jiao* are considered as pathways for qi and fluids.

Warm-heat pathogens often first invade the upper *jiao* of the body via the mouth, nose, (and lung). As the pathogens move more deeply, they enter middle *jiao* (the spleen and stomach), and further to the lower *jiao* (the liver and kidney). This is a general process of the disease going from superficial to deep levels as associated with a progression of mild to severe disease. If pathogens move from the lung to directly invade the pericardium, the condition will deteriorate. The transmission of disease is still determined by the relative strengths of the *zheng* qi and the pathogen. If a disease takes a turn for better, the pathogenic transmission may change direction, moving from the lower *jiao* to the upper *jiao*.

Upper *Jiao*

Pattern	Symptoms (all may have fever)	Pulse	Tongue	Notes
Dryness injuring the lung	dry cough with no sputum, dry throat	rapid, thready	red with no coating or peeled	no expectoration of phlegm
Wei level external attack	aversion to cold, headache, cough	superficial, rapid	normal	slight symptoms
Cold-damp attacking exterior	fever, heavy feeling in head and body	slow, soft pulse	wet	body aches

---

[1]   Will Maclean, Jane Lyttleton. *Clinical Handbook of Internal Medicine.* Sidney: Pangolin Press; 2010. p. 37.

Pattern	Symptoms (all may have fever)	Pulse	Tongue	Notes
Dryness affecting the head orifices	red eyes, sore throat, swollen gums	rapid	yellow, dry coating	
Toxic heat invasion	swollen face, sore throat, thirst, irritability	rapid, surging	red, yellow coating	
Heat in the lung	sweating, thirst, cough, asthma	rapid	yellow coating	may form dry phlegm
Heat injuring the pericardium	coma, agitation to the point of delirium	varies	dark red, stiff	may have "reversal cold" limbs

Middle *Jiao*

Pattern	Symptoms	Pulse	Tongue	Notes
Damp-cold jaundice	yellow skin and eyes, cold limbs	deep, slow, slippery	pale with white, thick coating	due to spleen yang deficiency or prolonged damp
Damp-heat jaundice	bright yellow skin, eyes, thirst, agitation, constipation	slippery, rapid, forceful	thick yellow coating	heat dries the fluid causing constipation
Dampness blocking the "mo-yuan"	alternating slight fever, severe chills, heavy sensations, retching, sweating	slow, slippery	"dirty" turbid coating	the "*mo-yuan*" (pleural space) becomes obstructed causing an intense struggle between *zheng* and *xie*
Damp retention in MJ	loose stool, nausea	soft, slow, slippery		full feeling in abdomen (*pǐ*)
Excess heat in *yangming* channels	high fever with profuse sweating, toothache, thirst	rapid, flooding	dry, yellow	irritability, frontal headache
Heat in *yangming* organ	constipation with water diarrhea, tidal fever	brown, yellow, dry coating	deep, strong	possible clouded consciousness, delirium
Damp-heat accumulation in MJ	fever even after sweating, nausea, irritability, yellow watery stool	soft, rapid, slippery	yellow thick coating	full feeling in abdomen (*pǐ*)

Lower *Jiao*

Pattern	Symptoms	Pulse	Tongue	Notes
Heat invading blood	spasms, inhibited urination, distension in LJ	thready, rapid, choppy	red, no coating	can cause agitation and mania
Heat in the *ying*	fever at night, poor appetite	deep, thready, rapid	red, no coating	
Yin deficiency creating wind	dry skin, palpitations, fatigue, shaking	soft, thready, rapid	deep red, no coating	
Heat impairing kidney yin	low grade fever, five palm heat, thirst, fatigue	rapid, thready	dry, deep red	

Pattern	Symptoms	Pulse	Tongue	Notes
Summerheat injuring heart and kidney	heat sensation in head, numbness, convulsions	wiry, rapid	yellow, dry coating	heat agitating the heart
Lower *jiao* sinking	incessant diarrhea and urination, fatigue, aversion to cold, cold limbs	soft, weak	pale	spleen and kidney deficiency
Cold-damp injuring kidney	edema, cold limbs, little urination	large, pale	deep, thready or wiry	cold-damp creating kidney yang deficiency
Damp-heat in LJ	fever, rigid muscles, hardness below waist, constipation		wiry	stagnant qi obstructing the flow of fluids

CASES

Review preceding chapters with your instructor and select relevant information that pertains to the following cases:

1. Your patient is a 58-year-old woman who contracted chronic hepatitis B several decades ago. Throughout her life she had been a heavy drinker. Recently, she began to feel tired all the time, and began to see purple spots on her abdomen. She feels more and more agitated and often has insomnia although she feels tired. She was always a bit overweight, and now has a prominent swelling in the stomach. Her tongue is purplish, and her pulse is wiry.

2. Your patient is a 63-year-old man who had surgery on his upper neck for disc bulges. Since that time, he has had pain in both arms that he describes as his "skin is on fire". The pain is usually a 6 on a scale of 1-10, with 10 being the worst. It gets a little worse at night, but is definitely there all day long. Narcotic painkillers do not seem to have any appreciable effect, although acupuncture treatment can take all the pain away temporarily. His tongue is red, and his pulse is wiry.

3. Your patient is a 28-year-old man who just off the plane from a short but stressful trip walks in the cold from the subway to his home in a southerly direction. As he returns to his house, his neck begins to hurt and that night he begins sneezing. The next day he has a reduced appetite, is somewhat nauseated by the sight of food, and is considerably fatigued. Over the next three days, he develops a fever and an aggravated toothache. He becomes very irritated with the situation, and despite the cold outside, he has to return to work. His pulse is slippery, and his tongue is red.

Chapter 6

Pathomechanisms

Pathomechanism means the mechanisms for the cause, development and progression of a disease. Pathomechanism reveals the nature and regularity of a disease and is the basis for disease prevention and treatment. For this reason, doctors throughout the ages have given great importance to pathomechanisms.

Any reader of this book, who has been faithfully following it front to back, should be running across familiar concepts and terminology. The progress or progression[①] of a disease is quite complicated. It may involve a localized part of the body or the entire body. Therefore, the study of pathomechanisms is necessary to view disease from a multi-level perspective. This chapter should solidify many of the proceeding chapters by grounding them more fully in the body and in particular, diseases.

Pathomechanism theory originated from *The Yellow Emperor's Inner Classic*. The famous "nineteen items of pathomechanism" established a basis for the pathomechanisms of the *zang-fu* organs and of the six pathogenic qi.

Basic pathomechanism is the most basic level to view because all diseases can be interpreted as having common laws. These basic laws or rules include the growth or decline of *zheng*/right qi and *xie*/pathogenic qi, yin-yang disharmony, disorders of essence-qi-blood-fluids. Pathomechanisms of a more "systematic nature" belong to the second level, which reveals the basic laws from viewpoint of the systems of the *zang-fu* organs or channels-collaterals. Pathomechanism of a category disease belongs to the third level, such as pathomechanism of the six channels, pathomechanism of *wei*-qi-*ying*-blood, and *sanjiao*. Disease pathomechanism, such as pathomechanisms of cold and asthma, belongs to the forth level, which studies the basic law of occurrence, development, change and outcome of a concrete disease. Syndrome pathomechanism looks at concrete syndromes, such as damp-heat syndrome in the spleen and stomach, and pathomechanisms of liver qi stagnation syndromes. Symptom pathomechanism belongs to a sixth level, such as pain and fever.

---

① (*cóng huà*, 从化) progression

Section 1 Basic Pathomechanism

ZHENG/UPRIGHT QI AND *XIE*/PATHOGENIC QI (SEE CHAPTER 4)

YIN-YANG DISHARMONY (SEE CHAPTER 4)

DISORDERS OF ESSENCE, QI, BLOOD AND FLUIDS (SEE CHAPTER 1)

THE FIVE INTERNAL PATHOGENS

The five internal pathogens are pathological conditions of wind, cold, dampness, dryness, and fire which involve dysfunctions of the *zang-fu* organs, channels and collaterals, essence, qi, blood, or fluids. These are internally-generated pathological changes with clinical manifestations similar to those caused by the same external pathogens of the same name. Patterns associated with the five internal pathogens generally involve deficiency, or complex patterns of deficiency and excess. Patterns caused by the six external pathogenic factors are usually exterior conditions of an excess nature.

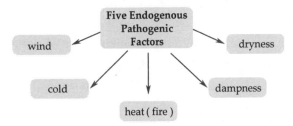

Internal Wind

Wind stirring internally comes from the interior of body, so it is also called internal wind. Internal wind is caused by unrestrained overactive ascending yang-qi creating turmoil of the yang qi. It can be caused by either yang exuberance or yin deficiency failing to restrict yang. Clinically, internal wind is characterized by dizziness, spasms, and tremors. The pathomechanisms include liver yang transforming into wind, extreme heat producing wind, stirring of wind due to yin deficiency, and blood deficiency generating wind.

Liver yang transforming into wind is caused by emotions and overstrain which damages liver and kidney yin. This creates excessive liver yang that transforms into wind due to the failure of deficient yin to restrain yang (called "deficient water failing to nourish wood"). The overactive liver yang causes tremors in the sinews and flesh, numbness in the limbs, dizziness, and deviations of the eyes and mouth. In severe cases there may be fainting or stroke due to the ascending movement of "blood following qi".

Extreme heat producing wind most often appears in the advanced stage of a febrile (heat) disease. Excessive fire dries the *ying*-blood and "cooks and burns" the fluids, which together causes wind. Internal fire scorches the liver channel, also affecting the sinews and vessels. Manifestations include convulsions, spasms, and in severe cases, high fever, coma, and delirious speech.

Stirring of wind due to yin deficiency usually appears in the late-stage of a heat disease. This pattern results from either a great loss of fluids and yin qi, or from deficiency of fluids in a prolonged disease. The pathomechanism involves an exhaustion of fluids with severe damage to yin qi where the sinews and vessels lose nourishment. This also results in a relative excess of yang qi with signs and symptoms of internal wind such as spasms of the sinews and flesh and contraction of the extremities. At the same time, signs of yin exhaustion include a periodic low fever, a tongue coating with little moisture, and a thready rapid pulse.

Blood deficiency generating wind is caused by impaired generation of blood, excessive bleeding, or damage to *ying*-blood in a prolonged disease. When a deficiency of liver blood causes malnourishment of the sinews and vessels, or when blood fails to nourish the collaterals, wind will move internally. Wind associated with blood deficiency is called deficiency wind. Other kinds of internal wind due to rising yang for example, do not have the implicit cause of deficient blood, but may also impact the blood over time. Manifestations of blood deficiency generating wind include numbness of the limbs, tremors of the sinews and flesh, and spasms of the hands and feet with impaired movement.

Internal Heat and Fire

The stirring of internal fire-heat can result from an overabundance of yang, yin deficiency with yang hyperactivity, stagnation of qi and blood, and/or stagnation of internal pathogens. The internal production and pathomechanism of fire-heat is characterized by both deficiency and excess.

Fire production from overabundant yang is one of the more extreme ways that internal fire is produced. Under normal conditions, yang qi in the body functions to warm the *zang-fu* organs and channels and collaterals. In Chinese medicine, this warming function is called the "minor fire[①]". However, under pathological

---

① (*shào huǒ*, 少火) minor fire

conditions, overabundant yang qi creates hyper-functioning that results in an increased consumption of substances with damage to yin-fluids. The pathological excess of yang qi is called "hyperactive fire".[1]

Generation of fire due to stasis of pathogens can occur in two ways. The first involves the stagnation of pathogenic factors that produce heat and fire; there may be stagnation of cold generating heat or stagnation of dampness generating fire. The second involves stagnation of pathological metabolic products such as phlegm, static blood, stones, food accumulation, and worms. The main pathomechanism of static pathogens generating fire also involves stagnation and constraint of yang qi which in turn generates heat and fire.

Generation of fire due to extreme emotion is also called the "fire of the five emotions". Extreme emotions impact balance among the organ-essence, qi, yin and yang, and results in the stagnation or counterflow of the movement of qi[2], where prolonged qi stagnation or qi counterflow can result in the generation of internal fire-heat. Injury by the emotions also often leads to liver constraint and qi stagnation where qi stasis generates liver fire. When rage injures the liver, the liver qi may quickly ascend to generate liver fire.

Yin deficiency resulting in intense fire[3] involves a deficiency-type fire that results in damage to yin qi and a deficiency of fluids that is so severe that yin qi fails to restrain yang qi. The relative excess of yang qi then generates intense heat and fire that further damages yin. Generally speaking, internal heat with yin deficiency often manifests deficiency heat symptoms such as night sweating, a red tongue with little coating, and a thready, rapid forceless pulse. Intense fire with yin deficiency commonly shows fire-heat symptoms in a localized part of the upper body, including toothaches, bleeding gums, sore throat, or flushed cheeks.

Internal Cold

Internal cold, or endogenous cold, is usually related to yang deficiency of the spleen and/or kidney. Spleen and kidney yang deficiency (especially kidney yang) results in a reduction in overall warming actions and leads to deficiency-type cold. Manifestations include frequent urination with profuse clear urine, thin and clear nasal fluids, phlegm-drool, diarrhea, or edema.

Internal cold is the result of yin abundance[4] with yang deficiency, while external cold results from exteriorly-contracted cold or from overconsumption of raw and cold foods. There are both differences and similarities between internal cold and external

---

[1] (zhuàng huǒ, 壮火) hyperactive fire
[2] (qì nì, 气逆) qi circulating in the wrong direction or "counterflow"
[3] (yin xū huǒ wàng, 阴虚火旺) yin deficiency with intense fire
[4] (shèng, 盛) fill, contain, abundance

cold. Clinically, internal cold is characterized mainly by deficiency accompanied by cold. External cold is characterized mainly by excess-type cold with deficiency (of yang) being secondary. The exogenous (externally-contracted) cold pathogen is prone to damage the yang qi of the body, resulting in yang deficiency and greater susceptibility to further cold invasion.

Dampness

Internal production of turbid dampness is a pathological state involving the retention and stagnation of turbid dampness due to the impaired transformation and transportation of water. Spleen qi is a main factor, with varied clinical manifestations according to the position of the pathogenic dampness. For example, if the dampness lodges in the channels, there can be a heavy or stiff sensations in the limbs and joints and body. When dampness invades the upper *jiao*, there may be chest distention, cough with phlegm, or a heavy sensation in the head as if the head is bandaged. When dampness obstructs the middle *jiao*, there can be distention and fullness in the abdomen, poor appetite, greasy or sweet tastes in the mouth, and a thick greasy tongue coating. When dampness stagnates in the lower *jiao*, there may be distending sensations in the abdomen, diarrhea, and difficult urination. If water-dampness diffuses into the skin, there can also be edema. Stagnation of dampness in the middle *jiao* is a common cause of nausea.

Dryness

Internal dryness results from damage to the fluids involving dryness and withering[1] of the tissues, organs, and orifices due to body fluids failing to nourish and moisten. Internal dryness may affect any of the *zang-fu* organs and tissues, but mainly the lung, stomach, and large intestine.[2] Exhaustion of fluids reduces the source of generation for yin qi, thus resulting in the production of internal heat. When yin qi becomes deficient, yang qi will become relatively excessive; therefore, internal dryness is often accompanied by manifestations of deficiency heat.

Manifestations of internal dryness include dry skin, dry mouth and throat, a dry tongue with no moisture, a dry nose, uncomfortable feelings in the eyes, brittle nails, constipation, and scanty dark urine. When affecting the lung, other signs and symptoms include dry cough with no expectoration of phlegm, or coughing of blood. When affecting the stomach, there may be poor appetite, anxiety, and a red tongue with no coating, and when the intestines are affected, there may be constipation.

---

[1]   (*kū hé*, 枯涸) dried and withered

[2]   The stomach and large intestine are both *yangming* organs and are thus prone to excess. The large intestine and lung are both metal elements and therefore tend to dryness.

Section 2　Eight Principles of Pathomechanisms (*Bā Gāng*, 八纲)

From the qualities yin and yang are derived the eight principle pairings of heat/cold, interior/exterior, deficiency/excess and yin/yang. The eight "principles" are in fact eight guidelines for diagnosis and treatment, as well as a way to understand and organize the basic pathologies and concepts involving the classification of disease. The eight principles allow the practitioner to view complex disorders under the large umbrella of yin and yang, thus providing an elegant method for categorizing both simple and complex conditions.

The eight principles of heat/cold, interior/exterior, excess/deficiency, and yin/yang combine with and interact with each other. Yin and yang categorizes the entirety of these dichotomies. Heat and cold describe the nature of temperature, excess and deficiency denote the relative quantity of pathogenic factors, while interior and exterior describe the general location of disease.

Qi in the body that assists and promotes normal bodily processes is called anti-pathogenic or upright qi, whereas that qi which disrupts normal processes is called pathogenic qi. Relative excesses or deficiencies of *zheng* qi and *xie* qi lead to pathology. The following dichotomies form the backbone of disease pattern identification in Chinese medicine: predominance and weakness, upright/*zheng* qi and pathogenic/*xie* qi, and excess and deficiency[①].

Among yin and yang's encompassing associations, none is so close as cold and heat. In appropriate situations, the qualities of yin and yang are indistinguishable from those of cold and heat. In treatment, excess and deficiency defines whether there is *xie*/pathogenic qi (excess) that needs to be eliminated, or whether *zheng* qi requires supplementation (deficiency). The disease process also involves close interactions between excess/deficiency and *zheng*/*xie* qi. (These pathological processes are discussed at length in this chapter.) Interior/exterior determines where in the body the pathogenic qi is located.

Due to the fact that these categories constantly interact and transform, they should not be thought of as existing independently. Their interconnections form a clinical pattern of disharmony which could, for example, involve a combination of "interior, deficiency, and cold", which together would create a yin pattern. Another example might be "exterior, heat, and excess", which create a yang pattern. Yet, there also

---

① *A Practical Dictionary of Chinese Medicine* defines excess, *shí* as "replete" and deficiency, *xū* as "vacuity".

exists the possibility of an "interior damp-heat" pattern, which is comprised of both yin and yang components. So again it must be understood that these pairings do not exist in isolation, and that they often manifest simultaneously in complex patterns.

Eight Principles

Yang	Yin
Exterior	Interior
Excess	Deficiency
Heat	Cold

EXTERIOR AND INTERIOR

Interior and exterior define the location of the disease. This is important because the location of the pathogenic evil will largely determine the required treatment. For example, interior-excess conditions are generally treated by draining through the urine or stools, while exterior-excess conditions can be treated through sweating. Interior-deficiency conditions are treated by supplementing or boosting qi, while exterior-deficiency conditions are treated by expelling the pathogenic evil and "consolidating" the exterior. If one mis-identifies the excess or deficiency nature of the pattern and the location of interior or exterior, one risks aggravating the disease with improper treatment.

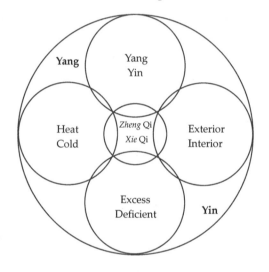

An exterior condition is one that is found on the surface of the body. Exterior conditions move from the surface to the interior. When this occurs, conditions generally worsen. Conversely, interior conditions generally become less severe when they move to the exterior of the body.

Exterior conditions enter through the skin, muscles and body hair, and first affect the lung and the upper parts of the body. The nose "opens to the lung", so sniffles and sneezing are often the first signs of an exterior attack. As *wei* qi rises to the surface to fight against the exterior pathogen, this gives rise to tight neck muscles, itching, headache, sore throat and fever. An exterior cold pathogen will close the pores of the skin causing body aches. An exterior heat-type condition will cause sweating and a higher fever than in a cold-type exterior condition. In biomedicine, these conditions can be compared to the common cold and the flu.

In Chinese medicine, a great amount of attention is given to preventing an external condition from penetrating into the interior.[①] Once interior, cold can easily transform into patterns of internal cold or internal heat.

Exterior conditions are best treated by "releasing" the exterior through sweating with pungent-acrid herbs, or by cupping therapy, or by *gua sha* (a method that employs scraping of the skin).

Interior conditions are considered as generally more serious and more chronic than those of the exterior. For this reason, preventing an exterior pathogen from progressing to the interior is very important. Interior conditions often affect the *zang-fu* organs and disturb the normal functions of qi, blood, and fluids. Internal conditions can follow the progression of an external condition, or result from internal causes. In some cases, an exterior pathogen can also "directly attack" the interior.[②]

	Internal	External
Pulse	generally deeper	more superficial
Tongue	changes with condition	no change
Location	*zang-fu* organs affected	channels and collaterals affected

COLD AND HEAT

Cold and heat reflect of the relative amounts of yin and yang within the body. Cold is a yin-pathogen, its movement is downward and inward, and it moves more slowly. Cold is produced by either a lack of yang, or by an excess of yin-pathogens. Yin-pathogens can come from the exterior, or they can be generated from within. Cold signs and symptoms include a lack of energy, cold body, a lack of thirst, white or clear saliva, a pale tongue and a slow pulse. Cold tends to contract the muscles, constrict blood vessels and cause pain. Therefore, any pain resulting from cold can be relieved by warmth.

A heat pattern may result from an excess of yang, or from a deficiency of yin. Also, many types of constraint can transform into heat, such as constrained internal dampness, food stagnation, and even emotions. Exterior cold can also transform into heat as it moves more deeply into the body. Heat signs and symptoms include red eyes, preference for cold drinks, irritability, constipation, a red tongue and a rapid pulse. If heat has damaged body fluids, the tongue will be dry. If there is sputum, it

---

① Before the advent of antibiotics, simple external conditions more often turned into life-threatening conditions thus one factor in Chinese medicine's attention to external conditions.

② Interior and exterior progressions are discussed more fully in Chapter 5.

will be yellow or yellowish-green in color.

Heat and cold often appear at the same time in different parts of the body. It is not uncommon to have internal heat with exterior cold, or vice versa. Similarly, there may be cold in the lower part of the body with heat above, or the opposite.

Cold can transform into heat, and heat into cold; this often occurs as heat or cold pathogens penetrate deeper into the body. Extreme heat and extreme cold can cause the "clumping" of either where one will "repel" the other. This is a more complex scenario involving heat and cold that will be discussed in the following section on yin and yang.

	Heat	Cold
Thirst	thirst with preference for cold drinks	no thirst
Complexion	red	pale
Tongue	red	pale
Body fluids	yellow	white, clear
Bowels	constipation	loose
Emotions	agitation, anger	apathy

YIN-YANG DISHARMONY

A yin-yang disharmony is an imbalance which may involve:
1) predominance of yin or yang
2) weakness of yin or yang
3) mutual decline
4) mutual impairment
5) repelling of yin and yang
6) collapse of yin and yang

These changes result in various pathogenic factors which can lead to the development of various disease patterns.

Predominance[①]

Yin moves slowly and downward and inward to manifest the qualities of coolness and material substance, whereas yang moves quickly and upward and outward, becoming heat. Under normal circumstances, yin and yang oppose and restrain these tendencies within each other. However, when the activation of yang becomes greater than the restraining action of yin, then yang becomes predominant. When the restraint

---

① (*piān shèng*, 偏胜) *Piān* (predominance) means slanting towards, and *shèng* is victory. Together they can be defined as a one-sided dominance, tendency, predominance or preponderance.

of yin becomes greater than the movement of yang, then yin becomes predominant. Therefore, predominance is a tendency of "leaning towards" yin or yang which can result from an overabundance[①] of either. (Again, it must be stressed that yin and yang are not "quantities", but rather abstractions involving the categorization of among other things: cold vs. heat and substance vs. function.)

Because yin is associated with cold, and yang is associated with heat, overabundant yin leads to excessive cold whereas overabundant yang leads to excessive heat. Heat and activity are yang properties, and if these properties become excessive, the overabundance of yang can damage structures and fluids, which are associated with yin; this pattern is called "yang consuming yin". The first stage of yang excess is considered as the primary cause, with the yin consumption and deficiency as the secondary effect. For example, this can be seen in an individual with a high fever who then also becomes very thirsty. So in this way, excess conditions can lead to deficiency conditions over time, and vice versa.

Yin predominance

At the beginning of yin predominance there is a growth of yin, but no change in the yang qi. Yin predominance in this case creates an excess-cold pattern. As the condition progresses, overabundant yin qi will consume and damage yang qi, thus changing the pattern from one of excess yin-cold to a pattern of "excess-cold complicated by weakness of yang-heat". When yang qi becomes even more damaged, the condition may transform from excess to deficiency to create a pattern of "yang deficiency". In all of the above stages, yang has failed to control and oppose yin, thus resulting in a predominance of yin.

Yin qi is characterized by coldness, quietness and dampness. Signs and symptoms of predominant yin include chills, cold limbs, lying with the body huddled up, a pale tongue with a moist coating, and a slow pulse. An excess-cold pattern presents with a pale complexion, a cold body, cold pain in the abdomen, loose stools, a pale tongue with a white coating, and a deep slow or deep tight pulse (coldness contracts the vessels thus giving rise to a tight pulse). Yang deficiency cold signs include a fear of cold, cold limbs, lying with the body huddled up and a deep slow pulse (yang deficiency gives rise to a slow and deep pulse). Causes of yin predominance include inactivity, exposure to cold weather, invasion of cold-dampness, or overconsumption of cold uncooked foods.

Yang predominance

Yang dominance creates hyperactivity and a surplus of heat with strong reactions

---

① (*shèng*, 盛) This term connotes energetic abundance, flourishing, filled.

of the body. This creates an excess-heat pattern of exuberant yang with normal yin. The main causes for yang predominance are invasion by yang pathogens, hot environments and overconsumption of hot spicy foods. Additionally, yin-pathogens may combine with yang, which then creates heat. For example, dampness is a yin-pathogen that, when it accumulates, often leads to pathogenic "damp-heat". Other factors that create internal heat include excessive emotion, qi stagnation, blood stasis, and food accumulation.

Yang qi warms, generates and activates. Yang dominance leads to patterns of excess-heat that generally present with a high fever, agitation, a red complexion, and a rapid pulse. When the growth of yang damages the yin qi, there will be yin deficiency signs and symptoms generally including dry mouth and lips, periodic heat rising to the head, and a red tongue with little moisture.

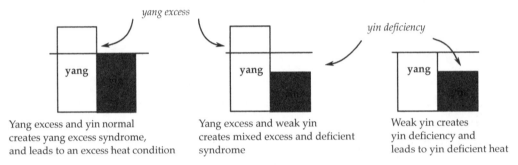

Three Forms for Yang-heat

Yin and Yang, Excess and Deficiency

A condition of excess yang or excess yin is relatively easy to identify. However, deficiency-type conditions seem to be more complicated because they manifest signs opposite to the corresponding yin-yang characteristics. For example, a pattern of yin deficiency can manifest with signs of heat, and a pattern of yang deficiency will show signs of cold. This is because when either yin or yang weakens[1] it will become unable to restrain its opposite, which then becomes relatively dominant (proportionally).

Excess patterns

When yin or yang is predominant and its opposite remains the same, the result is an excess-type pattern. Signs of yang excess may appear in an individual over-exposed to heat, following overconsumption of hot or spicy foods, or even following great anger, which also raises yang. Manifestations of yang excess are thus characterized by

---

① (*piān shuāi*, 偏衰) We have the same *piān* as in yang *piān shèng*, but *shuāi* means weakness or decline. So *piān shuāi* is a "leaning towards" decline.

heat, redness, symptoms affecting the head, and/or anger. As stated above, heat will eventually damage the fluids as well as impair the ability of yin to moisten and cool. Other signs and symptoms include pain with burning quality, a rapid pulse, and a red tongue with a thick yellow coating.

Signs of excess yin-cold may appear in an individual over-exposed to cold, following overconsumption of cold food and drink, or even after sitting on cold concrete or swimming in cold water. Signs and symptoms include pain with a stabbing-type quality, a slow tight pulse, and a pale tongue with a thick white coating.

Deficiency patterns

Although excess conditions are common, there is just as often a clinical scenario where yin or yang has become diminished or "deficient". This leads to a situation where the opposite yin or yang property appears as being relatively stronger, but where the true cause is actually deficiency. Differentiating an excess condition from a deficiency condition is of the utmost importance in diagnosis, and the distinctions are often quite subtle.

> "Deficiency heat" and "deficiency cold" conditions are most difficult for students to understand. It should be noted that "yin deficiency heat" and "yang deficiency cold" are both technical terms and not necessarily literal descriptions of the conditions. Keep this in mind as you read this section.

Lessened yang leads to a yang deficiency-type cold pattern, whereas lessened yin leads to a yin deficiency-type heat pattern. Yang weakness is characterized by a decline in activity, slowing of the metabolism, and a shortage of heat which results from declining yang actions of warming, promoting, and activating. This creates a pattern of yang qi deficiency. The main causes for relative yang weakness are: pre- and post natal essence deficiency, malnutrition, overwork, or yang qi decline in a prolonged chronic condition. Signs and symptoms include chills, cold limbs, cold pains in the stomach and abdomen, fluid retention, depression and apathy, lying with the body curled up, a pale face, clear profuse urine, loose bowel movements with undigested food, a pale tongue, and a slow pulse.

Yang deficiency cold often occurs over time as a person approaches old age or has a chronic illness. The patient may feel cold, sweat even without exercise, and have a pale complexion. Energy levels are often low, and there may be lessened libido. For older men, yang deficiency is often (but not always) a component of impotence and sexual dysfunction. A shortage of yang qi can manifest in any of the organs, but kidney yang deficiency is most prevalent. Because kidney yang is considered as the root of all yang in the body, kidney yang deficiency is usually involved in the pathomechanism of yang qi weakness.

Yang predominance (before any damage to yin qi) creates an excess-heat pattern. If the condition progresses, the excessive yang will diminish the yin qi. In this case, a purely excess-heat pattern changes into a pattern of excess-heat complicated by yin deficiency. As yin qi becomes severely damaged and diminished, the entire condition may transform from excess to deficiency, then giving rise to a pattern of deficiency heat.

Yin deficiency heat involves the appearance of more (predominant) heat even when there is no increase in the actual amount of heat in the body. The relative appearance of more heat is due to the insufficiency of yin qi with a subsequent failure to restrain yang qi. Again, this is important in treatment, because strongly clearing heat from the body can easily damage yin further and thus aggravate the condition. Therefore, the main treatment principle here is to supplement yin while also gently eliminating heat.

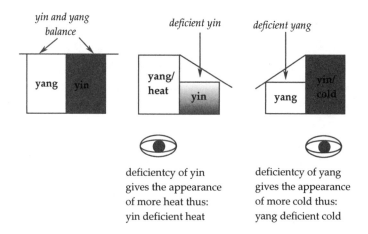

The main etiologies for the development of a relative yin weakness are damage to yin by an invasion of yang pathogens, damage to yin by fire-heat resulting from extreme changes in the five emotions, or damage to yin caused by a prolonged chronic condition. The patient may have signs and symptoms of deficiency heat such as a low fever, vexing (agitating) heat in the five centers[1] (chest, palms and soles of the feet), tidal fever with the sensation of steaming heat in the bones[2], night sweating, a red tongue with little coating, and a thready and rapid pulse.

The shortage of yin qi may occur in any of the five *zang*-organs or six *fu*-organs.

---

[1]   (*wǔ xīn fán rè*, 五心烦热) five-center heat
[2]   (*gǔ zhēng cháo rè*, 骨蒸潮热) bone steaming fever, also called hectic fever

However, because kidney yin is considered as the root of all yin in the body, patterns of kidney yin deficiency are most important.

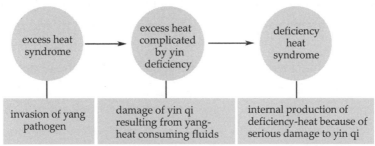

Progression of Excess Heat Syndrome to Yin Deficiency Heat Syndrome

Yin deficiency heat is created when yin declines and the yin properties of cooling and constraining are affected. To anyone observing (and to the patient themselves) there will be a greater relative appearance of heat signs. In other words, there is not necessarily an introduction of more heat in the body, but rather there is a reduced ability for cooling existing heat. Yin deficiency involves a lack of fluids, and because fluids cool the body, signs and symptoms of dryness and relative heat appear. Unlike the heat of an excess yang condition, however, the symptoms of yin deficiency-type heat generally appear in periodic waves, especially in the evenings (yin). This often happens when a younger person engages in too much activity such as over-exercising, working or worrying, and thus "burning up their yin".

For example, an active 40-year-old man may work at a stressful job, worry a lot, and also run for several miles each day. Unless he balances these yang-type activities with rest and plenty of fluids (yin), the yang will become predominant. He could maintain such an active lifestyle for many years, although he would be losing yin gradually over time. At 55, he may find that he has less energy and yet also feels agitated; his muscles may become so stiff that he can no longer run comfortably. This is a typical example of yang predominance leading to a deficiency of yin.

With a yin deficiency heat condition, the feverishness is usually less severe than in an excess condition, and it typically occurs periodically. Redness of the face may also be less red than as seen in an excess condition, and may be present only on the cheeks. The pulse is rapid (as in an excess heat condition), but it is also thinner in quality due to the lack of fluids. The tongue may be red, but also dry due to the lack of fluids.

Although menopausal symptoms are not always caused by yin deficiency, the classic signs of night sweating, hot flashes and agitation do generally correspond with the signs and symptoms of yin deficiency. With no signs of infection, nor a history of eating spicy hot foods- generalized anxiety, dryness, or heat are quite likely due to yin deficiency associated with aging.

Mutual Decline and Impairment of Yin and Yang

The mutual decline of yin and yang refers to a dual deficiency of both yin and yang. When either yin or yang decline to a certain point, yin and yang will both decline. This pattern is most common in old age or during a chronic condition. Although yin and yang can decline together equally, the decline of one can influence the other as described below.

Mutual impairment of yin and yang refers to a dual deficiency of both yin and yang which results from either yin deficiency or yang deficiency. As one condition progresses, the yin/yang counterpart is then affected. When yin deficiency leads to yang deficiency, this is referred to as yin impairment affecting yang. When yang deficiency leads to yin deficiency, this is referred to as yang impairment affecting yin.

Yin impairment affecting yang

Yin impairment affecting yang occurs as yin deficiency progressed to the point where yang is also affected. When there is a deficiency of yin qi, then yang cannot be sustained because it has no material substance(s) to draw upon. As yin fails to restrain yang, there will be both yin deficiency and yang hyperactivity. For example, when liver and kidney yin are both deficient, this initially causes liver yang to rise. There may be headaches, anxiety, a reddish face and a thready pulse. As the condition progresses, yang will also diminish (due to the lack of yin) and create a concurrent deficiency of kidney yang. Signs and symptoms would then include chills with cold limbs, a pale complexion, and a deep weak pulse. Because yin impairment has affected yang, the pattern then involves a dual deficiency of both yin and yang.

Yang impairment affecting yin

Yin is sustained by yang, thus when yang is impaired (deficient) there will eventually appear deficiencies of both yin and yang. For example, a pattern of kidney yang deficiency is characterized by declined warming and activating actions, which typically causes edema stemming from water stagnation in the skin. If the imbalance further progresses, due to the shortage of yang qi, yin can no longer be produced. The resulting deficiency of kidney yin would then give rise to restlessness and a flushed (reddish) face. Because yang impairment has affected yin, the pattern then involves a dual deficiency of both yin and yang.

Repellence of Yin and Yang

Although it is not often mentioned as a part of yin-yang theory, it does happen in the clinic that overabundant yin can "repel" yang and overabundant yang can "repel" yin. In the case of yin repelling yang, the signs and symptoms that at first seem like heat are actually part of an overabundant yin (cold) condition. When a predominance of yin or yang progresses to its extreme, yin and yang fail to communicate with each other; one aspect will stagnate inside the body and repel the opposite aspect to the surface of the body. This results in complex pathological changes associated with what is referred to as "true heat with false cold" or "true cold with false heat".

Overabundant yin repelling yang / cold repelling heat[①]

Overabundant yin repelling yang is a condition in which yin-cold forces yang qi to move outward to the surface of the body. As the abundant yin qi develops to an extreme amount, qi movement is obstructed inside the body, resulting in heat manifestations such as flushing of the cheeks, agitating heat, thirst, and a large pulse "without root". However, because they occur due to overabundant cold in the body, such manifestations are termed as "false heat" signs. The internal cold also produces signs of "true cold" such as a pale face, "reversal counterflow cold of the limbs" (cold limbs with cold moving proximally past the elbows and knees),

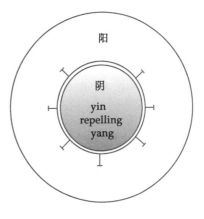

listlessness, a fear of cold with a curled-up body, and a faint and barely perceptible pulse. The pattern is called "true cold with false heat".

Overabundant yang repelling yin / heat repelling cold

Overabundant yang repelling yin is a condition in which overabundant yang-heat forces yin qi to move outward to the surface of the body. As overabundant yang qi

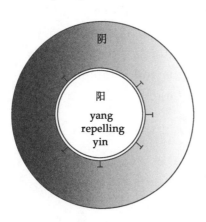

develops to an extreme amount, heat accumulates in the deeper levels of body. The first symptoms are high fever, a red face, rough breath and agitation, and "reversal counterflow cold of the limbs". The patient with reversal cold will have cold limbs but no desire for more clothing. Other signs and symptoms include burning heat in the chest and abdomen, diarrhea accompanied by dry feces, thirst with the desire for cold liquids, and a red tongue; the pulse is deep and thin, but rapid and powerful.

---

① (*yīn shèng gé yáng*, 阴盛格阳) yin repelling or resisting yang

The pattern is called "true heat with false cold".

Collapse of Yin and Yang

Yin collapse[1] and yang collapse are critical states in which the yin or yang qi of the body becomes suddenly and massively exhausted. The yin qi and yang qi of the body attach to, depend[2] upon and supplement one another. Therefore, yin collapse causes yang to lose its "attachment" (to substance), thus resulting in the collapse of yang. When yang collapses, yin loses its basis for production, thus resulting in the collapse of yin. Finally, essence-qi becomes exhausted as yin and yang separate from each other completely, which is a fatal condition.

Yang collapse

Yang collapse is a pathological state involving a sudden and massive loss of yang qi which results in a critical failure of whole-body function.

Generally speaking, yang collapse occurs in the following conditions: when *zheng/right* qi fails to resist extreme pathogenic qi, leading to sudden collapse of yang qi; when yang qi is depleted following a massive loss of body fluids; overconsumption of yang qi resulting from overstrain and a yang deficiency-type constitution; or prolonged damage to yang qi in a chronic condition which finally results in complete exhaustion of yang qi.

A case of acute yang collapse commonly shows critical signs and symptoms such as dripping cold sweat, palpitations, breathlessness, a pale complexion, "reversal cold" of the four limbs, aversion to cold with a curled-up body, fatigue, and a faint and barely perceptible pulse.

Yin collapse

Yin collapse is a pathological state involving a copious and acute loss of yin qi which results in a critical failure of whole-body function.

Generally speaking, yin collapse results from exuberant pathogenic heat with severe fluid depletion through excessive sweating which leads to collapse, although yin collapse may also result from prolonged consumption of fluids in a chronic condition.

A case of yin collapse commonly shows critical signs and symptoms such as copious sweating with warm limbs, restlessness, palpitations, difficult breathing, fatigue, and a rapid and racing pulse.

Treating A Patient with Yin and Yang

The basic cause of any condition involves an imbalance of the yin and yang. At

---

① (*wáng yīn*, 亡阴) yin collapse
② (*yī fù*, 依附) attach to, depend on

issue are yin and/or yang excesses, deficiencies and/or mutual impairments of both yin and yang. Here we imply that treatment is with herbs, acupuncture, moxibustion and physical therapies.

Eliminating surplus

Eliminating surplus[1] refers to the treatment of excess patterns according to the relative strengths of yin and yang. Specifically, an excess heat pattern caused by a predominance of yang can be treated with cold- or cool-natured herbs, and conversely, patterns of excess cold can be treated with herbs that are warm or hot in nature, thus "eliminating the surplus" of yin qi. As a generality, the first priority in treatment is to clear away excess, with any underlying deficiencies being treated secondarily.

Supplementing deficiency

Supplementing deficiency[2] refers to the treatment of a deficiency pattern that has resulted from a weakness of yin or yang. Patterns of deficiency heat are often due to deficient yin failing to restrict yang. A common mistake is to treat deficiency heat by clearing heat directly with herbs that are bitter in flavor and cold in nature; this approach drains qi and causes further damage. Because yin is deficient, proper treatment in such cases should act to nourish and supplement yin. In the same spirit, patterns of deficiency cold (due to deficient yang failing to restrict yin) generally should not be treated with herbs that are acrid in flavor and warm in nature. Because yang is deficient, proper treatment in such cases should act to strengthen yang.

Supplementing both yin and yang

In cases of mutual impairment of both yin and yang, yin and yang should both be supplemented. In patterns of yin impairment affecting yang, proper treatment should primarily strengthen yang while also nourishing yin. Conversely, if the pattern of dual deficiency of both yin and yang has prevalent yin deficiency, the pattern should be treated by primarily nourishing yin while also strengthening yang. In this way, yin and yang aspects can assist and promote and transform into one another.

A DISCUSSION ABOUT *ZHENG*/UPRIGHT QI AND *XIE*/PATHOGENIC QI

Chinese medicine divides the qi within the body into two large categories. *Xie*/pathogenic qi is that qi which impairs normal function or causes illness. *Zheng*/upright qi is that qi which maintains health and protects against illness. Excesses

---

[1] (*shí zé xiè zhī*, 实则泻之) eliminating (draining) surplus
[2] (*xū zé bǔ zhī*, 虚则补之) supplementing deficiency

and deficiencies within the body involve the balance of and interactions between the *zheng* qi and *xie* qi within the body. In order to fully appreciate the true nature of excess and deficiency, we need to fully explore the relationship between *xie* qi and *zheng* qi.

When illness occurs, there is a lack of rebalancing. We can visualize a perfect yin and yang relationship where when yin grows, yang declines, and vice versa. But how does the body become unhealthy and imbalanced? The answer is that any pathogens which are not repelled or overcome imply a deficiency of *zheng* qi. Thus the saying, "those who are invaded by pathogens must have a deficiency of qi."

When *zheng* qi "battles" or contends with a pathogenic evil, the result often manifests as an excess pattern, such as when a high fever appears following the contraction of an exterior pathogen. If the *zheng* qi prevails, then the body is quickly returned to balance and health. However, if the *zheng* qi is too weak to resist the evil, pathogens may enter the organs or channels and cause a more serious condition. If *zheng* qi remains deficient, organ functions will decrease as the distribution and metabolism of essence, blood and fluids also become abnormal. In this case, the likely outcome will involve a pattern of deficiency, or a mixed pattern of excess and deficiency. This example illustrates the importance of correctly differentiating signs of excess from those of deficiency in order to render a correct diagnosis.

Zheng qi acts to resist disease, expel pathogens, and create the conditions in the body for recovery, and yet the strength of *zheng* qi also depends on sufficient essence, blood and fluids within the body. Certainly, being "run down" or adopting an unhealthy lifestyle is a precursor to catching colds and flu and a host of other conditions. In fact, *zheng* qi deficiency can also result from inappropriate reactions to mental/emotional issues. Therefore, for problems such as anxiety, proper treatment

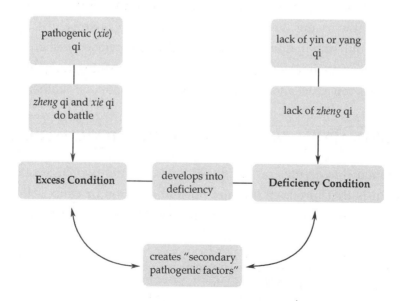

will involve both "calming the *shén*/spirit" and strengthening the *zheng*/upright qi.

MORE ON THE QUALITIES AND QUANTITIES OF PATHOGENIC QI

Xie/pathogenic qi refers to various pathogenic factors, often simply termed as "pathogens". These include the six pathogens (environmental factors), epidemic qi, external injuries, injuries by insects and animals, parasites, injuries from emotional factors, improper diet, phlegm and fluid retention, blood stasis, and stones. When a pathogen invades the body, the resulting imbalance of yin and yang in the body will disturb the metabolism and functioning of essence, qi, blood, fluids, organs and channels, and can also damage the skin, muscles, sinews and bones. A pathogen can also change the constitutional characteristics of an individual over time. For example, an invasion of a yin-pathogen may damage yang qi to the point where the individual constitution changes from its original type into a yang deficiency-type constitution.

The resistance of *zheng* qi to a pathogen has several aspects. The first involves resistance to the invasion itself. This resistance may act against environmental pathogens, pathogens which have already invaded interiorly, or those which have been created internally. When a pathogen is already within the body, *zheng* qi attempts to prevent the condition from exacerbating; with ample *zheng* qi, the condition will remain mild and temporary. *Zheng* qi therefore acts to correct any imbalance of yin and yang while also preventing the destruction of essence, blood and body fluids.

Zheng qi circulating in the organs, channels and collaterals is made up of organ-qi and channel-qi which drives and adjusts the functions of the organs and channels and collaterals to ensure their normal performance. This continuous flow promotes and regulates metabolism as well as the circulation and distribution of essence, blood, and fluids within the body. Smooth-flowing qi prevents stagnation[①] and thus the formation of phlegm and fluid-retention, blood stasis, and stones while also preventing the development of internal wind, internal cold, internal dampness, internal dryness, and internal fire.

If the body contracts a yang-pathogen, it is likely to give rise to a pattern of excess-heat. If the body contracts a yin-pathogen, it is apt to lead to an excess-cold or a cold-dampness pattern. If a patient is affected by a smaller quantity of pathogens or if the *zheng* qi is quite strong, the location of the condition will be more superficial and the condition will be relatively mild and of short duration. When a patient is affected by a larger quantity of pathogens or if the *zheng* qi is weak, the condition will affect deeper levels of the body and the condition will be more severe and chronic. Some conditions disturb the sinews, bones or channels, and others may intrude upon the organs; due

---

① (*yù zhì*, 郁滞) stagnation

to different disease locations, the presenting patterns will also vary.

Although we say that pathogens cannot attack where *zheng* qi is strong, there are notable exceptions. When the toxicity and strength of pathogenic qi is very strong, even the strongest *zheng* qi cannot resist it. Many kinds of epidemics, high or cold temperatures, car crashes, electrical current, gunshot wounds or insect and animal bites cannot be avoided even by the healthiest of people. However, the strength of the *zheng* qi influences how well the person will recover from such an attack.

We then see that there are several possible outcomes to the struggle between *zheng* qi and *xie* qi. An ample supply of *zheng* qi can drive pathogen out of the body, leaving the body uninjured with no appearance of clinical symptoms and signs. We see this in people who can easily bounce back from any number of conditions. (The quick response to disease in children is also a sign of strong *zheng* qi.) However, when the *zheng* qi is weak, pathogens can invade and enter deeply into the body, causing major imbalances of yin and yang and qi and blood. From this imbalance, there will be the appearance of clinical symptoms and signs. Older or weaker individuals in some cases may contract a disease from which they never seem to recover completely, and of course there are some conditions which can have devastating long-term effects no matter what the state of the *zheng* qi. One can also think of the number of pathogens that a person fights and conquers each day, but because the pathogens are so weak or because *zheng* qi is so strong, a person never even notices. Others with less abundant *zheng* qi may quickly fall ill to even the mildest of pathogens.

The nature of the pathogenic evils will cause different disease characteristics depending on the type of pathogen. For example, when confronted by sufficient *zheng* qi, conditions caused by external pathogenic factors are often quick to attack and have a shorter duration. However, the conditions caused by emotional factors are usually slower in their onset and their duration is more chronic. Some emotional conditions can attack the internal organs directly, quite often the heart, followed by other organs. This leads to disharmonies of qi and blood along with complex disturbances in the qi movement of the organs. As another example, problems caused by an improper diet often first damage the spleen and stomach and from there affect other *zang-fu* organs which leads to deficiencies of qi and blood. However, some emotions such as fright can have a sudden and lifelong effect on the spirit, *zang-fu* organs and other systems.

The qualities and quantities of invading pathogenic qi determine the severity and quality of the condition. Obviously, a patient who is invaded by a smaller quantity of pathogenic qi presents with milder clinical symptoms than one invaded by a larger quantity. The nature or qualities of the pathogen will also create different effects. For example, wind-pathogens are light and rising in nature. Wind attacks the yang aspects of the body (the upper back, neck and head) thus affecting the lung and *wei*/defensive qi. Pathogenic dampness tends to block qi movement, and often attacks the spleen.

The effects of epidemic qi can be dramatic at the onset and then transmit quickly throughout the body. Epidemic pathogens only remain in the superficial parts of the body for a short time, then move interiorly to attack the internal organs.

PATTERNS OF EXCESS AND DEFICIENCY

The struggle between *zheng* qi and *xie* qi influences the growth or decline of *zheng* and *xie* qi, the result typically being a pattern of either excess or deficiency. However, because many conditions involve more complex patterns, it is important to fully understand the full meaning of the terms involved.[1]

Excess[2]

An excess pattern involves an "exuberance"[3] of pathogenic qi. Often the pathogenic qi is strong but the *zheng* qi is also strong enough to resist it. This creates a strong or even violent conflict between *zheng* and *xie* qi in which there may appear an obvious series of acute signs and symptoms. This is called an excess pattern.

An excess pattern appears more commonly in the early and middle stages of a condition. Clinically, patients with strong constitutions and strong physical functions often present with excess patterns. An externally-contracted excess pattern displays symptoms such as a high fever, anger, a loud voice with rough breathing, abdominal pain aggravated by pressure, obstructed urination and defecation, strong pulse characteristics, and a thick greasy coating on the tongue. Excess patterns in internal damage conditions include abundant phlegm, food accumulation, qi stagnation, and blood stasis.

Deficiency[4]

Deficiency implies a deficiency of *zheng* qi[5]. A deficiency pattern appears more commonly in a person with a shortage of essence, qi, and/or essential substances. The pathogenic evil may have declined, or pathogens are barely present within. Therefore, there is no intense struggle between the *zheng* qi and a pathogen, nor the pathological reaction as seen in an excess pattern. Clinically, this results in characteristic signs and symptoms of weakness, decline and shortage, and is therefore called a deficiency pattern.

---

[1] In Chinese language, *shí* and *xū* are a commonly paired dichotomy. One image of *shí* is that of a bag filled to capacity.

[2] (*shí*, 实) full, substantial, real, replete

[3] (*qì shèng*, 气盛) qi overbearing, forceful qi

[4] (*xū*, 虚) deficiency, vacuous, empty

[5] (*zhèng qì bù zú*, 正气不足) *zheng* qi deficiency – lit. upright qi not enough

A deficiency pattern may occur as a result of an excess pattern. For example, after a condition of excess-heat, the body fluids and blood may be consumed, creating deficiencies in the advanced stage of disease or in a chronic condition. The result can involve deficiencies of *zheng* qi, blood, yin qi, yang qi, or fluids. Deficiency patterns can present with numerous symptoms typically including fatigue, a pale complexion, shortness of breath, spontaneous sweating, dryness, night sweating, fear of cold with cold limbs, and a weak deficient pulse.

Changes of Deficiency and Excess

Mixed deficiency and excess

This is a pathological state in which there is deficiency of *zheng* qi concurrent with an excess of *xie* qi. This can be a deficiency pattern complicated by excess or an excess pattern complicated by deficiency. Deficiency complicated by excess is when the primary condition involves a deficiency of *zheng* qi which is worsened by the presence of *xie* qi. Excess complicated by deficiency is when the major pathological change involves an exuberance of *xie* qi which is complicated by a deficiency of *zheng* qi, such as when high fever consumes yin qi and body fluids.

Examples of deficiency complicated by excess would include patterns of qi deficiency with blood stasis, or qi deficiency with phlegm stagnation. In the first case, qi is not able to move the blood, which then creates static blood (blood stasis and other pathological products are considered "excesses"). In the second example, *zheng* qi (in this case, primarily created by the spleen) is not strong enough to fully dispel or transform pathological products such as phlegm, water-dampness and retained fluids.

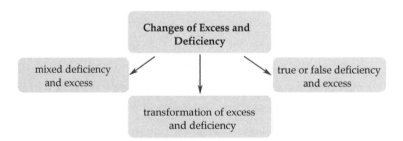

A case of mixed deficiency and excess might include exuberant *xie* qi which damages *zheng* qi, or an improperly treated condition that allows the *xie* qi to remain within the body for a long time which also results in damage to the *zheng* qi. A person with a weak constitution who is invaded by *xie* qi may not have enough *zheng* qi to resist or expel pathogens. Any of these factors can lead to co-existing deficiency and excess involving a deficiency of *zheng* qi with an excess of *xie* qi.

Formulas and Strategies, in a discussion on the formula *Zhū Shā Ān Shén Wán*

(Cinnabar Pill to Calm the Spirit, 朱砂安神丸) as used for insomnia and mental agitation: "this is vigorous heart-fire injuring the blood and yin. The scorching heart-fire depletes the blood and yin, which in turn deprives the heart of nourishment. The combination of heat and deficiency disturbs the serenity of the spirit, which manifests as insomnia and continuous palpitations."[1]

Transformation between deficiency and excess

Transformation between deficiency and excess refers to changes in the pathomechanism involving *xie* qi damaging *zheng* qi, or an accumulation of *xie* qi due to deficiency of *zheng* qi during the progression of a condition. This includes excess resulting from deficiency, and transformation from excess into deficiency. These changes are an extension of a mixed deficiency and excess pattern with the added factor of time where the yin and yang transformation becomes complete. Usually the progression is from excess to deficiency, although deficiency can create excesses for a limited time in that the end result of most chronic diseases will be a deficiency condition.

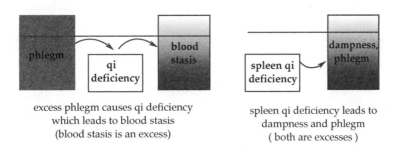

excess phlegm causes qi deficiency which leads to blood stasis (blood stasis is an excess)

spleen qi deficiency leads to dampness and phlegm (both are excesses)

Examples of Transformation of Deficiency and Excess

True or false deficiency or excess

True or false deficiency or excess is a condition characterized by pseudo-phenomena that are inconsistent with the nature of the true pathomechanism. This condition can be either true excess with false deficiency, or true deficiency with false excess.

True excess with false deficiency means that the nature of the pathomechanism is excess but with clinically "false/pseudo" phenomena of deficiency. This usually occurs as exuberant *xie* qi stagnates and accumulates in the body to block the channels and collaterals where normal qi and blood flow is impaired. For example, when heat accumulates in the gastrointestinal tract, a pattern of "heat retention with water discharge" can manifest as diarrhea with watery foul-smelling stools. Another example is profuse menstruation or spotting or bleeding between periods caused by

---

① Volker Scheid, Dan Bensky, Andrew Ellis, Randal Barolet. *Formulas and Strategies*. 2nd ed. Seattle: Eastland Press; 2009. p. 475.

blood stasis. In this case, the static blood blocks the normal free flow of blood. In both cases, the symptoms involve excessive amounts of fluid discharge, yet the cause is that of accumulation or stagnation.

True deficiency with false excess means that although the true nature of the pathomechanism is deficiency, there is also a clinical pseudo-phenomena of an excess nature. This is because deficient *zheng* qi leads to a shortage of organ-qi and channel-qi that leads to a decline in their nourishing and promoting functions. For example, such a condition could manifest with abdominal distention due to spleen qi deficiency, or it may appear as constipation resulting from the inability of qi to promote bowel movement. The abdominal distention would point to a pattern of excess, yet the true cause is that of qi deficiency. (Such conditions often require "paradoxical treatments" as discussed in later chapters.)

Zheng Qi and *Xie* Qi, and Prognosis

In general, with a predominance of *zheng* qi and a decline of pathogenic qi, any condition tends to improve as the patient recovers. On the other hand, with a predominance of pathogens and a decline of *zheng* qi, the condition deteriorates and the prognosis becomes poor. If pathogenic qi and *zheng* qi are equal in strength and neither tends to yield, the condition will become protracted or chronic.

The most common outcome in many conditions is that *zheng* qi is predominant and grows while the *xie* qi declines, in this case the condition turns to improvement and recovery. However, if in the elimination of *xie* qi the *zheng* qi recovers too slowly, this may lead to another pathological state involving *zheng* qi deficiency.

If in the course of a condition, *xie* qi is predominant and the *zheng* qi is too deficient to resist the pathogen, the condition can deteriorate to a critical condition, or even cause death. Following the exhaustion of *zheng* qi, the pathogenic qi flourishes exclusively. This can create yin collapse and yang collapse and a separation between yin and yang, all of which are potentially fatal conditions.

As stated above, *xie* qi and *zheng* qi can also be at a stalemate where they are equal in strength and neither has a tendency to yield. When *zheng* qi is deficient and *xie* qi has not been completely eliminated, or if it remains in a deeper position where it can cause damage to the *zheng* qi, the likely result is a chronic condition.

Chapter 7

Constitutional Theory

Section 1   General Concepts of Constitutional Theory

Constitution reflects and determines the differences in functional states among individuals, their reactions to external pathogens, as well as the specifics in the ebb and flow of yin and yang. In general, a person with a yang-inclined constitution is likely to be affected by yang pathogenic factors such as wind, heat and summerheat while being more resistant to yin-cold pathogens. Conversely, a person with a yin-inclined constitution is likely to be more affected by yin-factors such as cold and dampness while being relatively more resistant to pathogenic heat. [1]

In our daily lives we may observe that some people are tall and rotund, some smaller and energetic, some with larger abdomens and some extremely thin. Some people are generally quite healthy and rarely ill, while others frequently fall ill. Psychologically, some people can be characterized as open-minded, while others as more narrow-minded. In Chinese medicine, such characteristics may be viewed as constitutional traits, many of which can have diagnostic significance. For example, some people cannot eat watermelon because it causes them diarrhea, and in Chinese medicine, such a reaction points to patterns of deficiency-cold affecting the spleen and stomach. Some people cannot eat garlic because it causes them mouth sores, and this may point to patterns of damp-heat.

The concept of constitutional types is not only limited to Chinese medicine:
- In ancient Greece, Hippocrates described four types of constitutions: sanguine, phlegmatic, choleric and melancholic.

---

[1]   It should be noted that constitutional types as outlined in this chapter are not necessarily limited to a congenital and therefore unchangeable condition. People can change their constitutional type by proper and improper lifestyle choices such as diet, substance abuse and emotions. In addition, accidents, environmental causes and illness can change a person's constitution. Constitution is therefore seen as the underlying condition of a person as they present in a specific time with considerations to their history.

- Western medicine recognizes several different body types referred to as endomorphic, mesomorphic and ectomorphic.
- In India, Aryuvedic medicine uses constitutional types (*dosha*) referred to as *Vata, Pitta* and *Kapha*.
- Traditional medical systems in both Japan and the Republic of Korea have been deeply influenced by Chinese medicine. In the traditional medicine of the Republic of Korea, constitutional types are divided into *taiyang, taiyin, shaoyang* and *shaoyin* types.
- In some forms of traditional Japanese medicine, the individual constitution is classified into organ-toxic, detoxifying and blood static types.

The term, (*tǐ zhì*, 体质) or "constitution" was first recorded by Zhang Jie-bin in 1624 in the *Complete Works of* [*Zhang*] *Jing-yue* (*Jǐng Yuè Quán Shū*, 景岳全书). Although this is fairly recent in terms of Chinese medicine history, the idea of constitutional types that express the characteristics of an individual has a long history in Chinese medicine.

As early as 2500 years ago, *The Yellow Emperor's Inner Classic* stated, "understand the interior by observing the exterior", and "know the interior by examining the exterior". The classification of constitutional types also included five-phase constitutional types (wood, fire, earth, metal and water), as well as five yin-yang constitutions (*taiyin, shaoyin, taiyang, shaoyang* and balanced yin-yang). Also, in each type of person there are five possible kinds of mental disposition, thus creating a total of 25 psychological types. Another section divided the constitution according to physical features, and yet another section further recognizes overweight, greasy, and fleshy types. Other classifications were made according to skin color, courage, physical state, physical characteristics of the organs, and the emotional state.

Terms for Constitution in Different Dynasties

Classics	Author	Term	Dynasty
The Yellow Emperor's Inner Classic	Unknown	形 (*xíng*, form or shape), 质 (*zhì*, quality), 素 (*sù*, inheritance), and 态 (*tài*, state, form)	200 BCE
Treatise on Cold Damage and Miscellaneous Diseases	Zhang Zhong-jing	家 (*jiā*, lit: home or family)	Han Dynasty (AD 200)
Important Formulas Worth a Thousand Gold Pieces	Sun Si-miao	禀质 (*bǐng zhì*, intrinsic quality)	Sui and Tang Dynasties (AD 500)
The Complete Compendium of Fine Formulas for Women	Chen Zi-ming	气质 (*qì zhì*, intrinsic temperament)	Southern Song Dynasty (AD 1200)
General Essence of Formulas for Children's Health	Unknown	赋禀 (*fù bǐng*, inheritance)	Southern Song Dynasty (AD 1200)
Key Link of Medicine	Zhao Xian-ke	气禀 (*qì bǐng*, intrinsic temperament)	Ming Dynasty (AD 1600)
The Complete Works of [*Zhang*] *Jing-yue*	Zhang Jie-bin	禀赋 (*bǐng fù*, endowment) 气质 (temperament)	Ming Dynasty (AD 1600)

The concept of constitution in Chinese medicine has two basic characteristics. First, it emphasizes the impact of both prenatal endowment and postnatal care on the formation of the constitution, as prenatal factors determine the relative stability and other specificities of the individual constitution. The postnatal environment will affect the development of the prenatal constitution in both strength and in type.

Second, the body has corresponding physiological functions and psychological characteristics associated with the formation and development of the human constitution as conditioned by natural and social environments. Even in relatively affluent times, living under the pressures of modern life cannot help but influence the physical and psychological makeup of the individual and even groups of individuals. Individual adaptability to these social and natural environments is often determined to some degree by the constitution. However, through cultivation of the acquired constitution, the body can more fully actualize its innate prenatal potential and thus better adapt to the environment.

PHYSICAL STRUCTURE

The differences in human physical structure are an important component of constitutional characteristics, including both the external and internal structures. The external structure is directly shown on the body surface, directly observed as the physique and complexion. The internal structure mainly refers to the organs, channels and collaterals, essence, qi, blood and fluids. External structure is an external presentation of the constitution, while the internal physical structure is the inherent basis of the constitution.

Somatotype refers to the size and proportion of various parts of the body. In Chinese medicine, the main somatotypes involve height, weight, distribution of muscle and fat, and the complexion of the skin. For example, the *Spiritual Pivot* includes the characteristics of obese and thin persons, with the obese constitution again divided according to greasy, fat and fleshy types.

In *Further Discourses on the Acquisition of Knowledge through Profound Study* (*Gé Zhì Yú Lùn*, 格致余论), Yuan Dynasty physician Zhu Dan-xi further linked somatotype with pathogenesis with the well-known point of view that "obese people are characterized by internal dampness, while thin people tend to have internal fire".

PHYSIOLOGICAL FUNCTION

Physical structure is the basis to generate physiological function. The different characteristics of individual physical structures determine the difference in physiological function of the body and its reaction to stimuli. The personal trait in physiological function affects its physiological structure, causing a series of corresponding changes. Therefore, the difference in physiological function is also a component of the individual constitutional characteristic.

The body's physiological function depends on the internal physiological structure, and it is also the presentation of functions of the organs, channels and collaterals, essence, qi, blood and fluids. Therefore, the body's ability to prevent and resist disease, metabolic conditions, self-regulation, as well as the basic state being predisposed to excitement or inhibition, are all the physiological presentations of the organs, channels and collaterals, essence, qi, blood and fluids. And all these can be represented by the heart rate, cardiac rhythm, complexion, lip color, pulse condition, tongue manifestation, respiratory condition, voice, appetite, taste of mouth, body temperature, preference for or aversion to cold or heat, urine and feces, sexual function, reproductive function, female menstruation, bodily movement and activity, sleep, vision, audition, olfaction, pain tolerance, flexibility of skin and muscle, and the amount and luster of the hair.

PSYCHOLOGY

Psychology belongs within the scope of "spirit" in Chinese medicine. The functional activities of different organs are always expressed as specific emotional reactions and cognitive activities. For example, *Basic Questions* states that "a person has the five *zang*-organs to generate five kinds of qi and thus bring on joy, anger, sorrow, grief and fear." The essence-qi of organs and organ functions vary in each person, so the emotional activities of each individual are also different. For example, some people are predisposed to anger, some to sorrow, and some to timidity. Human psychological characteristics are related not only to shape and function, but also with the individual's life experience and social environment. Therefore, two people with the same physical structure may display unique psychological characteristics.

Section 2   Classifications of Constitutional Types

Constitutional classification divides people into several types based on individual characteristics. An overview of constitutional classification shows three basic methods of classification.

Yin-yang and five-phase theories are the philosophical foundations of constitutional theory. Each individual has a given tendency to yin or yang, and this leads an individual to tend towards a specific constitutional type; thus, the constitution can be seen as nothing more than two basic types as associated with yin and yang. Therefore, early medical experts first classified the constitution according to yin-yang theory, later considering the organs, channels and collaterals, and qi and blood. *The Yellow Emperor's Inner Classic* contains four and five yin-yang based categories of constitutional classification.

HARMONIZED YIN-YANG CONSTITUTION

The ideal constitution is the harmonized yin and yang-type constitution. *Basic Questions* states, "a person whose yin-yang are evenly balanced ... is of a healthy quality" and "only when yin is calm and yang is sound can the essence-spirit remain normal." However, the body's essence, qi, yin and yang are always in a dynamic state of growth and decline, so a normal constitution may also be in a yin- or yang-inclined state.

A harmonized yin-yang constitution manifests as an individual who is not easily attacked by external pathogens. Even so, when afflicted, such people will most often present with exterior- and/or excess-type patterns which can be easily cured, or a rapid recovery may occur without treatment. If such an individual has no traumatic injuries, chronic diseases or bad habits, he or she obviously has a better chance of living a long and healthy life.

YANG-INCLINED CONSTITUTION

A person with a yang-inclined constitution tends to be hyperactive, relatively hot, and constantly on the move; this type is generally extroverted with an aggressive personality and energetic movements, acute responses, and a strong libido. There may be a red complexion or oily skin, dry stools, dark urine, a preference for coolness with a general aversion to heat, a slightly higher body temperature, perspiration after slight exertion, frequent irritability, thirst, reddish lips, a red tongue with a thin yellow coating, and a rapid and slippery pulse.

This type is more susceptible to yang pathogens of wind, summerheat and heat. After a pathogenic attack, the person mostly presents with heat signs, excess patterns, and internally-produced dryness that damages yin. Patterns of exuberant fire or yang hyperactivity with yin deficiency often manifest with dizziness, headaches, palpitations, insomnia and bleeding. Because the yang qi of such a person is relatively hyperactive, yin is consumed so that over the long-term there will be a deficiency of yin. The depletion of yin is also bound to increase as a result of poor lifestyle habits. Typical presenting patterns include yang hyperactivity, yin deficiency, and phlegm-fire.

YIN-INCLINED CONSTITUTION

A yin-inclined person often presents with fatigue, a relatively cold body, a pale complexion, poor appetite and digestion, a general aversion to cold with preference for heat, a slightly low body temperature, a pale tongue and lips, and a slow or moderate pulse. There may be introversion, timidity, a lack of energy, slow movements and a reduced libido.

A person of this constitutional type is susceptible to invasion by yin-pathogens of cold and dampness. After a pathogenic attack, the person mostly presents with cold signs, deficiency patterns, or an exterior pattern that transmits into the interior creating internal dampness, edema and blood stasis.

Because this constitutional type is characterized by relatively underactive yang qi, the yang qi will weaken over time as organ function also declines. Typical presenting patterns include yang deficiency, phlegm-dampness and fluid retention.

NINE CONSTITUTIONAL CATEGORIES

After more than twenty years of research on both ancient and modern constitutional classifications, contemporary physician Wang Qi put forth an expanded version of constitutional classification, currently adopted by the Chinese Medical Association. Nine basic constitutional types are described below.

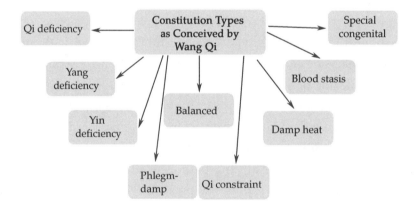

Balanced Constitution

A person with a balanced constitution is generally happy and of good health due to a harmony yin and yang with well-balanced qi and blood. Typically they are of moderate build with a good complexion and abundant energy. There is a moist and lustrous complexion, full hair with luster, bright sparkling eyes, an acute sense of smell, high energy levels, a tolerance to cold and heat, good sleep, appetite, defecation and urination, a light red tongue with a thin white coating, and a forceful moderate pulse. Psychologically, this type is easygoing with a cheerful personality, and they easily adapt to stimulation from the external environment.

Qi Deficiency-type

A person with a qi deficiency-type constitution often presents with *yuan* qi deficiency manifesting with tiredness, shortness of breath, weak muscles and spontaneous sweating. There may be a weak voice, shortness of breath, reluctance to talk, dispiritedness, excessive perspiration, a light red tongue with teeth marks on the edges, and a weak pulse. Psychologically, this type is typically introverted and not adventurous. There is greater susceptibility to diseases such as the common cold as well as a tendency to organ prolapse. This type is slow to recover from illness, and is intolerant of pathogenic wind, cold, summerheat and dampness.

Yang Deficiency-type

The yang deficiency-type often presents with a fear of cold, cold hands and feet and weak muscles, and is susceptible to pathogenic wind, cold and dampness. They may have a general fear of cold, cool hands and feet, preferences for hot food, dispiritedness, a pale tender tongue and a slow deep pulse. The general personality is sedate and introverted. There is greater susceptibility to phlegm-fluid retention, edema and diarrhea, and they are more susceptible to cold transformation following a pathogenic invasion. The person tends to feel better in the summer and worse in the winter.

Yin Deficiency-type

A person with a yin deficiency-type constitution often presents with signs of deficiency-heat such as a dry mouth and throat and feverish feelings in the palms and soles. The person is typically thin. There may be a dry nose, a preference for cold drink, dry stools, a red tongue with little moisture, and a thready rapid pulse. Psychologically, they may be dynamic and extroverted but with anxiety, insomnia, and even loss of essence. Following pathogenic invasion, the condition typically transforms into a pattern of internal heat. The person tends to well-tolerate cold and winter, but not dryness and summer weather.

Phlegm-dampness-type

The phlegm dampness-type individual often presents with an obese build with a fat abdomen, a sticky feeling in the mouth, and a greasy tongue coating. There may be oily facial skin, profuse and sticky perspiration, chest oppression, abundant sputum, a sweet taste in the mouth, preference for fatty or sweet foods, a greasy tongue coating, and a slippery pulse. They may have a stable and patient disposition. The person is more susceptible to diseases such as *xiāo kě* (wasting-thirsting, 消渴) or diabetes, stroke, and chest pain. There is poor adaptation to rainy and damp environments.

Damp-heat-type

The damp-heat constitution is characterized by internal retention of damp-heat manifesting with a dirty oily complexion, a bitter taste in the mouth, and a greasy yellow tongue coating. They have a medium or slightly heavy build. There may be acne, heavy sensations of the body, sleepiness, sticky or dry stools, scanty yellowish urine, a damp scrotum in men, leukorrhagia in women, a reddish tongue with a yellow greasy coating, and a rapid slippery pulse. Psychologically, this type tends to be temperamental and often upset. They are predisposed to sores, boils and jaundice. The damp-heat type finds it difficult to adapt to damp weather or high temperatures.

Blood Stasis-type

The blood stasis-type can have either a fat or thin physique, typically with a dark complexion and a dusky purplish tongue. There may be visible pigmentation or petechiae in the skin, dusky lips, a dark tongue with purplish or enlarged sublingual veins, and a choppy pulse. This type is irritable, forgetful, and often intolerant of cold. Internal masses and pain syndromes are most common.

Qi Constraint-type

Persons with constraint and stagnation of the qi mechanism often present with psychological depression, emotional vulnerability or anxiety. This type might have a thin physique, a normal light red tongue with a thin white coating, and a wiry pulse. They may be introverted with an unstable disposition, often sensitive and suspicious, and with excess mental stimulation they may become overwhelmed. They are predisposed to patterns of constraint or depression leading to organ agitation (*zàng zào*, 脏躁), plum-pit qi (the feeling of a foreign object in the throat), or lily disease (*bǎi hé bìng*, 百合病) (a specific type of mental disturbance). There is also a general intolerance to rainy weather.

Special Congenital-type

The congenital-type constitution refers to two types of inherited conditions, the first being allergies, rheumatic arthritis, diabetes, and other issues associated with inheritance. The second involves congenital disabilities, birth defects, deformities, and mental or physical retardation. Often times, people with these problems have trouble adapting to the external environment and thus may have special needs throughout their lifetimes. Special care is required to preserve the essence as much as possible.

Section 3 Applications of Constitutional Theory

Under normal conditions, within the human body there is an ebb and flow of yin and yang, qi, blood, and fluids. The constitution can be seen as the root (primary aspect), and the disease manifestations as the branch (secondary aspect). A pattern is an analysis and generalization associated with a certain stage of a disease or a certain type of pathology, where the constitution reflects an individual specificity as the basis for disease. The inherent constitution of the patient has a decisive role in the type of presenting pattern, especially in chronic disease. At this point, the name of the pattern and the name of the constitutional type may coincide, which indicates a close relationship between the individual constitution and the presenting clinical pattern.

INDIVIDUAL SUSCEPTIBILITY TO DISEASE

Constitutional factors often determine the manifestations and severity of illness at the onset. In general, children often suffer from cough, asthma, diarrhea, and food accumulation. Elderly people often show deficiencies of organ-qi, essence-qi, and a declining constitution, are thus more susceptible to conditions involving internal phlegm, fluid-retention, cough, asthma, dizziness, palpitations and diabetic symptoms. An obese person with excess phlegm-dampness is more susceptible to dizziness and stroke; a person with yin deficiency often presents with a dry cough; a person with constitutional yang deficiency and yin excess often presents with liver constraint and qi stagnation; and a person with qi stagnation is susceptible to emotional illnesses involving constraint, plum-pit qi, or organ agitation.

Genetics is also closely related with the individual constitution, most often associated with allergies and susceptibility to specific diseases. Those individuals with such a genetic background must be especially careful to nurture their postnatal qi.

PATHOGENESIS AND ONSET OF DISEASE

The strength of the individual constitution determines the onset of disease and how it manifests. Whether a disease occurs or not depends upon the strength of the *zheng*/upright qi in the body, with the constitution also being the basis of *zheng* qi. In general, a person with a strong constitution has a vigorous *zheng* qi and a powerful resistance to disease. This type is seldom invaded by pathogens and rarely becomes ill, whereas in a person with a weak constitution and weak *zheng* qi, pathogens will take advantage of the insufficient resistance and cause disease. However, due to the struggle between *zheng* qi and the internal pathogen, when a healthy patient does fall ill, the symptoms may actually be more severe than those of an afflicted patient with deficiency; often there will be excess signs and symptoms associated with heat and phlegm. However, when the *zheng* qi is strong, such heightened contention is often of short duration. On the other hand, although a deficient person may suffer fewer acute symptoms, the internal pathogens may produce deeper and more chronic conditions.

The onset of disease is closely related with the constitution in both exteriorly-contracted conditions and internal diseases. The *Golden Mirror of the Medical Tradition* (*Yī Zōng Jīn Jiàn*, 医宗金鉴) states, "All diseases caused by the nine kinds of qi (anger, joy, sorrow, fear, cold, heat, fright, strain and thinking) cannot appear in a person with a strong physique because the invading pathogenic qi is promptly removed; they can only appear in a person with a weak physique because the invading pathogenic qi is able to remain within." This indicates that the onset of disease is closely associated with both emotions and the physical constitution.

Occurrence of a disease is determined by the results of struggle between *zheng*/upright and pathogenic qi. Besides it is also affected by several other factors like the environment (including climatic, geographical factors and social factors), diet, nutrition, genetics, age, gender, emotions, work and rest, etc., all of which can induce diseases by influencing the state of human constitution to reduce the body's adjustability and adaptability.

UNDERSTANDING PATHOLOGICAL CHANGE

A Stick to Awaken Physicians (*Yī Mén Bàng Hè*, 医门棒喝) states, "The yin and yang of a pathogen changes according to the yin and yang of the human body." That is to say, the six pathogenic qi, because of their different yin and yang attributes, can cause diseases with qualities that vary, depending upon the yin and yang state of the body that they have invaded. A person with a harmonized constitution will contract a cold disease when invaded by a cold pathogen, and a dampness disease when invaded by a dampness pathogen. However, the same wind-cold pathogen invades a person with a yang-inclined constitution, it tends to transform into heat, and when invading a person with a yin-inclined constitution, it tends to transform into cold. Because of the different natural tendencies of yin or yang and relative strength of the organs, the pathogens of cold, heat, dampness and dryness will transform differently after invading the body. With constitutional yin deficiency and yang hyperactivity, there is commonly a transformation to heat after the pathogenic invasion. With constitutional yang deficiency with yin excess, there is commonly a transformation to cold when invaded. With constitutional blood deficiency, there is commonly a transformation to dryness when invaded by pathogens. With constitutional qi deficiency with damp-excess, there is commonly a transformation to dampness.

So the individual constitution has a definite role in how a disease will transform and transmit once a person becomes ill. A person with a strong constitution has sufficient *zheng* qi to fight against pathogens, and if disease does occur, the person can recover quickly as the signs and symptoms primarily reflect an excess pattern caused by the intense struggle between the *zheng* qi and the internal pathogens. The person may have acute symptoms, but they usually do not transform further. When a person with a weak constitution is affected, the same pathogens are able to move more deeply into the body, and the condition becomes more serious. In late-stage disease, although the strength of pathogen has declined, the weaker patient will have a difficult recovery because the *zheng* qi remains deficient.

Secondly, the transformation of pathogens also influences the transmission and direction of a disease. For example, with constitutional yin deficiency with yang hyperactivity, there is commonly a transformation to heat after invasion, which can be either excess-type heat or deficiency-type heat. With a constitutional yang deficiency and yin excess, the disease commonly transforms into patterns of excess-type cold or deficiency-type cold.

GUIDING PATTERN DIFFERENTIATION

The constitution forms a basis for pattern differentiation as well as influencing the manifestations of disease, and thus the same pathogenic factor can lead to different types of patterns (yin, yang, exterior, interior, cold, heat, deficiency, and excess types). For example, although attacked by a cold pathogen, a person with strong *zheng* qi which can resist the pathogen at the body surface will only develop an exterior wind-cold pattern, which is less severe. However, a person with constitutional yang deficiency who contracts a cold pathogen could soon after display signs of spleen yang deficiency. A person with a constitutional yang-heat will obviously show signs of heat when invaded by a heat pathogen. But when affected by wind-cold, the same person may again show signs of internal heat as the constrained cold transforms to internal heat.

TREATMENT METHODS AND CONSTITUTIONAL TRAITS

Treatment according to pattern differentiation is the basic principle of therapeutics in Chinese medicine. There is a clinical phenomenon that for a certain kind of disease, one specific method is effective for one patient, but for others the same method may be not only ineffective, but also harmful. This is in part due to the individual constitution. As examples, a person with constitutional yang deficiency will have a tendency to cold and dampness, and should be treated in accordance with that tendency.

A person with constitutional yin deficiency is predisposed to a "stirring of internal fire". After being invaded by a cold-dampness yin-pathogen, the pattern can transform into a yang pattern which consumes yin.

In a person with a yang-inclined constitution afflicted with an excess heat pattern, medicinal herbs with warm or hot properties are likely to damage yin.

In a person with a yin-inclined constitution with an excess cold pattern, herbs with cold or cool properties should be used with caution as they may cause damage to yang.

Acupuncture treatments are also performed in accordance with the patient's constitution. For those with a strong constitution, the drainage method is usually employed, whereas supplementation methods are generally used for those predisposed to deficiency due to a weak constitution. Older patients can become extremely fatigued from a twenty minute acupuncture treatment and blood-moving herbs may aggravate their pain. The elderly therefore often respond better to shorter acupuncture treatments and herbs that build blood and qi.

People with different constitutions also respond differently to herbal therapy.

- Generally speaking, those with yang-inclined constitutions respond well to herbs with sweet-cold, sour-cold, salty-cold and clear-moist properties, but not to those with acrid-hot, warm-dispersing, bitter-cold and descending-sinking properties.
- A person with a strong constitution can generally tolerate higher dosages, whereas a patient with a weak constitution may poorly tolerate even low dosages of herbs with moderate medicinal actions.
- Those with yin-inclined constitutions respond well to herbs that warm and supplement, but not as well to herbs that drain fire with bitter-coldness.
- Those with constitutional qi deficiency respond well to herbs that supplement qi, but not as well to herbs that disperse and drain.
- Those with harmonized yin and yang constitutions should be given moderate treatment without dramatic changes in the treatment principles.
- Those with constitutional phlegm-dampness respond well to aromatic dampness-eliminating herbs and those that strengthen the spleen, but not as well to herbs that are cold-cool or moist.
- Those with constitutional damp-heat can tolerate heat-clearing and dampness-draining herbs, but may be intolerant to herbs with enriching and nourishing functions.

- Those with constitutional blood stasis respond well to herbs that promote qi and blood flow, but not as well to consolidating and astringing herbs, which should be applied with caution.

AFTERCARE AND CONSTITUTIONAL TRAITS

When a person has just recovered from illness or is in the convalescent stage, it is very important to promote his/her health rehabilitation. The recuperating measures may include medications, diet, emotions and living habits. For the complete application of all these measures, the traits of the patient's constitution needs to be considered. For example, when a patient with a yang-inclined constitution has just recuperated from an illness, the warm-heat or hot-spicy food such as mutton, and longan fruit should be given with great caution. While a patient with a yin-inclined constitution has just recuperated from a serious, the moist and cloying medicinals like *guī jǎ* (Testudinis Plastrum, 龟甲), *biē jiǎ* (Trionycis Carapax, 鳖甲) and *shú dì* (Rehmanniae Radix Praeparata, 熟地); as well as the sour and astringent medicinals such as *wǔ wèi zǐ* (Schisandrae Chinensis Fructus, 五味子) and *wū méi* (Mume Fructus, 乌梅) should be cautiously taken.

HEALTH PRESERVATION

Health preservation in Chinese medicine considers all the basic factors involved in living a healthy lifestyle; these include the daily diet, regular moderate exercise, balanced periods of work and rest, practices that cultivate the spirit in harmony with the seasons, etc. When a person is in convalescence, it is very important to promote his or her recovery through consideration of constitutional factors along with various lifestyle factors.

For example, in dietary therapy, a person with a yang-inclined constitution should eat cooler foods and avoid hot foods, while a person with a yin-inclined constitution should eat warm foods and avoid cold foods. A person with an obese build and constitutional phlegm-dampness should eat light bland foods and avoid fatty and sweet foods.

A person with constitutional yin deficiency should eat sweet moist foods in order to generate fluids while avoiding fatty, spicy or dry foods. A person with constitutional yang deficiency should eat warming and supplementing foods.

In cultivating the spirit, various methods can be taken in accordance with the constitution so as to maintain psychological balance and enhance mental health.

For example, a person with constitutional qi constraint often has mental depression, introversion, melancholy, anger and frustration. In such cases, once patterns of liver constraint and qi stagnation are resolved, many physical and emotional complaints often disappear. A yang deficiency-type is typically dispirited with an apathetic look, low self-esteem, and a lack of courage; this type of person may also require psychological and/or spiritual counseling.

CASES

Review the following cases with your instructor:

1. Your patient is a 27-year-old woman with back pain in her upper thoracic spine. She was born with scoliosis of the back, and wore a back brace from ages eight to seventeen. She has pain that runs from her shoulder to the ends of her fingers on both arms. She says that she is always angry unless she smokes marijuana to relieve the pain. Her pulse is wiry and the tongue red. She often lashes out at her friends and worries constantly about the future.

2. Your patient is an 18-year-old man who had run in a marathon. In the last hours of the race, it started to rain gently, and the next day he felt very tired as if he had caught a cold. He took several over-the-counter medicines and ate a "healthy raw food diet" for a week after the race. In addition, he continued to train for a few hours a day. Six months later, he developed a stomach pain and pains in the legs. He often felt nauseous and was tired. He attributed the leg pain to the fact he hadn't had enough energy to train more. He continued on a raw food diet and often felt stomach pains a few hours after each meal. He had three bowel movements a day. His tongue is pale with teeth marks on the edges, and his pulse is slow and slippery.

3. Your patient is a 55-year-old man of robust build. His chief complaint is nervousness and "paranoia" with a fear of authority figures whom he feels are video taping every aspect of his life. He has an insatiable appetite and eats often through the day. He was an "intellectual worker" as an artist and journalist for most of his working life. Yet 6 years ago he witnessed a major earthquake. He himself was not hurt but is haunted by traumatic images of what he saw. For exercise everyday he does 20 minutes "free style" dancing which he says relieves tension. His tongue is covered with a greasy yellow coating and his pulse is slippery.

4. Your patient is a 36-year-old man who has difficulty sleeping. He had been addicted to heroin and methamphetamines for several years, but stopped over ten years ago. He is now a yoga instructor who works out for several hours each day in addition to teaching yoga classes for six hours. Since childhood he has felt agitated, and for the last five years has a hard time falling asleep, often waking up during the night. He has constipation some days and loose stools on other days. He often has heart palpitations. His face is pale and his tongue is red, dry, and pointed at the tip. His pulse is thready and deep.

Chapter 8

Prevention, Principles and Methods of Treatment

Section 1   Prevention of Disease

PREVENTING DISEASES FROM OCCURRENCE

The concept of preventing disease by "treating the un-diseased" was raised very early in the history of Chinese medicine. For healthy people, the aim of prevention is to maintain the body's normal constitution whereas for patients who already ill, the aim is to prevent progression of the disease by transformation and transmission, and to then eventually effect a complete remission.

The invasion of *xie*/pathogenic qi is a major cause of disease. In the course of a disease, depending on the relative strengths of the *zheng*/upright qi and the *xie* qi, the development of the disease may transmit from the shallow to the deeper, from mild to severe, or from simple to complex. At the beginning of a disease, an effort should be made to diagnose and treat early so as to prevent a more complex condition. It is of primary importance then to prevent pathogens from passing more deeply into the body.

The broadest form of health preservation can be seen as preventative medicine that enhances the constitution and strengthens the *zheng* qi, because the onset of a disease is largely related to the relative strengths of *zheng* qi and *xie* qi. Therefore, the basic principle of preventative medicine is to increase *zheng* qi and thus prevent the contraction of pathogens. The goal is obviously to enhance the quality of life while also increasing longevity.

The best way to resist disease and maintain health is through lifestyle choices such as diet and exercise combined with regular acupuncture and other treatments and the taking of proper herbs even when healthy. The resulting increased immunity is especially helpful when there are colds, flu and other diseases present in the general population. Wind often combines with other pathogens, so it is often said that "external pathogens like wind should always be avoided". This means we should be especially vigilant toward pathogenic summerheat in the summer season, dryness in the autumn, and the cold in the winter.

Kidney-essence is of the utmost importance for maintaining life quality and longevity. Essence can transform into qi which then produces the spirit, and in turn the spirit acts to protect the qi of the body. Essence is therefore the material basis for the body, qi and spirit. We have no decision as to the prenatal qi that we have inherited, yet all of the processes in this chapter can be seen as guidelines that benefit the postnatal essence which "nourishes the prenatal". To preserve kidney-essence, one should maintain a healthy lifestyle with appropriate amounts of exercise, leisure time, sexual activity, friendship, music and art, meditation, massage, and nutritious foods combined with acupuncture, moxibustion and herbal medicine.

The Natural World

Human life is closely related to the variations in the natural world, thus a person benefits from living in harmony with nature and its rhythms. The Chinese medicine principle of following the laws of nature is expressed as "obeying the waning and waxing of yin and yang". This involves "promoting yang in the spring and summer, and nurturing yin in the autumn and winter". Concepts of the seasons are often expressed in terms of an agricultural agrarian culture in that springtime is for renewal and planting, summer is for continuing work, and autumn is the time to collect what has been cultivated. Winter is a time for rest and renewal, and would naturally involve more sleep and less work. Ideally, on a day to day basis this means rising with the sun and finishing work as the sun goes down. Although following the rhythms of nature may seem archaic, outmoded and/or difficult to follow in a modern society, they do in fact remain clinically relevant in terms of maintaining good health and avoiding disease.

Emotions

Chinese medicine highly regards the relationships between emotional activity and physical health. There are seven emotions that are considered natural yet also destructive: anger, sadness, over-joy, grief, fear, melancholy, and pensiveness. When these seven emotions become uncontrolled, they can injure the organs directly, impair normal qi movement, and also weaken the ability of *zheng* qi to ward off diseases.

These destructive emotions are created internally in conjunction with the external environment. We cannot always control whether we have a pleasing natural environment, a peaceful and just society or harmonious family surroundings, yet we do our best to react well to what is given and to what we have chosen. If not, extreme or prolonged mental stimulation and agitation may become pathological factors when they exceed the extent of our regulatory abilities. The capacity to absorb this stimulation is related to our temperament, constitution, background, experience and age. In addition, extreme events, both physical and emotional, may register within the body, and while not immediately recognized consciously at the time, may surface in physiological dysfunction years or even decades later. Acupuncture and herbs can help us cope with immediate tensions as well as gently releasing past "body memories", which can result in a return to health in many cases. The Chinese medical paradigm seems particularly suited to such a claim because of the way that emotions are related to the processes of qi.

Sexual Life

Chinese medicine holds that the kidney-essence can be preserved by "maintaining an appropriate sexual life". An appropriate sexual life is of course subject to any number of discussions, and may change according to age, or cultural or religious backgrounds. Yet, however defined for the individual, sexual behaviors are a normal aspect of a physical and mental health. Different people obviously have different psychological and physiological needs; that being said, Chinese medicine has always maintained that overindulgence in sex will consume kidney-essence and make one more susceptible to disease[1]. The appropriate amount of sexual activity is not constant throughout a lifetime, and it often transforms as a person ages. No less important (if less talked about) is how the repression of sexual needs and desires can cause a disordering and stagnation of qi which leads to its own set of psychological and physical problems.

Physical Body

Chinese medicine stresses the importance of the union between "an active body and a peaceful spirit". An active body refers to physical movement that strengthens the muscles, bones and tendons, promotes the circulation of qi and blood, and enhances the functioning of the organs. Moreover, an active body can contribute to peacefulness of the spirit that promotes both well-being and longevity. Traditional exercises like tai ji quan, qi gong, *yi jin jing* (muscle-bone strengthening exercise), *ba duan jin* (eight pieces of brocade), and martial arts are all beneficial in moderation; all physical exercise should be appropriately limited according to the physical capabilities of the individual. Physical exercises should begin gradually and continue with regularity, and any overstrain should be avoided.

Acupuncture, acupressure and moxibustion create stimulation at acupoints on the body through the channel and collateral system. Such therapies act to regulate the yin and yang and qi and blood of the body in order to regain a new and more well-balanced system.

---

① Senility is often mentioned as one of those diseases caused by "over-sexuality".

Tui na is a Chinese therapeutic method somewhat akin to a mixture of massage and chiropractic care. The practitioner manipulates regions on the body surface in order to regulate physiological processes and treat pathological conditions. Tui na can correct anatomical abnormalities while also optimizing the functions of the internal organs.

Diet

It goes without saying that one should eat and drink regularly and in proper amounts; unfortunately, many people eat quickly and often at irregular times. For some, this means eating while watching television, at work, in noisy fast food restaurants or even in a car while driving! Eating at irregular hours or late at night wreaks havoc with blood sugars and our energy levels. In Chinese medicine, poor eating habits harm the spleen qi. Most importantly, food should be eaten only until 75% full so that the stomach qi can effectively move and digest the food. Obviously, at the other end of the spectrum, not eating enough, either through starvation or extreme diets should be avoided. Food should be nutritious, grown locally and free from preservatives whenever possible, and the daily diet should contain balanced amounts of all five flavors (sweet, sour, bitter, pungent, salty). Preferences for any special kind of food or flavor should be avoided so as to prevent the overwhelming the associated organ. Eating a small amount of sweet foods after a meal can stimulate the spleen to assist digestion.

Eating while relaxed in a harmonious environment among friends and family is considered ideal, as well food prepared in one's own kitchen with fresh ingredients. Chinese texts often mention avoiding foods that are spoiled, and although modern refrigeration makes this less likely to occur, we still should generally avoid foods that are overly-processed or those shipped from great distances. One modern guideline in a supermarket is to "shop in the perimeter" where the fresh and perishable foods are located, while generally avoiding the canned and frozen food areas. For the modern Western consumer, a farmer's market is perhaps the closest many will come to grow their own food and certainly has many benefits.

Foods, just like medicinal herbs, also have cold, cool, warm and hot properties. Therefore, it is best to eat foods with properties that benefit the individual condition and/or physical constitution. For example, warm or hot foods should be avoided by people with heat-inclined constitutions, and those foods with cool or cold properties should be taken. Chinese medicine emphasizes, "The five grains nurture[1] the body, the five fruits assist,[2] the five food animals benefit,[3] and the five vegetables

---

① (yǎng, 养) raise, nourish

② (zhù, 助) assist

③ (yì, 益) benefit

supplement[①]. If the natures and flavors of foods are harmonized, the essence and qi of the body will be strengthened."

Yet, even with all these precautions, some people do fall ill from the food they eat. Sometimes food carries bacteria or viruses, so many people have allergic reactions to specific foods while others are intolerant to entire classes of foods. Gluten and soy, for example, can cause many types of unpredictable and devastating effects in some people, with relief only appearing after they remove them from the diet completely. However, those with ever-increasing multiple foods sensitivities are often seen as having organ deficiencies (usually spleen), and these individuals can often be treated successfully with Chinese medicine.

There is a long tradition of using foods themselves as therapy, and many Chinese herbs are everyday foods in the Asian diet, so using herbs is not always limited to times of illness. Many soups will contain herbs that correspond with the time of year; in fact, some restaurants will provide medicinal meals for their patrons. Although it may not be practical to visit such a restaurant, there are a number of written resources for identifying the best foods for our patients and ourselves[②]. In all cases, a proper balance of foods is required, thus the medicinal properties of certain foods should not be used to justify extreme or mono-food diets.

CONTROLLING THE DEVELOPMENT OF EXISTING DISEASE

At the beginning of a disease, an effort should be made to diagnose and treat it early so as to prevent its development, or transmission and/or transformation.

Early Diagnosis and Treatment

In the course of a disease, because of the *zheng*/upright qi and the *xie*/pathogen, the development of a disease may transmit from shallow to deeper, from mild to severe, or from simple to complex.

Generally speaking, in the early stage of a disease, the location is superficial and/or the condition is mild, and/or the *zheng*/upright qi is not seriously damaged. So diagnosis and treatment in the early stage contributes to the elimination of the pathogen and protection of the *zheng*/upright qi and the disease seldom transmits and is usually easy to recover from. On the contrary, if no timely diagnosis and treatments are given, the pathogen will go deeper progressively, and thus make the condition deteriorate and become complex, as the result, the cure of the disease will be more difficult.

---

① (*chōng*, 充) supplement
② Two such books are *Healing with Whole Foods: Oriental Traditions and Modern Nutrition* by Paul Pitchford and *The Tao of Nutrition* by Maoshing Ni and Cathy McNease.

The opportune moment of early diagnosis and treatment lies in grasping the rules of occurrence, development and change of a disease, so as to make accurate diagnosis at the very beginning of the onset, and then apply a timely and effective treatment.

For instance, for a patient with exogenous contraction of wind-cold syndrome, the pathogen invades the body surface through the skin and fine hair, which is clinically manifested as a floating pulse, headache with rigid neck and back, and aversion to cold. This is a stage of *taiyang* channel pattern; therefore the proper treatment should be to expel the exogenous pathogen by the dispersing method. If the treatment is delayed or mistaken, it may induce the pathogen to go into the interior, and then the pattern will turn into *yangming* channel characterized by high fever and extreme thirst with a desire for drinking fluids.

Stopping the Progression of Disease

Prevention of the disease from developing needs early diagnosis and treatment on the basis of grasping the law of onset and development, and the transmission pathways.

Blocking the pathway of transmission

The transmission of a disease has certain laws and pathways. For example, in terms of the six channels transmission in cold damage diseases (*shāng hán*, 伤寒), at the beginning, the location of the disease is usually in the *taiyang* channel. However if the disease progresses, it will transmit to the other channels. So the *taiyang* stage of cold damage is the key for early diagnosis and treatment. A warm disease (*wēn bìng*, 温病), often begins at the *wei* level pattern, so this stage is the key for early diagnosis and treatment of warm diseases. It thus can be seen that after invasion of pathogens into the body, an early diagnosis and treatment determined based on the progression law can block the pathway of transmission, and thus prevent the deterioration of the disease. Therefore a correct and effective therapy is the best measure to prevent a disease from developing.

REINFORCING THE UN-INVADED FIRST

To enhance the un-invaded first one may take the laws of generation, restriction, over-restriction and counter-restriction among the five phases, integration of the five *zang*-organs, and transmission among channels as guidance. For example, in visceral diseases, because of the different nature of the disease, there are such five-phase transmission types of involvement of a child by its mother disorder, involvement of a mother by its child disorder, over-restriction, and counter-restriction. So, according to the transmission law of different diseases, some preventive treatments are used to check pathological transmission. An idea in Chinese medicine is that, "For a liver disease one should know it can affect the spleen so that the spleen must be replenished in advance." That is, clinically at the same time of treating liver disease the remedies to regulate and strengthen the spleen and stomach are commonly taken so as to make the spleen qi strong enough to resist pathogens, therefore a better effect can be achieved. For a warm-heat disease, when the stomach yin is injured, further progression will affect the kidney yin. So according to the principles to enhance the un-invaded first, it is advised to add kidney yin-replenishing medicinals with salty-cold properties to an herbal formula for nourishing stomach yin, in order to prevent the consumption of kidney yin. These are examples of the application of "controlling the development of an existing disease".

Section 2   Therapeutic Principles & Methods of Treatment

Therapeutic principles and methods of treatment are closely related in that there are general therapeutic principles (treatment principles) or theories that direct the actual treatment methods. The therapeutic principles are more theoretical and broad in scope than the specific treatment methods. The treatment method follows the therapeutic principles, yet they are more concrete, specific and more flexible. With a clear sense of the general principles, the treatment method which follows can be both specific and creative. Because herbal medicine has such a long and rich written history, many of these principles are described by referring to an associated herbal formula name as an example. However, many of these principles are equally applied to acupuncture techniques as well.

A disease occupies a position somewhere between the *xie*/pathogenic qi and *zheng*/upright qi, depending on the relative strength of each; therefore, "reinforcing the upright and dispelling the pathogen" is the basic therapeutic principle for any disease. From a general therapeutic principle, one can employ one or several specific methods of treatment such as invigorating qi, nourishing blood, enriching yin, strengthening yang, etc.[①]

---

① There are 3 ways to look at treatment methods. There are "fundamental methods", "common methods", or "curative measures" and each treats diseases and patterns with a given treatment principle. The "fundamental methods" are broadly oriented to the pattern that has been diagnosed. For example, in a cold disease, the treatment method is to warm. The "common methods" are a specific treatment of a particular clinical pattern, such as to release the exterior or to fortify the spleen and drain dampness. Finally, "curative measures" are specific techniques and modalities such as herbs, acupuncture or moxibustion.

Treatment of the root is a primary concept in the treatment of any disease. Other general principles of treatment such as routine treatment and paradoxical treatment, treating branch and root, reinforcing *zheng* qi and dispelling pathogens, adjustment of yin-yang, regulation of essence-qi-blood-fluids, and treatment "in accordance with the three factors", for example, are all governed and guided by this fundamental concept.

THERAPEUTIC PRINCIPLES OF TREATMENT

Treating Root and Branch

To treat the root of a disease means that one must first differentiate the etiology and pathomechanism in order to discern the root of the disease. The etiology and pathomechanism include the causes, nature, and location of disease, the relationship between *zheng* qi and *xie* qi and the patient's constitution. Therefore, "to seek the root" is actually to determine the etiology and pathomechanism and the presenting pattern of disharmony. The application of pattern differentiation in order to discover and then treat the root is the ideal approach to clinical treatment.

Root (*běn*, 本) and branch (*biāo*, 标) describe two aspects of disease. The root and branch are relative to one another, so an understanding of their relationships is also important. The metaphor of a tree is used to demonstrate their relationship; the roots of the tree form a primary foundation, while the branches are a secondary phenomenon or manifestation. The designations of branch and root will also vary under certain conditions. For example, in terms of *xie* qi and *zheng* qi, the *zheng* qi is the root, while the *xie* qi (pathogen) is the branch. To compare pathomechanisms with signs and symptoms, the clinical manifestations are the branch, while the pathomechanism is the root. In the sequence of diseases, older or chronic conditions are the root, while newly-acquired diseases are the branch. In terms of location, disorders of the organs and essence-qi are the root, while disorders on the body surface are usually the branch.

As an example, in a heart disease patient with kidney yang deficiency who has been subsequently weakened by an attack of wind-cold, the original heart condition is the root, while the newly-contracted wind-cold is the branch. This is not to say that the branch can be ignored, especially in consideration of this patient's serious condition. Because branch manifestations may easily combine with the root condition (or with other branches), neglecting the branch may cause complications involving the root condition. During the course of complex diseases with chronic and acute aspects, different branch and root conditions can appear over time. Root and branch may also intermingle or at times even switch places during the course of disease.

Rules for treating root and branch

1) Treating the root in a chronic condition is often used for mild conditions or when the stage of a disease has no critical symptoms. Because the branch condition directly originates from the root cause, after the root cause is addressed, the branch condition will improve accordingly. For example, for a cough due to lung yin deficiency, yin deficiency of the lung (and kidney) is the root pattern and the cough is a branch manifestation. To treat the root in this case is to nourish the yin of the lung; once the root condition has been successfully treated, the coughing will be relieved. Another example is a case of spontaneous sweating due to qi deficiency; in this case the root pattern is qi deficiency while the sweating is the branch manifestation. Astringing the sweat will not be effective, because the branch is directly associated with the root; in this case one should treat the root by supplementing qi. With sufficient supplementation of qi, the manifestation of sweating will be controlled as well.

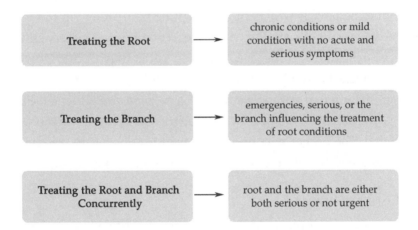

Treating the Root	→	chronic conditions or mild condition with no acute and serious symptoms
Treating the Branch	→	emergencies, serious, or the branch influencing the treatment of root conditions
Treating the Root and Branch Concurrently	→	root and the branch are either both serious or not urgent

2) Treating the branch is important when the condition is critical. If the branch symptom is urgent, and especially an emergency, obviously it should be treated first. For example, for an acute pain with a definite cause, it should be treated by stopping the pain first, and then by treating the root cause. As for a patient with ascites swelling in the abdomen due to liver disease, the liver-blood stasis is the root cause, and the ascites swelling is the branch. Thus, if the ascites is not serious, the disease should be treated by mainly resolving the root of blood stasis while promoting urination secondarily. However, if the ascites becomes serious, with abdomen distention and fullness and rapid breathing, the branch has emerged as an acute problem and the branch aspect of ascites needs to be treated first. After the ascites is relieved and the condition becomes stable, the liver disease can be treated. As another example, heavy bleeding may endanger a patient's life, so the treatment should be to stop the bleeding first regardless of the cause of bleeding. After the bleeding is stopped and the condition gets milder, the root cause can be treated.

In addition, in the relationship between branch and root, sometimes the branch condition of a disease is not urgent. However, if the branch is not treated, it will influence the treatment plan of the disease, and the branch aspect needs to be treated first. Using again the case of the heart disease patient, if the patient catches a mild cold, the cold should be treated first, and then the treatment plan for the primary aspect of heart disease can be implemented.

3) Treating branch and root concurrently would seem to be the best way to treat a disease, but this approach is not always applicable method of treatment. However, when neither the branch nor root is a severe condition, they can be treated concurrently. For example, in the course of a heat disease, exuberant heat can damage the fluids and yin qi to create constipation with bowel dryness. In this case, the root cause involves an internal accumulation of pathogenic heat, with the consumption of fluids and yin qi as the branch manifestations. This can be treated by gently draining heat and moving the bowels while at the same time nourishing yin to increase fluids and promote defecation. As another example, if the body is persistently deficient with a lowered resistance to disease, repeated colds may occur. However, when such a patient contracts an excess wind-heat condition and a treatment is given to supplement qi, the internal pathogens may also become strengthened. Furthermore, if sweating is promoted to dispel the pathogen, the *zheng* qi of the patient may become damaged. The proper method of treatment in such a case is to boost qi while concurrently releasing the exterior, thus addressing both root and branch.

Summary of root and branch

Disease patterns vary from mild to serious, from chronic to acute, and they also have a certain sequence and impact the body differently. Distinguishing the chronic from an emergency or the primary aspects from secondary aspects of disease is a highly valued skill. The methods of treating root and branch also distinguish the experienced doctor. While some may be able to easily relieve symptoms, treating the root often takes superior talents. An experienced practitioner may give herbs to be taken over a period of weeks or months to correct a very deep seated and chronic condition. Although the symptoms may not change dramatically at first, the overall condition improves and thus prevents future and more serious problems.

Strengthening *Zheng* Qi and Eliminating Pathogens

Generally speaking, in the early stage of a mild disease, the *zheng* qi is not seriously damaged, thus early-stage diagnosis and treatment is the best way to protect the *zheng* qi while eliminating the pathogens. With early diagnosis and treatment, the disease is often prevented from further inward transmission, and the patient will more easily recover. On the other hand, if diagnosis and treatment is not given at an early stage, the pathogen may move more deeply inward and result in a condition that is more difficult to treat.

Chinese medicine holds that transmission of disease follows specific patterns and progressions within the body. For example, in terms of six-channel transmission, at the beginning of a "cold damage disease", the disease location is usually the *taiyang* channel, but as the disease progresses it may transmit to other channels. In any event, following a pathogenic invasion, early diagnosis and treatment can block further transmission and prevent a deteriorating condition.[①]

As a clinical example, in an external wind-cold pattern, the pathogen invades the body surface through the skin. The patient may have a floating pulse, a headache with a tight neck and back, and an aversion to cold. This describes the initial stage of a *taiyang* channel pattern, so treatment should be given to disperse the pathogen from the surface of the body. If the treatment is delayed or in error, the pathogen may move inwardly to create a "deeper" *yangming* channel condition characterized by a high fever with thirst.

The relative balance of *zheng* qi and pathogens

The balancing of *zheng* qi and pathogenic *xie* qi is seen in their opposition and struggle, with the outcome determining the frequency, development and prognosis of the disease. When the *zheng* qi is able to overcome the pathogens, the condition will improve. When the pathogens prevail, the condition will deteriorate. Therefore, one basic principle of treatment is to adjust their relative balance through supporting *zheng* qi and eliminating pathogens.

1) Strengthening *zheng* qi means to build up the body's power to resist pathogens and promote recovery. This method of treatment applies to all kinds of deficiency patterns and is called "supplementing what is deficient". Strengthening *zheng* qi will assist the body in eliminating the pathogens; thus the saying, "as *zheng* qi strengthens, pathogens will go away on their own." Methods for strengthening *zheng* qi include: boosting qi, nourishing blood, enriching yin, warming yang, replenishing essence, supplementing fluids, and supplementing and nourishing the qi, yin and yang, and essence-qi of the organs.

2) Eliminating pathogens helps to reduce the effect of pathogenic factors and inhibit pathological responses. Eliminating pathogens will also reduce damage to the *zheng* qi; it is said that "when pathogens are eliminated, the *zheng* qi will recover on its own". This method of treatment applies to all kinds of excess patterns and is called

---

① What is being described here are *Shāng Hán Lùn* and *Wēn Bìng* theories as applied to certain types of externally contracted diseases.

"draining what is excessive". Specific methods for eliminating pathogens include: sweating, emetic therapy, promoting digestion, resolving phlegm, invigorating blood, dissipating cold, clearing heat, and eliminating dampness.

Strengthening *zheng* qi and eliminating pathogens are dependent upon and complementary to each other. The rules for doing so are as simple as strengthening *zheng* qi in a deficiency pattern, and eliminating pathogens in an excess pattern. In a pattern of mixed deficiency and excess, one needs to carefully assess the branch and root and make intelligent decisions based on them. The overall principle remains to strengthen *zheng* qi while not allowing the pathogens to remain, and to eliminate pathogens while not causing injury to the *zheng* qi. More specific applications of this idea are as follows:

Specific applications

1) Strengthening *zheng* qi is used for both deficiency patterns and patterns of true deficiency with false excess. In strengthening *zheng* qi, one should first identify the affected organ(s) and channels and then evaluate any decline in yin or yang, essence, qi, blood, and/or fluids. Generally, the treatment approach for a deficiency pattern is slower and mild rather than using an aggressive approach that could result in side-effects. Deficiencies are often chronic in nature, and rebuilding the *zheng* qi usually requires a significant period of treatment.

2) Strengthening *zheng* qi before eliminating pathogens is also called "treatment with supplementation before attacking". This method is used when there is a prominent deficiency of *zheng* qi where the body cannot tolerate attacking or purging methods. If in this scenario one attempts only to eliminate pathogens, the *zheng* qi may become further damaged. We therefore need to first strengthen *zheng* qi and later eliminate the pathogens. Strengthening *zheng* qi also enables the body to resist the pathogens internally.

3) Eliminating pathogens is used for excess patterns or in patterns of true excess with false deficiency. To eliminate pathogens, one should first identify the nature and the strength of the pathogenic factors and their location. To avoid injury to the *zheng* qi, such treatment is often withdrawn as soon as the signs of excess are eliminated. At this point, deficiency issues can be addressed and root treatments can be applied to prevent recurrence.

Simultaneous usage

When there is a mixed pattern of combined deficiency and excess, we use a strategy of strengthening *zheng* qi while eliminating pathogens at the same time. This treatment is called "both attacking and supplementing". Because of the more complex nature of the condition, treatment in this manner takes a higher degree of sophistication.

1) The first strategy in simultaneous usage is to primarily strengthen *zheng* qi while secondarily eliminating pathogens. This method is applicable for patterns of mixed deficiency and excess, but where a deficiency of *zheng* qi is most prominent.

2) Eliminating pathogens and strengthening *zheng* qi together first eliminates pathogens as the primary action and strengthens *zheng* qi secondarily. This method is used for patterns of mixed deficiency and excess but where the pathogenic excess is most prominent.

Strengthening *zheng* qi and eliminating pathogens is a commonly used method for both herbal and acupuncture treatments. No treatment should be either 100% yin or yang, nor should they employ elimination or strengthening methods exclusively. This idea may seem easy enough in simple cases, but improper treatment in serious cases can cause real harm to a patient. This approach is certainly needed in more serious or entrenched cases of HIV/AIDS, chronic hepatitis, and among the aged with chronic and deep-rooted medical issues. The principles here should be applied flexibly according to the clinical presentation rather than only according to theoretical constructs. This concept of strengthening and eliminating together is especially important in the practice of herbal medicine where overuse of cloying or sticky supplementing herbs can result pathogens being trapped internally. Many would argue that this is less of a problem in acupuncture treatment.

Adjusting Yin & Yang

The basic pathomechanism of any disease involves a fundamental imbalance of yin and yang, so "adjusting yin and yang" is another way to state the basic principles for the prevention and treatment of any disease. Adjustment of yin and yang means to correct the predominance or weakness of yin or yang so as to restore their relative balance. This is achieved through either reducing the surplus or supplementing the deficiency.

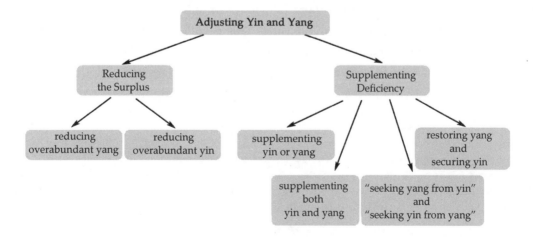

Reducing the surplus

Reducing the surplus, or draining what is excessive, is used for excess patterns caused by a relative overabundance of either yin or yang.[①]

1) Reducing overabundant yang

According to the principle of opposition and restriction between yin and yang, an excess-heat pattern due to "yang overabundance causing heat" should be treated with cold- and cool-natured herbs. This acts to drain the overabundant yang-heat by "cooling what is hot". Yang overabundance "makes yin suffer" thus creating yin deficiency, so treatment for this condition should not only clear yang-heat directly, but also clear heat by nourishing yin. This method eliminates pathogens primarily with the strengthening of *zheng* qi as the secondary aim.

2) Reducing overabundant yin

For an excess-cold pattern, warm- and hot-natured herbs should be used to resolve cold caused by overabundant yin, i.e., "heating what is cold". With concurrent yang deficiency, because "yin overabundance makes yang suffer", the use of yang-supplementing herbs is also required. This method also eliminates pathogens primarily while secondarily strengthening the *zheng* qi.

Supplementing deficiency

Treating deficiency with supplementation is used for patterns of deficiency of either yin or yang. There are four ways to supplement deficiency. The first involves the mutual restraint of yin and yang and the second involves the interdependence of yin and yang. In cases of yin and yang dual deficiency, the third principle is to supplement both yin and yang. The fourth method is to restore yin and yang from collapse.

1) Because of the mutual restraint between yin and yang, the first principle is to supplement yin or supplement yang. For a deficiency heat pattern characterized by the relative appearance of yang where deficient yin fails to restrain yang, treatment should nourish yin in order to inhibit yang. This is called "nourishing the origin of water to check the hyperactivity of yang", and "treating a yang disease through yin". For patterns of deficiency cold where deficient yang fails to restrain yin, thus causing a relative excess of yin qi, treatment should supplement yang in order to inhibit yin.

---

① This section deals with the very basic concepts of "excess" and "deficiency". Although these would seem to be very simple words, they do merit a short discussion from the source text. "Reducing the surplus" and "draining what is excessive" are used synonymously in many texts. The word denoting surplus is *yōu yù* (优裕) or "having enough (to spare), affluence" or "have more than enough". In the second phrase, excess is drained. The word for drain is *xiè* (泻) which also appears in the term for draining as well as in diarrhea or in "losing qi wantonly".

This is called "supporting the source of fire to expel yin" and "treating yin diseases through yang".

2) When treating patterns of deficiency heat or deficiency cold, the principle is to supplement yin or supplement yang according to the principle of the interdependence of yin and yang; this is called "seeking yang from yin" and "seeking yin from yang". Seeking yang from yin means that when supplementing yang, one should also include some yin-nourishing herbs. Seeking yin from yang means that when nourishing yin, one should also include some yang-supplementing herbs. The purpose of this is to assist yin and yang to promote one another while also restricting side effects that could appear when administering only yang-supplementing or yin-nourishing herbs.

3) Supplementing both yin and yang

Supplementing both yin and yang is applied for cases of dual deficiencies of both yin and yang. However, in some cases one may have to differentiate which deficiency is predominant and which is secondary. For example, in a case where yang deficiency is predominant, correct treatment will primarily supplement yang while enriching yin secondarily.

4) Restoring yang and securing yin

This method is suitable for yin collapse or yang collapse patterns. For a case of yin or yang collapse, treatment should restore and secure yin or yang as soon as possible. Since both yang collapse and yin collapse involve a sudden massive loss of the general qi of the body, qi is greatly supplemented. *Rén shēn* (Ginseng Radix et Rhizoma) is commonly used for this purpose.

For a case of repellence between yin and yang, the treatment method involves "treating coldness with cold" or "treating hotness with heat". A pattern of true heat with false cold is essentially an excess-heat pattern with accompanying signs of cold, and the treatment is to clear and drain yang-heat, thus "treating coldness with cold". A pattern of true cold with false heat is a pattern of excess cold with accompanying yang deficiency but with some signs of heat; the treatment principles are to warm yang and dispel cold, thus "treating heat with heat".

Regulating Essence, Qi, Blood and Fluids

Essence, qi, blood and fluids are the material basis for the activities of the organs and channels and collaterals. Although their physiological functions are different, they depend upon one another.

Regulating essence

1) Replenishing essence/*jīng*

Replenishing essence means to supplement the kidney-essence in order to support

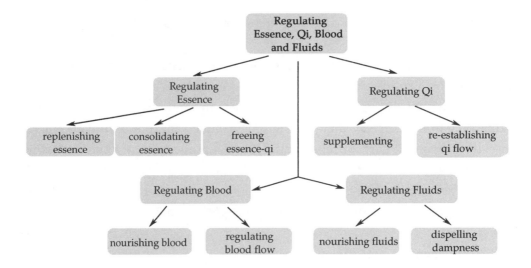

the general essence of the body, including both the prenatal and postnatal essence. Diseases involving essence generally involve deficiency. Replenishing essence is a long process which would probably include lifestyle changes in addition to therapy.

2) Consolidating essence

The essence-consolidating method is used for the overall pathomechanism of the insecurity of kidney qi (*shèn qì bú gù*, 肾气不固). Standard examples include premature ejaculation or an otherwise persistent loss of semen where treatments that supplement and boost kidney qi are applied.

3) Freeing the essence-qi

Essence stagnation in males is often characterized by obstructive ejaculation with turbid semen which results from obstruction of the sexual organ vessels. This is caused by constraint and stagnation of the qi mechanism which results when the liver fails to maintain the free flow of qi, or in some cases involving blood stasis. The treatment is to free the essence-qi and dissipate masses by unblocking the collaterals. As a possible cause of infertility in males, essence stagnation can result from trauma through sports or bicycle riding, or even from qi gong practices that involve semen retention.

Regulating qi

1) Supplementation is appropriate for deficiencies of qi. The production of qi depends upon the actions of prenatal qi as transformed from the essence stored in the kidney, food qi as transformed and transported by the spleen and stomach, and the clear qi inhaled into the lung. Therefore, qi supplementation usually involves methods that reinforce and nourish the lung, spleen and kidney. The generation of *wei* qi, *ying* qi, *zong* qi and *yuan* qi are all related to the qi produced from water and food as transformed by the spleen and stomach. For this reason, it is particularly important to supplement and boost the spleen qi in many cases.

2) Re-establishing qi movement is the treatment principle used for patterns of qi stagnation, qi counterflow, qi sinking, qi block, and qi desertion. For qi stagnation, treatment should move qi; for qi counterflow, treatment should descend qi; for qi sinking, treatment should supplement and raise qi; for qi block, treatment should smooth the flow of qi; and for qi desertion, treatment should boost qi to rescue desertion. To re-establish qi movement, one must follow the normal descending and ascending qi movements of the involved organs. For example, spleen qi mainly ascends, whereas liver qi ascends and disperses. Stomach qi is mainly characterized by descent, whereas lung qi is associated with purification and descent.

Regulating blood

1) Nourishing blood is the principle of treatment for simple blood deficiency. The production of blood is closely related to the functions of the spleen, heart, liver, kidney and other organs. Therefore, when supplementing blood, the functions of the organs must also be regulated. Supplementation of the spleen and stomach is emphasized because the spleen and stomach are the "foundation of the acquired constitution" as well as the "source of qi and blood production".

2) Regulating blood flow is the principle of treatment for blood circulation disorders such as blood stasis, bleeding, etc. The main pathomechanisms of bleeding include blood heat, qi deficiency and blood stasis, while congealing internal cold and qi stagnation is a main pathomechanism for blood stasis. The treatment for blood stasis is to invigorate blood to resolve stasis, whereas treatment for blood stasis due to congealing cold is to warm the channels. The treatment for bleeding is to stop bleeding by clearing heat, supplementing qi, or invigorating blood, depending on the pathomechanism.

Regulating fluids

1) Enriching and nourishing fluids is used to treat a shortage of fluids. For impairment of fluids due to excess heat, the treatment is to clear heat and promote the production of fluids.

2) Dispelling treatment for water-dampness and phlegm-fluid retention is to eliminate or drain (*lì*, 利) dampness. For cases of edema or ascites, the principle of treatment is to relieve swelling by promoting urination. For phlegm and fluid retention, the treatment principles are to dissolve phlegm[1] and expel retained fluids[2]. Water metabolism disturbances are mostly caused by dysfunctions of the lung, spleen,

---

① (*huà tán*, 化痰) dissolve phlegm
② (*zhú yǐn*, 逐饮) expel dampness

kidney and liver, thus treatments usually focus on the lung, spleen, kidney and liver.

Regulating Relationships of Essence, Qi, Blood and Fluids

Regulating the relationship between qi and blood

Because of the interdependent and mutually promoting relationship between qi and blood, they often impact on each other pathologically as well; for this reason, qi and blood both require simultaneous regulation in most cases.

For blood deficiency caused by qi deficiency, the primary treatment is to supplement qi while supplementing blood secondarily, or to supplement both together. For blood stasis caused by deficient qi failing to move blood, the primary treatment is to supplement qi while invigorating blood to eliminate stasis secondarily. For blood stasis caused by qi stagnation, the treatment is to move qi while invigorating blood to eliminate stasis secondarily. For deficient qi failing to contain blood, the treatment is to supplement qi and stanch bleeding while employing astringent or channel-warming agents secondarily.

If blood is so deficient that it cannot nourish qi, qi deficiency may result; the treatment in this case is to supplement blood primarily while boosting qi secondarily. However, for a case of qi desertion following blood loss, treatment should first rescue desertion by boosting qi; this is because "visible blood cannot be quickly produced so the 'intangible' qi should be quickly consolidated in an emergency". Only after the condition improves should blood-supplementing herbs be used as a primary treatment.

Regulating the relationship between qi and fluids

Qi and fluids promote each other, but they are also influenced by each other when diseased. Therefore, qi and blood treatments focus on regulating the relationship of the disorders between them. For under-production of fluids caused by qi deficiency, the treatment is to supplement qi to produce fluids. When qi fails to move fluids, water-dampness and phlegm-fluid retention are the result; the treatment is to supplement and move qi, which will then move the fluids. When qi fails to contain fluids, the treatment is to supplement qi. Fluid retention can also cause qi obstruction; in this case, the treatment first focuses on eliminating the water-dampness and retained phlegm-fluids, after which treatment are given to move qi and remove stagnation. For qi desertion following fluid desertion, the treatment is to supplement qi to rescue it from collapse.

Regulating the relationship between qi and essence

Physically, qi maintains the free flow of essence because qi and essence produce and promote one another. Pathologically, qi stagnation can lead to the obstruction of essence; the treatment is to promote the free flow of both essence and qi. If deficient essence fails to transform into qi, qi deficiency can result, while if deficient qi fails to transform into essence, essence deficiency can result. In both cases, methods that supplement qi and supplement essence should be used together.

Regulating relationships among essence, blood and fluids

"Essence and blood are from the same source." Therefore, in some cases of blood deficiency, one should supplement the blood while also replenishing essence and marrow. "Fluids and blood are from the same source", so disorders involving both fluids and blood are common; in such cases, treatment should supplement blood while enriching fluids and moistening dryness.

Using the Five Phases

To enhance prevention, one may employ five-phase laws and principles including the controlling and restricting relationships among the five phases, integration of the five *zang*-organs, and transmission between the channels. For example, when treating liver disorders, regulating and strengthening the spleen and stomach acts to strengthen spleen-earth in order to help resist an invasion by liver-wood. For a warm-heat disease where stomach yin is injured, kidney yin will also become affected as the disease further progresses. In this case, one would add kidney and stomach yin-replenishing herbs in order to prevent damage to either or both. These are examples of "controlling the development of an existing disease".

Treatment principles for five-phase imbalances

Five-phase principles offer an elegant method for solving many clinical problems, but they cannot be always used effectively as a primary method of diagnosis. Attempting to force a five-phase solution onto any given case is generally not warranted. However, there are a number of practical clinical scenarios in which five-phase principles of treatment are often applied.

1) **Checking wood to bank up earth** is a method of soothing or calming the liver while also strengthening the spleen; it is used to treat patterns of liver and spleen disharmony, or hyperactive liver qi attacking the stomach. When liver hyperactivity is prevalent, the primary treatment method is to soothe and calm the liver. When spleen deficiency prevails, spleen-strengthening methods should be emphasized.

2) **Banking up earth to dam water** is a method for strengthening the spleen to promote the flow of water. It is used for patterns of water-dampness accumulation resulting from spleen deficiency with failure to transport water, as often in cases of edema with distention and fullness.

3) **Assisting metal to subdue wood** is a method of nourishing the lung and

clearing liver fire, also called "nourishing the lung and draining the liver". The associated pattern involves both lung yin deficiency and liver fire attacking the lung.

4) Draining the south and supplementing the north is used to subdue heart fire and replenish kidney water in patterns of "heart and kidney not communicating", also known as disharmony between water and fire. This pattern involves both kidney yin deficiency and overactive heart-fire. The heart is in charge of fire and the south is attributed to fire, while the kidney is in charge of water and north is attributed to water. Therefore the method is called "draining the south and supplementing the north" as well as "cutting down fire and replenishing water" or "enriching yin and subduing fire".

TREATMENT METHODS

Based on the general therapeutic principles, a treatment method is a more specific therapeutic application that may be employed following a proper diagnosis.

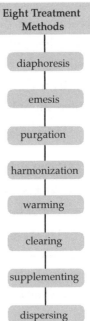

The Eight Treatment Methods

Diaphoresis is a treatment method for relieving exterior patterns by leading pathogens outward from the lung and skin through sweating. Indications include externally-contracted conditions such as aversion to cold, fever, headache, coughing and generalized pain, as well as rashes, edema, and diarrhea.

Emesis is a method of inducing vomiting to remove phlegm-damp accumulation, mistakenly ingested toxic substances or undigested food from the stomach. Obviously this method is unpleasant and thus rarely used, but it can be very effective when applied for the right condition.

Purgation is a method for relieving the gastrointestinal tract by purging the stomach and intestines through the discharge of feces. Indications include constipation, food accumulation, blood stasis, phlegm-fluid retention, and parasites.

Harmonization is a method for regulating two or more systems or organs and to coordinate their actions. There may be a disharmony between two organs, of yin and yang, or of the exterior and interior. Indications include *shaoyang* patterns, liver-spleen disharmony, mixed signs of cold and heat, and diseases involving both exterior and interior.

Harmonization is an interesting category for a number of reasons. Because it involves more than one system or organ and actions, a certain degree of sophistication in treatment beyond the other categories is required. Harmonizing is obviously a more subtle method of treatment than emesis or purgation. It has also been addressed over the years in different ways; from narrow interpretations associated with *shaoyang* conditions to more complex disease patterns. Although harmonization is not confined to the spleen or liver, modern Chinese herbal medicine often utilizes "earth school" methods, those which "harmonize" the spleen-stomach and liver. Harmonizing has become particularly relevant to the complexity of modern diseases which often include psychological stress. In addressing formulas that harmonize, *Formulas and Strategies* states, "For complex historical reasons, contemporary Chinese medicine in East Asian and the West associates psychosomatic disorders with conditions of the Liver or Gallbladder, or with Liver-Spleen disharmony. Diseases due to emotional problems or to the stresses involved in coping with the rigors of modern life are therefore often treated with formulas selected from this category."[①]

The **warming** method dispels internal cold through warming actions. Indications include cold-fluid accumulation or internal cold-dampness with prolonged organ coldness and a decline of yang qi.

The **clearing** method removes internal heat by means of heat-clearing, fire-draining, and blood-cooling actions. Clearing can be seen as the opposite of the warming method and is often called "cooling method" in some texts. This method is applicable for patterns of excess heat, deficiency heat, internal fire, and toxins with extreme heat.

The **supplementing** method recovers the *zheng* qi of the body through nourishing actions and is suitable for all kinds of deficiency patterns.

The **dispersing** method dispels or resolves the substantial pathogens from stagnation or accumulation by means of promoting digestion and resolving stagnation, moving qi and invigorating blood, dissolving phlegm and promoting urination, and expelling worms. This method is applicable for food accumulation, qi stagnation and blood stasis, abdominal masses, retention of water-dampness, phlegm-fluid retention, infantile malnutrition with accumulation, and worms.

Routine Treatment (*Zhèng Zhì*, 正治) and Paradoxical Treatment (*Fǎn Zhì*, 反治)

In complex diseases, some conditions are consistent with their presenting signs and symptoms, and yet there are others with roots that are inconsistent with their clinical manifestations (branches). While this review of routine and paradoxical treatments may seem obvious and simplistic, in the clinic it often means the difference between successful treatment and utter disaster. Mistaking excesses for deficiencies,

---

① Dan Bensky, Randall Barolet. *Formulas and Strategies*. Seattle: Eastland Press; 1990. p. 104.

cold for heat, or yin for yang can obviously cause big problems in both diagnosis and treatment.[①]

Routine treatment

Routine treatment is the most commonly used approach to clinical treatment, and refers to the use of herbs whose nature is opposite to that of the disease pattern. Because the nature of the treatment is opposite to that of the disease pattern, this approach is also called "allopathic treatment"[②]. As an example, routine treatment addresses a heat pattern by using cold-natured herbs.

Routine treatment is applicable for diseases with signs and symptoms that are consistent with their natures, i.e. a heat pattern that presents with heat signs, a cold pattern with cold signs, a deficiency pattern with deficiency signs, or an excess pattern with excess signs. Routine treatment applies the methods of "cooling what is hot", "heating what is cold", "supplementing what is deficient", and "draining what is excessive" respectively.

Heating what is cold uses warm and hot herbs to treat patterns of cold presenting with signs and symptoms of cold.

Cooling what is hot uses cold and cool herbs to treat patterns of heat presenting with signs and symptoms of heat.

Supplementing what is deficient uses supplementing and nourishing herbs for treating deficiency patterns. For example, yang deficiency is treated with herbs that act to warm yang, yin deficiency with herbs that nourish yin, qi deficiency with herbs that boost qi, and blood deficiency with herbs that nourish blood.

Draining what is excessive uses purgation and dispelling methods to treat excess-type pathogens. For example, food accumulation is treated with herbs that promote digestion and resolve stagnation, retained water-fluid with herbs that expel water, blood stasis with herbs that invigorate blood and dissolve stasis, internal dampness with herbs that eliminate dampness.

Routine Treatment

using treatment methods opposite to the problem

cooling what is hot: treating cold syndrome with heat-natured herbs

heating what is cold: treating heat syndrome with cold-natured herbs

supplementing what is deficient: treating deficiency syndrome with nourishing herbs

draining what is excessive: treating excess syndrome with pathogen-eliminating herbs

---

① These methods are particularly important for herbal treatments because their effects are so direct and side effects can be drastic. Arguably, this is not always the case with acupuncture and other therapies.

② The term "allopathic" was first used by the inventor of homeopathy, Samuel Hahnemann. Homeopathy uses "like for like" for example, minute amounts of bee venom for a bee sting. Allopathic is using cold to treat heat, dryness to treat damp, etc. So although Chinese medicine is considered "holistic", it shares with biomedicine aspects of being allopathic.

Paradoxical treatment

Paradoxical treatment uses methods that match the (false) signs and symptoms, used in such cases of "false cold" and "false heat" or fatigue where the true problem is stagnation[①] and not qi deficiency. Paradoxical treatment of heat and cold is applied at the extremes, when yin and yang repel each other. Such cases of cold and heat are less common than those of excess and deficiency, yet paradoxical treatment remains an important method for many difficult and complicated cases. Although the approach is counter-intuitive to the presenting symptoms and signs, it is also important to remember that all of these treatments are in fact aimed at the root of the disease.[②]

1) Treating heat with heat means to treat a disease pattern of true cold with false heat with warm- or hot-natured herbs. True cold with false heat occurs when exuberant yin repels yang; as yin-cold fills the inside, it forces the yang qi outward thus giving the appearance of heat at the extremities. Yin-cold excess is the root of the disease and there are signs of true cold such as diarrhea with undigested food, extremely cold limbs, a faint pulse, and a pale tongue with a white coating. Therefore, a prescription comprised of warm-hot herbs is applied to treat the root.

2) Treating coldness with cold means to treat a disease pattern of true heat with false cold where exuberant yang repels yin. For example, in heat stroke, yang qi is blocked inside the body by extreme internal heat. As yang cannot go outward to the four limbs, there appear false cold signs such as cold of the four limbs[③] (cold limbs below the elbows and knees) and a deep hidden pulse. However, careful examination may find the trunk of the patient being warm or hot; other signs and symptoms include an aversion to heat, thirst with a desire for cold water, scanty dark urine, and a dark red tongue with a yellow coating. Therefore, a prescription comprised of cool-cold herbs is applied to treat the root by clearing the internal heat.

3) Treating excess with supplementation[④] is used when there is a deficiency pattern with some signs and symptoms of excess such as stagnation, such as when there is a lack of urination due to a deficiency of kidney yang. Warming the kidney yang will promote the formation and excretion of urine, thus normalizing urination, whereas simply promoting urination through draining may harm the kidney qi. In

---

①   Stagnation is considered an excess.

②   One often looks to the tongue (and to the pulse) for a determination of the true nature of the condition.

③   This phenomenon of "reversal" cold at the four limbs is a very important and widely used term throughout Chinese medical theory.

④   "Treating excess with supplementation" is often termed "treating obstruction with supplementation" and "treating deficiency with drainage" is often termed "treating openness with purgation". Obstruction and stagnation are considered excess conditions. Openness refers to diarrhea, excessive bleeding, etc.... and is considered as a deficiency condition. It is sometimes treated in a paradoxical manner with moving and draining herbs and techniques, and in some cases, purgatives.

a case of constipation with distention (bloating) due to spleen qi deficiency, it is best to strengthen the spleen and boost qi in order to regain the normal ascending and descending of the qi mechanism. To apply purgation in this case might only damage the *zheng* qi. As another example, pain is often treated as an excess of qi and blood stagnation, but for many older patients, chronic pain conditions are best treated by nourishing while concurrently moving qi and blood. Using only blood-moving herbs (and acupuncture) may further scatter qi and blood and actually aggravate the pain.

4) Treating deficiency with moving and draining is suitable for patterns of true excess with false deficiency. Usually diarrhea, menstrual "flooding and spotting", and frequent urination are treated by arresting diarrhea, securing the *chong mai*, and reducing urination respectively. However, if these signs and symptoms appear in a disease pattern characterized by deficiency, they should be treated according to the principle of "treating openness by draining". For example, a case of diarrhea (openness) might occur due to the partial blockage of the gastrointestinal tract caused by food stagnation. This diarrhea cannot be treated by simply stopping the leakage, but on the contrary should be treated by promoting bowel movements in order to resolve the stagnation and accumulation. The diarrhea will then cease as the blockage is removed.

As another example, some cases of excessive menstrual bleeding may be due to blood stasis. If in such a case hemostatic herbs are employed, this may create more blood stasis and aggravate the condition. A better approach is to invigorate the blood and dissolve stasis so that blood can circulate normally inside the vessels.

• Paradoxical Treatment-Herbal Formula Examples (only to be used with appropriate presentation)		
	Signs, Symptoms, Disease	Formula
Heat with Heat	irritability, sore throat	*Sì Nì Tāng*
Excess Symptoms with Tonics	edema, reduced urination	*Zhēn Wǔ Tāng*
	headache	*Dāng Guī Bǔ Xuè Tāng*
	chest pain, acid reflux	*Yī Guàn Jiān*
Deficiency Symptoms with Moving and Draining	diarrhea	*Huáng Qín Tāng, Sháo Yào Tāng*
	profuse menstrual bleeding	*Sì Wù Tāng*
	leukorrhea	*Lóng Dǎn Xiè Gān Tāng*

Suiting Treatment to the "Three Factors"

Chinese philosophy believes that "man exists by the interaction of heavenly and earthly qi". This means that the human body and its diseases are inevitably influenced by yin and yang and their expression as seasonal, climatic, rhythmic, geographical and environmental factors. The patients' differences in gender, age, and constitution also influence the frequency, development and conversion of disease to a certain degree. Therefore, in treatment of disease, all these specific factors must be analyzed so that an appropriate treatment can be made according to time, locality and the individual. These are termed the "three factors".

Suiting treatment to locality

Older Chinese texts emphasized the difference between persons living in the various geographic regions of China. Up until recent times, there had been relatively little migration and movement between people within and outside of their home regions and countries. Although people from all nations are found throughout the world today, some generalizations about location still often apply. For example, where the climate is generally warm and humid, the surface of the body is open, yang qi tends to escape outward, and the body is susceptible to wind invasion. Climates now include not just geographic areas, but are also associated with modern influences of artificial heating and cooling systems; a person living in a hot and damp climate often works in an air conditioned office all day and then goes outside to suddenly confront a hot environment or in winter when people go from heated buildings out into the cold.

Suiting treatment to the time

To formulate an appropriate principle according to the seasons and climate is known as "suiting the treatment to the time". Here "time" has several meanings. The first refers to the seasons, and the second can refer to years, months, days, or even the time of day.

Just as the time factor of a year, month, season, day and night can affect climatic features in the natural world, they can also to some degree influence human physiological activities and pathological changes. For example, yang qi is abundant during the hot summer, and the body sweats because the pores are open. Under these conditions, even for a case of pathogenic wind-cold, acrid-warm herbs with a dispersing action should not be overused. In the cold of winter, the body's yin prevails while yang qi astringes and the pores of the human body tighten and contract. Under these conditions, one should use cool- and cold-natured herbs or foods with great caution while also being cautious in the use of warm- and hot-natured foods or medicinals in the hotter seasons. Again, summerheat pathogens often combine with dampness, so in mid-summer one should focus on clearing summerheat and eliminating dampness. In the dry season of autumn, one should focus on gentle dispersion as well as the moistening of dryness.

In terms of lunar time, one concept is that the drainage method should not be used as the moon begins to grow from new to full (waxing), supplementation should not be applied when the moon is full, and as the moon is waning (becoming smaller) no treatment can be used. Some Chinese medicine practitioners still consult the waxing and waning laws of the moon phases, especially as applied in the treatment of menstrual disorders.[①] Others will apply moxibustion at the new moon, and bleed the collaterals on full moons. Many of these practices are not applied for the most part, but continue with some classical traditions and practitioners.

Within a day, signs and symptoms can change dramatically. Yin deficiency signs tend to arise in the evening, qi deficiency signs in the afternoon, and yang deficiency signs in the morning. The internal organs also are assigned time periods though out the day in which their qi strengthens and weakens.

Suiting treatment to the individual

To formulate an appropriate treatment according to the patient's characteristics of age, gender, constitution, etc. is known as "suiting treatment to the individual".

1) Age

The physiological functions and pathological responses of an individual vary with age, so treatment should also be varied accordingly. For example, children are very energetic, but their qi and blood is not fully developed and their organs are delicate. Children's diseases move quickly from cold to heat, deficiency to excess, interior to exterior and vice versa. Thus, in the treatment of children, the dosage of herbs should be reduced with a shorter course of administration and any drastic measure should be avoided. The blood and qi of young adults is relatively strong, so diseases in this group often present as excess patterns because of the vigorous struggle between the *zheng* qi and *xie* qi. Treatment can focus on attacking the pathogens and draining the excess, while the herb dosages can be higher. Elderly people often have declining qi, blood, and organ functions. Therefore, the diseases of this group more often involve patterns of deficiency, or complex patterns of deficiency mixed with excess. In treatment, supplementation is common, or simultaneous supplementation and drainage. Senior adults and children respond very strongly to acupuncture and herbal treatment, and leaving the needles in the body for too long or using too many needles can tire an older patient. Although a young child may respond quickly to acupuncture, some will find it hard to remain still for the duration of the treatment. Shorter acupuncture treatment times are therefore often quite effective and appropriate for both the elderly and the young.

2) Gender

In Chinese medicine, men and women are for the most part treated the same, although some practitioners will distinguish the left and right sides as associated with each gender when using acupuncture or taking pulses. Blood is considered as

---

① There is a system of using the Chinese calendar and clock (stems and branches) to find the most appropriate acupuncture points for a given treatment on a given day and hour. In addition, some systems use astrology to find the acupuncture points based on the patient's chart.

the main substance in women, while qi is the main substance in men. Obviously, in gynecology and fertility issues, gender is the central factor, but a particular focus on gender is generally absent from theory and treatment.

3) Constitution

Prenatal endowments and postnatal living environments are different for each person. In a patient who tends to yang overabundance, warm- and hot-natured herbs should be used with caution. For a patient who tends to yin overabundance, cold-natured herbs should be used with caution. When a patient has a strong physique, the dosages of attacking and purging herbs may be larger, while for a patient with a weak physique, more supplementing and boosting treatments may be needed. Although the principles of treatment should be primarily based on pattern differentiation, the three factors of seasonal climate, geographical environment, and the individual constitution should still be taken into consideration.

CASES

1. Your patient is a 50-year-old man who has had a chronic cough with copious phlegm for several years. Ten years ago, he moved into a new house that faces the ocean. Before this, he lived in a dry climate and lived a relatively sedate lifestyle. In the new location, he has a high stress job and he manages the stress by running on the beach and drinking "one or two" glasses of wine a night. He has several small children who always seem to be ill. He is slightly overweight, has a red complexion, his pulse is rapid and slippery, and his tongue has a thick yellow coating.

2. Your patient is an 84-year-old woman with sciatic pain for the last six months. She takes several prescription pain medications, and you had previously given her a strong acupuncture treatment to move qi and blood. The next week she reported that her pain was relieved for about 3 hours but then became worse. She also said that she was "wiped out" and that she had slept for most of the day after the treatment. Her tongue was pale and dry, and her pulse was weak, thready and deep.

Chapter 9

Diagnosis

This chapter contains a relatively brief introduction to the methods of Chinese medical diagnosis. Some diagnostic tools and methods of Chinese medicine are relatively easy to understand, while others, such as pulse examination, can take many years to fully master. The process of diagnosis requires the clinical skills of observation and inquiry along with a firm grasp of Chinese medical theory. Because a correct diagnosis leads to the correct method of treatment, diagnostic ability is fundamental to any medical practice. A correct diagnosis can hinge upon the smallest clinical detail, or in some cases, a diagnosis may be easily rendered according to clearly observable signs and symptoms. However, many times the presenting signs and symptoms will differ from the textbook description due to the complexities of an individual case; furthermore, clinical experience also shows that diagnostic signs (such as the tongue and pulse) will not always match the actual pattern of disharmony. In order to correctly diagnose the clinical pattern and formulate an effective treatment, a practitioner must become adept first at listening and then at gathering and interpreting any number of signs and symptoms at the time of examination.

The Chinese word for diagnosis has two components, *zhěn duàn* (诊断), where *zhěn* refers to the examination, with *duàn* being a judgment of the disease and pattern[1]. Diagnosis is an acquired skill which involves a differential analysis of the patient's presenting signs and symptoms, any one of which may be the key to a correct diagnosis. Symptoms refer to abnormal changes in a patient which may be associated with illness, especially those issues as perceived by the patient subjectively. Clinical signs refer to objective indications of the patient's condition as observed and noted by the practitioner. Proper differentiation of signs and symptoms requires careful consideration and great skill in many cases.

Clinical Reasoning in Chinese Medicine states, "Generally speaking, the more solid the doctor's theoretical foundation, the broader his knowledge and the richer his clinical experience will be, the more competent he will be at drawing inferences, and the better he will be at understanding the internal pathological correlation between isolated symptoms. His intuition and ability to use imagery

---

① Yi Qiao. *Diagnosis Study Guide*. Seattle: Eastland Press; 2008. p. 2.

will also be enhanced."[1]

The final diagnosis will identify and include both a "disease name" as well as the Chinese medical "pattern" of disharmony. For a person with insomnia (the disease name) for example, there can be a number of associated clinical patterns, and conversely, one pattern can be associated with many different diseases. For example, treating a pattern of "liver blood deficiency" can cure the "diseases" of both insomnia and amenorrhea. So any one disease may fall under different patterns, and one pattern may be associated with many different diseases. Jiao Shu-de writes, "... the disease symptoms are processed by 'separating the grain from the chaff, by distinguishing the true from the false, by proceeding step-by-step, and from exterior to interior'. After that, what emerges in any specified stage of disease observable at that moment is the synthesized result that we recognize as the pattern." [2]

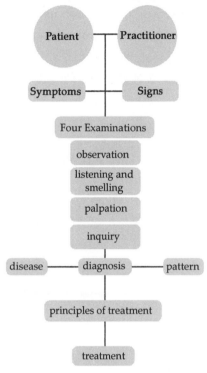

DISEASE AND PATTERN

There are over 4000 diseases in Chinese medicine, with each disease name describing particular qualities as they occur through time[3]. Diseases are dynamic processes resulting from yin and yang imbalances as well as the interactions of *zheng* qi and *xie* qi. Knowing the disease name allows the practitioner to predict the future course of the condition, while a pattern is found only at one particular point in time; it is from this point in time that one creates the treatment plan. Therefore, both disease identification and pattern differentiation are required. Qiao and Stone write, "... the full course of pathological and predictable changes of a disease cannot be grasped through pattern identification alone. On the other hand, if one identifies only the disease, but not the pattern, treatment cannot be undertaken since the treatment

---

① Hu Zhen, Dong Fei-xia. *Clinical Reasoning in Chinese Medicine*. Beijing: People's Medical Publishing House; 2008. p. 40.

② Jiao Shu-de. *Case Studies on Pattern Identification*. Taos: Paradigm Publications; 2006. p. 225.

③ Many "Chinese diseases" closely resemble those of biomedicine. In recent times, various attempts have been made to correlate the two systems. As a famous example, *xiāo kě* is widely known to correlate to late-stage diabetes. However, many scholars and practitioners have complained that making these direct translations is incorrect as Chinese diseases and patterns have their own distinct qualities that do not reflect the depth of traditional Chinese medicine.

principle is based on the differentiation of the particular pattern, and not the overall disease."[1]

The pattern diagnosis can be based on a *zang-fu* diagnosis, on the channels and collaterals, levels (such as in the *Treatise on Cold Damage* or *Warm Disease*), qi and blood, or simply yin and yang. Additionally, some herbal formulas are so clearly associated with specific signs and symptoms that their names are used in the diagnosis, such as a *Xiǎo Chái Hú Tāng* pattern or a *Yī Guàn Jiān* pattern.

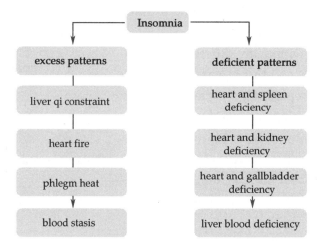

Disease Diagnosis and Pattern Diagnosis

EIGHT PRINCIPLES

Misinterpretation of complex and contradictory signs and symptoms may lead the practitioner to false conclusions. In a previous chapter we discussed the eight principles of yin/yang, heat/cold, exterior/interior and excess/deficiency, which are the broadest categories to which we apply diagnosis. Although a proper diagnosis may consider a vast amount of information, when faced with a difficult case, even the most experienced practitioner will return to the eight principles. The following chart shows the basic categories which serve as broad markers for diagnosis using the eight principles.

① Yi Qiao. *Diagnosis Study Guide*. Seattle: Eastland Press; 2008. p. 7.

Eight Principles

Sign	Internal Disease	External Disease
pulse	generally deeper	more superficial
tongue	changes with disease	no change
location	attacks *zang-fu* organs	affects channels and collaterals
Sign	**Heat**	**Cold**
thirst	thirst with preference for cold fluids	no thirst or preference for warm fluids
complexion	red	pale
tongue	red	pale
body fluids	yellow	white, clear
bowels	constipation	loose stool
emotions	agitation, anger	apathy, depression
Sign	**Excess**	**Deficiency**
time of disease	generally more acute	more chronic
treatment	clears, drains, purges	boosts, tonifies, raises
constitution	underlying strength	underlying weakness
pain	worse with pressure	better with pressure
voice	strong	weak
pulse	forceful	weak
tongue	thick coating	little coating
Sign	**Yang**	**Yin**
fluids	dryness	dampness
direction	raises, expands	lowers, contracts
temperature	heat	cold
voice	loud, shout	low, weak
color	red	pale
nature	excess	deficiency
position	exterior	interior

FOUR PILLARS

Chinese medical diagnostics employs the "four pillars" of diagnosis: observation, listening and smelling, touching (palpation) and inquiry. In 1556, Xu Chun-fu wrote, "the four words 'to look', 'to smell and to listen', 'to ask', and 'to press' are the basic theme running through medicine. If one has grasped the meaning of these four words, he may be called accomplished in the medical teachings."[1]

1) Observation includes looking at the entirety of the body and sometimes even

---

[1] Xu Chun-fu. *The Complete Compendium of Ancient and Modern Medical Works* (*Gǔ Jīn Yī Tǒng Dà Quán*, 古今医统大全). From *Chinese Life Sciences*, compiled and translated by Paul Unschuld, p. 144.

the clothing that the patient is wearing. Typically, the practitioner will be looking at the overall body shape, the color and texture of the skin, posture, body language and other particular diagnostic markers on certain areas. For example, redness on a particular channel can indicate heat within the corresponding organ. The physical signs often parallel the pathology; for example, redness indicates heat, paleness points to blood deficiency, etc.

The tongue is a major diagnostic indicator and is divided into several sections according to the three *jiao* and the internal organs. A large tongue can be a sign of spleen deficiency. A tongue with teeth marks or scallops on the sides also shows a deficient spleen that cannot adequately constrain the flesh of the tongue. A red tongue shows internal heat, while a dusky (pale purple) color would reflect constrained qi or blood. A darker purple tongue is most often caused by blood stasis, and viewing the veins under the tongue often confirms this. A yellow coating on top of the tongue itself is often a symptom of internal heat and dampness. A tongue with small cracks can be a sign of yin and/or fluid deficiency, and a tongue with purple spots may indicate blood stasis (although this can also be natural pigmentation for those of African or South Asian ancestry). Below are some of the indications used in tongue diagnosis.

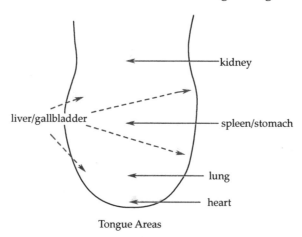

Tongue Areas

Tongue Color	
pale red (pink)	normal
pale	yang deficiency or blood deficiency
pale and wet	yang deficiency
dry, pale, orange sides	blood deficiency
red	heat
red with yellow coating	heat and damp-heat
red with no coating	deficiency heat
deep red	severe heat
purple	blood stasis, cold
red or purple spots	blood stasis
black	extreme heat or cold

Tongue Shape	
thin	blood or yin deficiency
shortened	cold, phlegm, heat or deficiency
swollen	dampness
stiff	internal wind, heat
flaccid	yang deficiency
deviated	wind
quivering	qi and/or yang deficiency
scalloped (teeth marks)	spleen qi deficiency
Tongue Coating	
white	cold
yellow	heat
"dirty" grayish, brown	cold, dampness, food stagnation
cracked, dry	yin, fluid deficiency
wet	yang deficiency
thick	retained pathogens such as food, heat, cold, etc.
black	extreme cold or heat

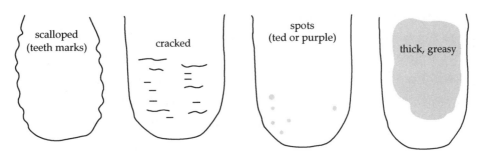

Some Tongue Examples

The eyes can also be used in special cases as a diagnostic tool. For example, it is said that drooping eyelids point to spleen qi deficiency. The state of the *shén* is most often observed through the amount and of "spirit" in the eyes, as well as in the quality of eye contact with the patient. The area

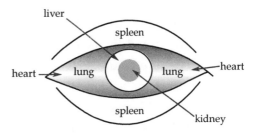

associated with the heart is at the inner and outer canthus, the liver area in the cornea, the lung area at the whites of the eyes (sclera), the kidney area at the pupil, and the spleen area at the upper and lower eyelids.

2) Listening and smelling includes listening both to the words spoken by the patient as well as how they are delivered. Hesitation, raspiness, mumbling, disjointedness, and loud or soft voices can be as or more important to diagnosis as the actual content of the spoken words. An overly loud voice points to excess, whereas an overly soft voice can indicate deficiency. Listening to the quality of a cough can reveal how much dryness or dampness remains in the lung. In addition, practitioners may listen to the heartbeat either through modern devices or by putting their ears to the chest.

Although not emphasized as a diagnostic tool, the smell of the patient's body, stool, urine, vaginal and other discharges can often tell us more about the patient's condition and the prognosis. For example, a strong foul smell is often associated with damp-heat, while slight fishy odors can be associated with cold.

3) Touching (palpation) is very important in two ways; a thorough examination of the body and the channels can reveal signs of heat, cold, pain, tender or tough spots, knots and other diagnostic indicators, while the second type of palpatory examination involves examination of the pulse. Chinese pulse diagnosis is considered an art form with many unique schools of thought from within China and other countries as well. Practitioners and teachers over the millennia have refined, and adapted the practice of pulse diagnosis in various ways. When examining the pulse, one must consider the pulse rate as well as depth, size, rhythm, tension, and other qualities.

In the original texts, pulses were taken at the neck, wrist, ankle and other locations, although the current standard of pulse-taking employs examination of the radial artery with three fingers on both the left and right wrists. The positions closest to the fingers (*cùn*) represent the lung on the right hand, and the heart on the left. In the middle positions (*guān*), the right hand represents the spleen, and the left the liver. The positions furthest from the wrist (*chǐ*) represent various aspects of the kidney. In addition, different qualities can be found depending on how hard one presses at each position. Again, pulse examination can be a highly involved process with many variations depending on the teacher or family lineage.

Subhuti Dharmanda writes, "The classic Chinese pattern of pulse-taking is based on touching the wrist with three levels of pressure: superficial palpation (almost no pressure, to feel the bounding of the pulse up to the skin surface); intermediate palpation (light pressure, to feel the basic pulse form); and deep palpation (somewhat heavy pressure, to feel how the pulse is able to emerge from the physical constraint). In addition, the changes in pulse feeling as one moves from less to more pressure, and again from more to less pressure, can also give some information about the resilience of the pulse. In essence, there are nine pulse takings on each wrist: one for each of the three pulse taking fingers at each of the three levels of pressure."[1]

---

[1]   Subhuti Dharmanda. http://www.itmonline.org/arts/pulse.htm

Simple Pulse Positions

closer to fingers (distal)		
	Left	**Right**
Cùn	heart	lung
Guān	liver	spleen
Chǐ	kidney yin	kidney yang
closer to elbow (proximal)		

The table below is adapted from the book *Li Shi-zhen's Pulse Studies* by Li Shen-qing and William Morris[1]. These pulses can be combined, and are found at different positions on the wrist and at different depths. In these various configurations the indications will change as well as the diagnosis. The first step in learning the art of pulse-taking is to memorize the descriptions and indications associated with the pulses listed below.

Name			Brief Description	Brief Indications
choppy	*sè mài*	涩脉	uneven, thready, slow, rough, comes and goes with difficulty	blood stasis, essence deficiency
deep	*chén mài*	沉脉	sunken, soft, slippery, strongest in the depths	qi and yang deficiency, interior, chronic conditions
deficient	*xū mài*	虚脉	with light pressure slow and large, yielding, floating	deficiency of essence-qi
drum skin	*gé mài*	革脉	hollow and wiry, superficial, tense	deficiency of yin, *jīng*, blood, qi
excess	*shí mài*	实脉	large and long at superficial and deep, hardness and excess	heat or deficiency or healthy
faint	*wēi mài*	微脉	light, soft, feeble	deficiency of blood, qi, yin or yang
firm	*láo mài*	牢脉	wiry, long, excess, deep, forceful	yin-cold, qi blockage, heat, blood stasis, food accumulation
floating	*fú mài*	浮脉	moves at superficial level	exterior conditions, deficiency of blood or yang
hasty	*cù mài*	促脉	rapid, irregular with occasional rest, yang on verge of yin collapse, fire in *sanjiao*	heat or healthy constitutionally
hidden	*fú mài*	伏脉	hidden, deep, close to the bone	often serious or normal in pregnancy
hollow	*kòu mài*	芤脉	floating large, excess outside empty inside, distinct "sides"	blood or fluid deficiency
intermittent	*dài mài*	代脉	missed beats at regular intervals	trauma, wind, cold, pain, emotions, deficiency of blood and qi
knotted	*jié mài*	结脉	slow and irregular, missed beats in chaotic intervals	stagnation of qi, blood, phlegm or food
long	*cháng mài*	长脉	extending beyond all three positions	excess or normal
moderate	*huǎn mài*	缓脉	no extremes, ideal	normal by itself
rapid	*shuò mài*	数脉	urgent arrival	heat

---

[1] Li Shen-qing, William Morris. *Li Shi-zhen's Pulse Studies*. Beijing: People's Medical Publishing House;2011.

Name			Brief Description	Brief Indications
scattered	*săn mài*	散脉	uneven rate, coming and going	depletion of essence, qi, blood
short	*duăn mài*	短脉	does not extend, sinks at both ends	deficiency or excess, stagnation
slippery	*huá mài*	滑脉	moves quickly and smoothly under fingers	excess
wiry	*xián mài*	弦脉	forceful, long, flat, taut	stagnation, excess, normal in springtime
slow	*chí mài*	迟脉	feels slow	slow, qi and yang depletion
soggy	*rú mài*	濡脉	floating, thready and soft, like a thread on water	qi, yin, blood deficiency, dampness
surging	*hóng mài*	洪脉	arrives with force and departs with force	*yangming* excess heat, normal in summer
thready	*xì mài*	细脉	small diameter, also called thin	qi, blood, yin deficiency
throbbing	*dòng mài*	动脉	short, urgent, shaking, slippery, forceful	struggle between yin and yang

4) Inquiry includes the gathering of information regarding the patient's medical history, lifestyle, desires and goals, all of which can be the key to making an accurate diagnosis. Specific questions include inquiry about chills and fevers, sweating, pain, symptoms of the body, ears and eyes, diet, defecation and urination, sleep, and conditions affecting women and children when applicable. A complete medical history is extremely important. Family history, past biomedical and Chinese diseases, old injuries, lifestyle choices, living situations and even prescribed medications from years or decades past can have relevance to the current situation. Especially important is establishing a timeline to assess the precipitating factors.

TEN QUESTIONS[①]

The "ten questions" or "ten asking songs" was a poem devised by Zhang Jing-yue during the Ming Dynasty. Since that time, practitioners have adapted the ten songs as a convenient way to focus the questioning of the patient. Questioning should not be applied mechanically, but should follow the contours of the problems and the comfort levels of the patient.

1) The practitioner should inquire as to any pain, itching or other physical discomfort. For all questions, it is important to know when the issues arise, for what length of time, any precipitating factors, and the areas affected. It is often useful to establish a "pain scale" with 0 being minimal or nonexistent and 10 being excruciating. In this way, aggravating factors can be identified and pain levels can be tracked from

---

① The original 10 Asking Songs has several ambiguous passages that have been adapted to more practical uses. Following is one version of the original: 一问寒热，二问汗，三问头身四问便，五问饮食六问胸，七聋八渴俱当辨，九因脉色察阴阳，十从气味章神见。见定虽然事不难，也须明哲毋招怨。

treatment to treatment.

Pain due to qi and blood stagnation can often be treated most effectively with acupuncture; pain not easily relieved with acupuncture may have a component of deficiency.

Pain	Diagnosis
dull	qi stagnation
stabbing	blood stagnation
very sharp (knife-like)	cold (improved with heat)
burning	heat (improved with cold)
pins and needles	blood deficiency
moving	qi stagnation or wind
dull, worse when tired	qi deficiency
worse after eating	food retention
chronic pain, especially lower back	kidney deficiency

2) Factors of heat and cold are important, such as if the body or an area of the body feels hot or cold or if the patient feels better or worse in the presence of either. Ask the patient if there are feelings of fever or chills, and again, the time frame should be established. The simplest conclusion is that if any pain or discomfort is alleviated by heat, then the cause is cold, and vice versa. However, many acute pain conditions can be temporarily relieved by cold; for this reason, just as in Western medicine, sprains and strains are often first treated with cold and later with heat as needed.

Chills and Fever	
acute illness with more chills than fever	wind-cold
acute illness with more fever than chills	wind-heat
alternating chills and fever	*shaoyang* disease
low grade fever in afternoon or evening	yin deficiency
chronic low grade fever	damp-heat

3) The presence or absence of sweating is important. In Chinese herbal medicine, issues of sweating are particularly important for both diagnosis and treatment. Sweating which occurs spontaneously or after slight exertion is often the result of qi deficiency, and may also be a key indicator for heart qi deficiency. When there is an exterior condition, sweating indicates a deficiency of *wei* qi, while the absence of sweat may indicate a cold condition causing contraction of the pores. Sweating that occurs at night or on the palms, soles of the feet and the center of the chest (five-heart heat) is an indication of yin deficiency. Clammy and often foul-smelling perspiration may indicate damp-heat, while oily sweat points to yang collapse, which is a serious condition.

Sweating	
easily sweats or spontaneously	qi deficiency
with an exterior condition	deficiency

Sweating	
oily sweating	yang collapse
at night	yin deficiency
palms, soles, chest	yin deficiency
overall	damp-heat
no sweating	exterior cold

4) Inquiry should include all of sense organs of smell, taste, hearing and vision. Dizziness, headaches or stiffness should also be noted.

Headache	
chronic	internal
severe	excess
dull	deficiency
sharp	blood stasis
worse with fatigue	qi deficiency
heavy, like a wet towel around the head	dampness
vertex	liver

5) If there are problems with a particular area of the body, the associated channels and collaterals and their internal divergences should be closely examined for clues as to the specific location of the disease.

Location		Location	
lower body	yin predominance	redness in face, upper body	heat
upper body	yang predominance	broad areas of body	tendino-muscular channels

6) The practitioner should inquire about defecation and urination. Constipation may be indicative of food and qi stagnation, heat, yin deficiency and/or qi deficiency. Foul-smelling stools may indicate internal heat, while loose stools usually indicate spleen qi deficiency. Deep-yellow urine indicates heat, while profuse clear urine indicates cold. Frequent urination can be a symptom of kidney deficiency.

Urination	
incontinence	kidney qi deficiency
incomplete urination	qi deficiency, yang deficiency or dampness
painful urination	damp-heat in the bladder, blood stasis
pale urine	cold
yellow urine	heat
frequent urination	kidney deficiency
Defecation	
constipation with heat	heat in the stomach and large intestine
small stools	liver qi constraint
alternating loose stools and constipation	liver qi constraint

Defecation	
chronic diarrhea	yang deficiency
foul-smelling stools	heat
early morning diarrhea	kidney yang deficiency
improvement after defecation	excess condition
diarrhea after meals	spleen qi deficiency
dry stools	blood deficiency, heat, yin deficiency
diarrhea with odor	damp-heat

7) Ears, eyes, tastes and smells

Eyes		Eyes	
twitching	liver wind	redness	heat
yellow sclera	damp-heat	itching	blood deficiency
Ears		**Ears**	
muffled sounds	phlegm	gradual chronic tinnitus	kidney deficiency
sudden deafness	excess		

Tastes in the Mouth	
bitter	liver-gallbladder heat
sweet	spleen qi deficiency or dampness
sour	food retention
salty	kidney yin deficiency
pungent	lung heat
metallic	intestinal problems
lack of taste	spleen deficiency
Thirst	
dry mouth with desire to drink	yin deficiency
thirst with no desire to drink	dampness
strong thirst for cold fluids	heat
lack of thirst or desire for warm fluids	cold
Body and Excretion Smells	
foul	heat
odorless	qi stagnation or deficiency
sour and foul	stomach heat, food stagnation
mild fishy odor	cold and dampness

8) One should ask about any special circumstances regarding the health of the mother during the person's gestation, the mother's labor, and breastfeeding. Inquiry may include vaccinations and infectious diseases contracted during childhood and adulthood.

9) Inquiry into sleep is very important for assessing the overall state of qi and blood and the yin/yang balance. Sleep quality can be a direct reflection of heart and kidney function.

Sleep	
nightmares	liver constraint, heart fire, food stagnation
waking often	kidney or heart deficiency
difficulty falling asleep	heart blood deficiency, liver stagnation

10) Women's questions

For a woman, the regularity, quantity, consistency and color of the menses and the length of the cycle, as well as concurrent symptoms such as cramps, headache, constipation or diarrhea, insomnia, moodiness, etc. can reflect the functional state of the blood and the liver. Premenstrual syndrome (PMS) is generally associated with liver qi stagnation, pain before menstruation is a sign of blood stasis, and fatigue following menstruation points to blood deficiency.

Menstruation and Gynecology (妇科, *Fù Kē*)	
early menstruation	heat in the blood or spleen deficiency
late menstruation	blood stasis, deficiency, cold
irregular menstruation	liver qi stagnation
profuse menses	heat in the blood or spleen deficiency
scanty menses	blood stasis, qi constraint, deficiency, cold
premenstrual headaches	blood stasis
headaches after menstruation	blood deficiency
Menses	
bright red	heat
dark red	heat and/or stasis
clots	blood stasis or cold
Leukorrhea and Vaginal Discharge	
white	cold
yellow	heat

Associated symptoms

Sexual Function	
no desire	yang deficiency, qi stagnation
rapid sexual desire and quick excitation	yin deficiency
strong desire but not satisfied	yang excess
adequate desire but inadequate performance	qi stagnation
Emotions	
agitation	yin deficiency
anger	fire
frustration	qi stagnation
apathy	qi deficiency
sadness	lung qi deficiency
confusion	phlegm

CHIEF COMPLAINT

The chief complaint is interpreted as the patient's main reason for coming to the clinic. Often times the chief complaint will be the same as the disease itself, as with diarrhea for example. Some patients will have many specific complaints, some will describe only a vague discomfort or emotional difficulties, and others feel fine and simply want to maintain their well-being. Often times there will be two or more "chief complaints". If there is a litany of complaints, the practitioner will either endeavor to tie them together under a single cause or try to focus the treatment approach upon one or two main issues. With multiple complaints, it is often unrealistic to expect them all to be addressed within a single acupuncture session or with a single herbal formula. However, multiple complaints are many times the result of a single condition with various complications. For example, food stagnation may result in constipation, fatigue, insomnia, depression, breathlessness and/or headache.

The patient's chief complaint and signs and symptoms are not always the same as the root of the disease. Treating the symptoms may satisfy the patient in the short-term, yet the disease will recur if the root is not treated as well. Of course, some complaints are not serious in nature, i.e. there is no ongoing pathology and they can be cured relatively easily. Other symptomatic complaints may seem superficial, yet they can reveal other underlying and potentially serious diseases and patterns. In such cases, the root of the disease should be treated simultaneously along with the symptoms (branch).

Clinical Reasoning in Chinese Medicine says, "On the basis of the patient's complaint and the doctor's understanding of the disease condition, the doctor should first inquire about the main symptom with a well thought out plan in mind, and then make a complete analysis of the collected information and form an initial judgment, which is of course, still subject to reconsideration. Afterward, the doctor should form a second conclusion on the basis of the patient's chief complaint and accompanying symptoms that are revealed in the pulse, tongue and facial complexion through careful examination. Finally, the doctor should combine the two assessments and make a general diagnosis. Sometimes the first and second conclusions are consistent, and sometimes they are not."[1]

In accordance with the scope of this book, this chapter has touched only briefly on the many aspects of Chinese medical diagnosis. However, an understanding of the origins and progression of illness as introduced here is required before any diagnosis or treatment can be rendered. Furthermore, the material in this chapter serves as an essential prerequisite for the advanced study of diagnosis as a major part of any comprehensive Chinese medicine curriculum.

---

[1] Hu Zhen, Dong Fei-xia. *Clinical Reasoning in Chinese Medicine.* Beijing: People's Medical Publishing House; 2008. p. 20.

Chapter 10

Channel and Collateral Theory

The theories of channels and collaterals touch on all aspects of human physiology, pathology, diagnosis, prevention and treatment of disease. Being associated with theories of the organs, essence-qi-blood-fluids, etiology, and pathomechanisms, it explains the physiological activity and pathological changes of the human body. For these reasons, an understanding of the theories of the channels and collaterals is essential for various Chinese medical clinical practices and not only for acupuncture and moxibustion, tui na or qi gong.

This system is known in Chinese as the *jīng luò*. *Jīng* (经), connotes the warp or the long threads of the fabric on a carpet loom. *Luò* (络) means net or network. The sense is that the *luò* extends across and ties together the *jīng*/channels. The *jīng* run vertically while the *luò* run crossways. One image is of cloth with the weave and warp of fabric.

Channel and collateral theory concerns the relationships between the organ system, the nine orifices (nostrils, eyes, ears, mouth, anus and urinary opening), essence-qi-blood-fluids, and the spirit. The channels consist of several interlocking systems while the collaterals are smaller branches coming out of the main channels. The 12 main channels of the channel system (and the *du* and *ren*) are those most often pictured on acupuncture charts. The collateral system is less well known and understood even if ancient writings about it predate those of the 12 main channels. While it would seem the physicality of the channels and collaterals should make them easier aspects of fundamental theory to understand, the opposite is often true. The understanding of the channels and collaterals comes from ancient and often obtuse phrases dated to the first Chinese medical writings and the 12 main channels have only for the last 1200 years been (more or less) agreed upon. *The Spiritual Pivot* states, "The beginners start at the twelve channels and the masters end up there. To beginners, it often seems easy but the masters know how difficult it can be. "

Introduction

To set the stage, we should introduce the components of the channel-collateral system, called the "*jīng luò*" (经络). The 12 main (*zhèng*, 正) channels are the "*jīng*" (经). Parts of these channels (along with the midline *ren* and *du*) are what is being pictured in a simple acupuncture chart. The 12 main channels each have branches coming off of them to go to their and other organs to spread their influence throughout the body. Therefore, related to the 12 main channels are a set of channels called "divergent" channels (*jīng bié*, 经别) that explicitly communicate between the *zang* and *fu* related organs themselves. They are grouped into 6 pairs (convergences) to match their related *zang-fu* organs (such as the lung to the large intestine).

The collaterals (*luò*, 络) are major networks of the body and can often be seen on the surface of the body. As an example, some types of collaterals are thought to be what can be viewed on the feet and hands as veins. The collaterals have 3 types: 1) The "fifteen collaterals" branch out from the 12 main channels (these are not the same as the branches of the main channels), the *du mai* and the *ren mai* and a special "major collateral of the spleen"; 2) The superficial collaterals run on the surface of the body and 3) other "minute" collaterals are the smallest of the collaterals.

In addition to the above channels, there are the sinew channels (*jīng jīn*, 经筋) and the cutaneous regions (*pí bù*, 皮部) which cover large areas of the main body. The sinew channels (often called "musculo-tendinous channels") connect and move the bones and joints of the body. Neither the sinew channels nor cutaneous regions have their own acupuncture points.

The eight extraordinary channels/vessels (*qí jīng bā mài*, 奇经八脉) have larger influences on the body. These are referred to as "vessels" and encompass and run between the other channels to serve as "reservoirs" of qi and blood. The *ren mai* and *du mai* extraordinary vessels run on the center of the front and back of the body and are vital enough to be pictured on all acupuncture charts. Because of their importance, we often refer to the "14 main channels".

All of the above constitute what is called the "channels and collateral system".

Deadman and Al-Khafaji write, "Whilst a typical chart of the acupuncture channels, therefore, illustrates only the superficial pathways of the twelve primary channels, we should remember that the channel network is considerably more complex than this, and there is no part of the body, no kind of tissue, no single cell, that is not supplied by the channels."[1]

---

[1] Peter Deadman, Kevin Baker, Mazin Al-Khafaji. *A Manual of Acupuncture*. East Essex:Journal of Chinese Medicine; 1998. p. 11.

Section 1   Channels and Collaterals

THE THEORY OF CHANNELS AND COLLATERALS

The channel and collateral system facilitates communication between the organs, the different areas of the body and the five sense organs.[1] It establishes communication between the upper and lower parts of the body as well as from the interior to the more external areas of the body. It enables information from the environment to be transmitted inwards to the body as well as to allow reactions to these stimuli. The meridian system is made up these channels and collaterals which link all parts of the body.

The channels are the major passageways to transport qi and blood, and the collaterals are branches of the channels that function to distribute qi and blood to all the various body locations. In order to function well, channels and collaterals themselves also need to get their nourishment from qi and blood. It is this transporting and distributing action that makes it possible for qi and blood to nourish the organs internally as well as moisten and nourish the surface of the body. When these physiological functions are working well, the body has its own natural power to resist invasion of external and internal pathogens.

Like the trunk of a tree or a river, the channels form the main route of a vast system and the major passageway of information and nutrients. Collaterals mean liaison and network. Being the branches of channels, they criss-cross to network the body.

It is important to remember that the channels and collaterals are not just lines on an acupuncture chart. Not only do the channels dip deep into the body, the channels can be described as areas of influence of body processes. Others may try to conceive of the channels not as tubes or pipes that carry qi but as "qi itself" or the process of carrying information which also facilitates the carrying of blood.

Dr. Wang Ju-yi talks about two ways to look at the channels. His first concept is of "spaces within the fibrous connective tissues of the body". His second insight expands on the river and canal paradigm that is often used for acupuncture. He describes the channels as "like a river in that it includes the riverbanks and also the complexity of life within the water itself held by those banks".[2]

Although different, the channels and collaterals are closely connected and together they form a complex system which functions to circulate qi and blood,

---

[1] 五官 —the ears, eyes, nose, tongue and lips - together they are referred to as *wǔ guān* or the five officials.

[2] Ju-yi Wang, Jason D. Roberston. *Applied Channel Theory in Chinese Medicine.* Seattle: Eastland Press; 2008.

communicate with the five-*zang* and the six-*fu* organs, the four limbs and the skeleton, the five sense organs and the nine orifices, the skin, sinews and vessels. Therefore, they are what is needed to create the conditions for a fully integrated, well-functioning person.

The Channels as a "Communication System"

The channel and collateral system can react to and conduct information from all kinds of stimuli (including acupuncture, acupressure and moxibustion). Channel qi is a kind of qi that is distributed into the channels and collaterals. The function of channel qi is to accept, carry and transmit information. By accepting and conveying the information of channel qi, various therapeutic stimuli and information can regulate disharmony. For example, needling the acupuncture point, ST 36 (*zú sān lǐ*, 足三里) on the foot *yangming* stomach channel can regulate the function of gastric peristalsis and secretion. A slight stimulation when there is gastric under-functioning may enhance the constriction of stomach and increase the concentration of gastric juice. A heavy stimulation when there is a hyperactive condition of the stomach may produce an inhibiting effect. As another example, needling PC 6 (*nèi guān*, 内关) may accelerate the heart beat for treating bradycardia (slowed heart rate) under some conditions, and inhibit the heart rate for treating tachycardia (fast heart rate) under other conditions. It thus can be seen that the actions of the channel and collateral system can regulate what was hyperactive to be inhibited and what was inhibited to be excited. This is a beneficial dual regulation, and has important significance in acupuncture and moxibustion, and tui na massage therapy.

The reaction and conduction induced by stimulation of the points is generally called the "arrival of qi". This can be a sensation of aching, numbness and distension that may transmit along the channel. The channel and collateral's reactions are made possible through the reception and conveyance of information from channel-qi. The channels run and distribute among the organs like an information network. They can transmit and accept information throughout the body, according to the nature, characteristics and qualities of the relevant organs and body areas.

This conduction of information occurs both between the organs and orifices and between the body surface and the organs, so as to coordinate every process of the activity of human life. When the body surface is stimulated by moxibustion, acupuncture or massage, the information will be accepted and carried by the channel-qi, and transmitted to the relevant organs along the channels, producing an effect based on the differences of the information in nature and intensity. The information on functional activities and pathological changes of the organs may also be accepted and transmitted to the body surface along the channels, collaterals, channel sinews, and cutaneous regions, presenting different symptoms and signs. This is the chief physiological basis for the phenomenon of internal changes that manifest externally and for the basis of acupuncture treatment.

The Channels and Acupuncture

It would be impossible to fully describe the importance of channels in one book, let alone one chapter. The channels are an obvious cornerstone to all aspects of Chinese medicine including acupuncture, tui na massage and acupressure as well as to herbology. The earliest books concerned themselves with channels if only in rather generalized terms. The Mawangdui manuscripts from 200 BC says, "Foot Great Yang (*yangming*) vessel. It emerges in the hollow by the outer malleolus. Ascending, it penetrates the calf and emerges by the poples. A branch at the lower part of the center of the forehead goes to the ear. The direct path penetrates the inner canthus of the eye and goes to the nose."[1]

The channels are pathways for the use of acupuncture points and the functions of the points and their practical usage have evolved over the thousands of years[2]. Early treatments consisted mainly of bleeding points or "cauterizing" them using direct heat moxibustion on the body. As technology improved, metal needles evolved from stone ones. There are countless contemporary acupuncture techniques used today but modern acupuncture treatments, no matter what their tradition, have undoubtably evolved significantly from their roots.

An acupuncture treatment can be as varied as there are acupuncture practitioners. In general, we can say that a single treatment may employ as few as one needle to more than fifty. These points can be selected by the function or the indication of the acupuncture points. The function might include "descending liver yang" while the indication may be "for headache and pain". A treatment may be based on the channels where, for example, ST 44 (*nèi tíng*, 内庭) on the foot is needled for toothache because the stomach channel passes through the area of the teeth. No less important are the channel sinews that cover large areas of the body but have no distinct acupuncture points themselves. They are commonly used in the treatment of muscular pain.

Some points have specialized indications. For example, GB 37 (*guāng míng*, 光明) on the lower leg is used for many eye problems. "*Yi shu*" on the back is a special point that treats diabetes, no doubt because its physical location is located near the pancreas.[3] SP 6 (*sān yīn jiāo*, 三阴交) is a widely used point on the lower leg because it treats a number of *zang*-organ issues, no doubt because the liver, kidney and spleen

---

① *Early Chinese Medical Literature, the Mawangdui Medical Manuscripts*, Donald Harper. p. 193.

② Acupuncture, acupressure, massage and moxa points are in the same locations and share the names.

③ *A Manual of Acupuncture* states, "This point, nowadays known as "*yí shù*" (Pancreas Shu) was first mentioned in the Thousand Ducat Formulas. It was recommended by Sun Si-miao for wasting and thirsting disorder (i.e. diabetes mellitus) and the accompanying symptoms of dryness of the throat."

channels cross here. As stated above, most acupuncture treatments use several points together. Randy Barolet in the *Journal of Chinese Medicine* writes, "For constipation within the context of Deficiency of both Qi and Yin, we may choose REN-6, *Qi hai* along with Sanyinjiao (Spleen 6) in order to reinforce the Qi and nourish the Yin, thus 'increasing the water to move the boat'."[1] The ability to choose elegant point combinations that decrease the number of needles is the goal of many practitioners.

COMPOSITION OF THE CHANNEL AND COLLATERAL SYSTEM

The connections between the organs and the orifices are achieved through the channels and collaterals. For example, the hand *yangming* channel "goes by the mouth" and the foot *yangming* channel "runs by the mouth", and curves around the lips. The *chong mai, ren mai* and *du mai* all "descend and emerge at the perineum". Thus the channel system helps the organs to communicate with the orifices through the channels and collaterals so as to form a whole. The physiological functions (and pathologies) of the organs also manifest at the orifices because of the channel system.

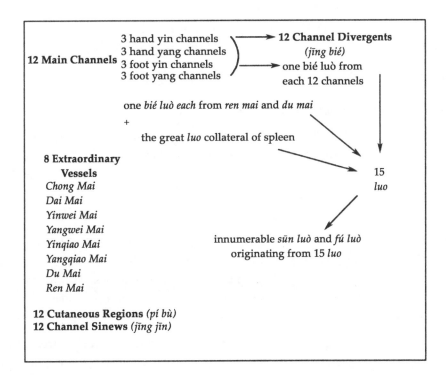

---

① Randy Barolet. The Clinical Application of the Point Sanyinjiao. Journal of Chinese Medicine. Sept 1983;3.

We see that the foot *shaoyin* kidney channel is not only affiliated to the kidney and connects with the bladder, but through its branches also passes through the liver, enters the lung, links with the heart, and goes into the thorax to link with the pericardium. The foot *jueyin* liver channel, besides being affiliated to the liver and connecting with the gallbladder, again runs by the stomach, and goes into the lung, etc. In addition, there are channel divergences that supplement the main channels. For example, the divergences of the foot *yangming*, *shaoyang* and *taiyang* channels all pass through the heart.

Twelve Channels (*Shí Èr Jīng Mài*, 十二经脉)

The twelve channels are the core of the channel and collateral system. The twelve channel divergences and collaterals in the system all branch out from them and communicate and cooperate with each other. More information about the twelve channels are described in Section 2 of this chapter.

Eight Extraordinary Vessels (*Qí Jīng Bā Mài*, 奇经八脉)

Although not directly connected with the main channels, the eight extraordinary vessels form "reservoirs" of surplus qi and blood of the main channels. These vessels are the *du mai, ren mai, chong mai, dai mai, yinqiao mai, yangqiao mai, yinwei mai,* and *yangwei mai*. They communicate with the twelve channels and regulate the qi and blood within them. More information about the twelve channels are described in Section 3 of this chapter.

Channel Divergences (*Jīng Bié*, 经别)

The twelve channel divergences (divergents) are major branches which diverge from their associated channels at the arms and legs. They enhance the connection and supplementation of the external-internally related channels in the twelve channels after entering the body cavities.

> Because of their names, students often become confused about the difference between the channel divergences (*jīng bié*, 经别) and the divergent collaterals (*bié luò*, 别络). The channel divergences are considered "deeper" of the two and through the channels meet the organs themselves. The divergent collaterals are more superficial and tie together channels.

The channel divergences originate in the superficial or exterior areas and then plunge deeply into the body to meet with the organs. Most of the channel divergences, after entering the thoracic and abdominal cavities, also link with the organs of their own and those of their interior-exterior related channel. For example, the foot *shaoyang* gallbladder channel divergence "links with the gallbladder and spreads in the liver".

As another example, the foot *yangming* stomach channel divergence "links with the stomach and spreads in the spleen".[①]

The six yang channels travel to the head and face but the six yin main channels do not go directly to the head. Instead they join through the divergences with the yang channels. The divergences of the three foot yin channels ascend to the head after they join yang channels, and the divergences of the three hand yin channels all pass through the throat, then join the yang channels and then run up to the head and face.

The channel divergences of both the three foot yin and yang channels run up through the abdomen and chest. Besides strengthening the communication between the *zang-* and *fu-* organs in the abdominal cavity, they all link with the heart in the chest.

The pathways of the twelve channel divergences make the distribution of the twelve channels more extensive, thus enlarging the indication range for the points of the twelve channels. For example, the foot *taiyang* bladder channel does not reach the anus (large intestine organ), but its divergence does. Therefore points of the bladder channel, such as BL 57 (*chéng shān*, 承山), found on the leg calf, can be used to treat hemorrhoids. The divergences explain many of the more perplexing and esoteric functions of certain acupuncture points.

Collaterals (*Luò Mài*, 络脉)

Collaterals are branches and are divided into divergent collaterals (*bié luò*, 别络), superficial/floating collaterals (*fú luò*, 浮络) and minute collaterals (*sūn luò*, 孙络). Divergent collaterals are larger and travel from the main channel into the adjacent channel, to reinforce the connection between the two external-internally related channels. They also serve to supplement the main channels by communicating with the other yin and yang collaterals. The superficial collaterals lie below the skin while the minute collaterals are the smallest of all the collaterals. Thus the collaterals as a whole go to places where the main channels do not reach and thus extend the influences of the main channels.

Divergent collaterals (*bié luò*, 别络)

Divergent collaterals are the largest of the three types of collaterals. The twelve main divergent collaterals branch from the main channels to go to their interior-exterior related channel. For example, the lung divergent collateral travels to the large intestine main channel. These collateral connections between the yin and yang (interior-exterior) related channels may occur near the surface of the body but then continue and often travel deeper into the body.

---

① Note that there is a specific vocabulary here of "linking", "communicating" and "spreading" etc... that will be largely unexplored in this fundamentals book.

The divergent collaterals mainly distribute on the surface of the body. There are 15 of divergent collaterals made up of the 12 main channels and the *ren mai* and *du mai* plus the large collateral of the spleen channel. (In addition, some texts include the stomach great collateral making 16 in total.)

The divergent collateral of the *du mai* spreads over the back and its qi also spreads over the head, and connects with the *taiyang* channel. The divergent collateral of the *ren mai* spreads over the abdomen. The larger collateral of the spleen channel spreads through the thoracic and hypochondriac region.[1]

Huang-Fu Mi in *The Systematic Classic of Acupuncture and Moxibustion (Zhēn Jiǔ Jiǎ Yǐ Jīng*, 针灸甲乙经) states, "The (main) channels typically cannot be seen… The vessels which can be seen are the network vessels (*luò mài*). None of these network vessels pass through the major joints. They travel along paths which are inaccessible (to the channels), coming and going (to connect with the primary channels) and spreading throughout the skin. The places where these (network vessels) meet one another may be observed on the exterior of the body."[2]

Minute collaterals (*sūn luò*, 孙络)

The minute collaterals branch out from the divergent collaterals and are the thinnest and smallest of the collaterals. They distribute throughout the body and are innumerable. The minute collaterals function to dispel external pathogens and to regulate the *ying* and *wei*.

Superficial collaterals (*fú luò*, 浮络)

Superficial or "floating" collaterals, as the name suggests run superficially on the surface of the body. They distribute widely and do not have fixed regions. The superficial collaterals communicate with the channels and transport qi and blood to the surface of the body.

The minute and superficial collaterals, branch again and again, to become increasingly thinner. Their channel qi also gets weaker gradually and are distributed in a network throughout the body. By the distributing action of the qi and blood circulating in the channels, channel qi flows into the minute and superficial collaterals, and further moistens and nourishes the body.

Convergences (*Hé*, 合)

The six pairs of externally-internally related channels are grouped in what

---

[1]   In many texts "the large collateral of the stomach channel" is omitted making the "fifteen divergent collaterals".

[2]   Huang-Fu Mi. *The Systematic Classic of Acupuncture and Moxibustion (Zhēn Jiǔ Jiǎ Yǐ Jīng*, 针灸甲乙经) trans: Shou-zhong Yang and Charles Chace. Boulder: Blue Poppy; 1994. p. 49.

is called the 6 "convergences". The convergences tell us where exactly channel divergences meet with their interior and exterior channels. Each pair of divergent external-internally related channels consists of "a confluence" or a joining of two channel divergences, thus the twelve channel divergences are divided into six pairs of the hand and foot channels.

The First Convergence - foot *taiyang* and *shaoyin* divergents (bladder and kidney)

The Second Convergence - foot *shaoyang* and *jueyin* divergents (gallbladder and liver)

The Third Convergence - foot *yangming* and *taiyin* divergents (stomach and spleen)

The Fourth Convergence - hand *taiyang* and *shaoyin* divergents (small intestine and heart)

The Fifth Convergence - hand *shaoyang* and *jueyin* divergents (*sanjiao* and pericardium)

The Sixth Convergence - hand *yangming* and *taiyin* divergents (large intestine and lung)

Sinew and Cutaneous Systems (*Jīng Jīn Pí Bù*, 经筋皮部)

Channel sinews

The channel sinews are the systems of the tendons, muscles and joints where the qi of the twelve channels "gather, converge, distribute and connect." They are affiliated with the twelve channels and link the four limbs and bones, communicate throughout the body, and control the motion of the joints. They are nourished and regulated by the qi and blood of the twelve channels.

The channel sinews often attach to the bones and the joints and link the bones together and control the motion of the joints. As the *Basic Questions* said, "All sinews are in charge of linking up the bones and controlling the smooth motion of the joints." The channel sinews also distribute over the trunk and the superficial parts of the four limbs and therefore playing a certain role in protecting the organs and other tissues throughout the body.

The distribution of the twelve channel sinews follows the routes of the twelve channels on the body surface. They generally travel to the limbs, going from the ends of the limbs to the trunk and head. They travel on the body surface and gather in the regions around the joints and bones. The channel sinews of the three hand and foot yang channels distribute themselves on the lateral aspects of the limbs, while the channel sinews of the three hand and foot yin channels distribute on the medial aspects of the limbs. Some of them also enter the thoracic or abdominal cavity yet they usually do not enter the organs. Their pathways can be summarized by "gathering, converging, distribution and connection". This means the twelve channel sinews start at the ends of limb and gather around the joints, distribute in the chest and back, and terminate at the trunk or head.

Cutaneous regions

Cutaneous regions are the superficial regions of the body and reflect the functional activities of the twelve channels. Qi from the channels spread over the body through the cutaneous regions. The areas of the twelve cutaneous regions are based on the areas at which the twelve channels distribute in the body surface. The surface of the body is divided into twelve parts based on the twelve channels. The channel sinews and cutaneous regions do not have their own acupuncture points and are often used for relieving muscle pain and strains.

The cutaneous regions depend upon nourishing and moistening by the qi and blood of the twelve channels and their collaterals. The skin is the most superficial part of the body and is directly exposed to the outside environment. The skin regulates the body to adapt the changes of outside environment, and plays a role to resist external pathogens by *wei* qi which spreads over the body surface. Inspecting the color and luster, and physical change of the cutaneous regions of the skin is helpful for diagnosing disorders of the organs and channels and collaterals. Therapeutic methods like moxibustion, cupping, *guasha* and plum-blossom needling[①] used on the skin are then often used for diseases of the internal organs.

APPLICATIONS OF CHANNEL AND COLLATERAL THEORY

Functions of Channels and Collaterals

Channel and collateral theory not only explains body functions, but is also valuable in explaining pathological changes, and guides the diagnosis and treatment of disease. The channel and collateral system can communicate, regulate, react and transport information. By this we mean that the system can circulate qi and blood to nourish the organs, body areas and orifices. Pathogens can also transmit along these channels and collaterals and it is through this same channel system that the body

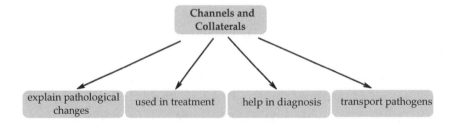

---

① Plum-blossom needling groups a number of very small needles on a stick which is then lightly tapped on the skin to produce small spots of redness and/or bleeding.

resists pathogens.

When pathogenic evils (*xie* qi) invade the body surface, they can go through the channels and collaterals from the exterior to the interior, from the superficial parts to the deeper parts and transmit inwards until they eventually invade the organs. For example, at the beginning of an invasion of an external pathogen on the body surface, a patient can have fever and aversion to cold, body pains and headaches. These are some general symptoms of invasion of the *taiyang* bladder channel. If the external pathogen is not eliminated, it can penetrate into the lung and create cough, chest distress and pain. Because of the connection between the lung and the large intestine channels, the patient may also have abdomen pain, diarrhea or constipation. The treatment at the beginning of a *taiyang* invasion might be to use points on the *taiyang* channel as well as use cupping and *gua sha* (scraping) on the upper back where the *taiyang* channel travels.

Organ disorders can also manifest externally to the channels and collaterals. For example, the foot *jueyin* liver channel curves round the external genitalia, goes to the lower abdomen, spreads over the rib region, and links with the eyes[1]. Therefore, "liver qi constraint" can cause pain below the rib-sides (hypochondrium), or "liver fire flaming upward" to cause red eyes, or create "damp-heat in the channel" which can cause pruritus of the vulva. Another example would be that the foot *yangming* stomach channel which goes into the upper gums of the mouth and the hand *yangming* large intestine channel into the lower gums. Gingival swelling and pain may show up in these channels when heat accumulates in the gastrointestinal tract. This is what allows us to use acupuncture points on the foot *jueyin* liver or foot *yangming* stomach channels in the above cases.

Because the channels of the organs also communicate with each other, a disorder from one organ may transmit into another organ through the channels. For example, the foot *jueyin* channel is affiliated with the liver and runs by the stomach, so a liver disorder may affect the stomach. The foot *jueyin* liver channel also enters the lung, so fire from the liver can invade the lung. As another example, the hand *shaoyin* heart and hand *taiyang* small intestine channels are connected by interior and exterior organs and heart heat may transmit down to the small intestine to cause yellow or bloody urine.

The channels begin and end at definite regions of the body then pass through their related organ, so a disorder of an internal organ may be reflected in these corresponding regions. Many acupuncture practitioners are adept at the art of palpating (touching) the channels to find problems of the corresponding organs. These practitioners feel for tenderness and tightness, temperature or look for

---

[1] Certain cancers of the eyes correlate to a high propensity for liver cancer.

changes of color on the pathway of a channel. These pathological changes may be helpful to diagnose disease as well as guide where the needles should be used.[1]

Often diagnosis begins by differentiating the channel where the problem occurs. A headache on the forehead is usually associated with the *yangming* stomach channel, pain of the lateral sides with the *shaoyang* gallbladder, a pain in the occipital region and nape with the *taiyang* urinary channel, a pain on the vertex with the *jueyin* liver channel. As a further example, a pain of the upper tooth indicates a foot *yangming* channel disorder, and pain of the lower tooth indicates a hand *yangming* channel disorder. In addition, six-channel pattern differentiation in *Treatise on Cold Damage* is also based on channel and collateral theory.

There are other applications of channel theory in diagnosis, such as collateral examination, pediatric inspection of the fingers, and inspection of the ears. Cold or heat, deficiency or excess may also be judged through examination of the channel. For example, red spots often appear on the channel route of an organ that has heat.

Clinical Applications

The channel and collateral theory is widely used to guide the treatment of diseases of various clinical departments; it is the theoretical basis for acupuncture, moxibustion, tui na and prescribing herbs.

The principles of combining acupuncture points in a treatment are also guided by the channel and collateral theory. Since the channels create a complicated network, there are many versatile and complex principles for selecting points. The commonly used are: selection of points based on the channel affected, combining points from the interior-exteriorly related channels, combining "back-*shu*" and "front-*mu*" points, transporting points, as well as some special point combinations.

Points that are most commonly used are those on the channel on which the problem is diagnosed. It would be rare to have a treatment of the spleen, for example, that did not use some spleen points. In treating pain and especially musculoskeletal pain, following the channel is almost always used. If there is shoulder pain we can use a point exactly on the site of the pain, called an *ashi* point. We might then follow the musculo-tendo channel down the arm, "downstream" to lead the pain out. If the shoulder hurts more on the back, we might use the *taiyang* small intestine channel but if on the front, then the *yangming* large intestine channel. If the pain is muscular, we

---

[1] Wang Ju-Yi writes, "... the process of channel palpation provides a measuring stick by which patient progress can be gauged: as the patient improves, the channels will change. Thickness and hardness will soften, weakness may become more firm, and nodules may dissipate. " Ju-yi Wang, Jason D. Roberston. *Applied Channel Theory in Chinese Medicine*. Seattle: Eastland Press; 2008. p. 45.

are not as concerned about named acupuncture points but rather appropriate spots on the muscular level on the broader sinew channels.

We can treat a headache by local points but if the headache is on the side of the head and on the *shaoyang* gallbladder channel, then we can also use GB 41 (*zú lín qì*, 足临泣) which is towards the end of the channel on the foot. A special point for generalized pain conditions is LI4 (*hé gǔ*, 合谷) on the hand. If the headache is due to stress caused by liver qi constraint then a point or two on the liver channel may also be used. We can see that just one symptom can quickly build a "point formula" of several acupuncture points.

In English language texts, we often write about the channels as organs. For example, we say the "large intestine channel" while in Chinese texts this is more often expressed as the "hand *yangming* channel". This channel designation gives a more direct rationality to needling the foot *yangming* (stomach) channel for issues that involve the large intestine organ and channel (hand *yangming*). Students are therefore, once again, encouraged to learn the channel designations by the hand *yangming*, foot *shaoyang*, foot *taiyang* etc…

Points may also be used that are on the opposite channel of the interior-exterior (yin and yang) relationship. The most obvious example of this is using stomach foot *yangming* points for issues of the spleen organ since the stomach is the "exterior" organ to the "interior" spleen. The interior-exterior relationship is hardly arbitrary and we see many diseases that are closely related by this pairing. Some symptoms of anxiety for example, can be related to the gallbladder but are effectively treated by using liver channel points.

Special Points on the Channels

The organs also have special front and back acupuncture points called front-*mu* and back-*shu* points. The back-*shu* points are located on the back on the foot *taiyang* bladder channel. For example, the heart back-*shu* point is located at BL 15 (*xīn shù*, 心俞) on the back at the level of the heart. The front-*shu* points are located on the front of the body except one (GB 25, *jīng mén*, 京门). The front-*shu* points also treat the organs to which they are related but not especially the channel to which they belong.[1] The back-*shu* and front-*mu* points can therefore be seen as more directly targeting the organs and often have powerful effects.

---

[1] Peter Deadman, Kevin Baker, Mazin Al-Khafaji. *A Manual of Acupuncture*. East Essex: Journal of Chinese Medicine; 1998. p. 42.

Organ	Time	Channel	Source	Luo-connecting	Xi-cleft	Front-mu	Back-shu
LU	3-5 AM	Hand *taiyin*	LU 9	LU 7	LU 6	LU 1	BL 13
LI	5-7 AM	Hand *yangming*	LI 4	LI 6	LI 7	ST 25	BL 25
ST	7-9 AM	Foot *yangming*	ST 42	ST 40	ST 34	RN 12	BL 21
SP	9-11 AM	Foot *taiyin*	SP 3	SP 4	SP 8	LV 13	BL 20
HT	11-1 PM	Hand *shaoyin*	HT 3	HT 5	Ht 6	RN 14	BL 15
SI	1-3 PM	Hand *taiyang*	SI 4	SI 7	SI 6	RN 4	BL 27
BL	3-5 PM	Foot *taiyang*	BL 64	BL 58	BL 63	RN 3	BL 28
KI	5-7 PM	Foot *shaoyin*	K 3	K 4	K 5	GB 25	BL 23
PC	7-9 PM	Hand *jueyin*	PC 7	PC 6	PC 4	RN 17	BL 14
SJ	9-11 PM	Hand *shaoyang*	SJ 4	SJ 5	SJ 7	RN 5	BL 22
GB	11-1 AM	Foot *shaoyang*	GB 40	GB 37	GB 36	GB 24	BL 19
LV	1-3 AM	Foot *jueyin*	LV 3	LV 5	LV 6	LV 14	BL 18

Xi-cleft points (xī xué, 郄穴)

Xi-cleft points are used to move blood and stop pain on the channels in which they are found. For example, LV 6 (*zhōng dū*, 中都), the *xi*-cleft point of the liver channel, can be used to stop hernia pain.

Transporting points (*wǔ shū xué*, 五输穴)

Transporting points were mentioned in the five phases section of this book. Each of the channels has points with one of the five phases attached to it. These points are generally located on the fingers, arms, toes or leg. This group of points has been translated in various ways and includes transporting, antique, 5 element and *t'sing* points. This is a very complex system but some principles can be stated briefly.

Each of the transporting points has a designation of well, spring, stream, river and sea. The well points are located on or towards the ends of the fingers and toes while the sea points are located nearest the body when compared with the others, usually near the knees or elbows. The well points on the yin channels are wood and on the yang channels are metal. The element moves in order of the generating cycle so that the second spring point of a yin channel will be "fire", the stream is earth, the river is metal and the sea is considered water. On the yang channels, the well point is metal, the spring is water, the stream is wood, the river is fire and the sea point is earth. When a point is the same element on the same channel, then this is usually referred to as a "horary" point (for example, if a metal point is on a metal channel). Horary points are considered particularly powerful.

In addition, there are a few "lower *he*-sea" points that help directly connect the large intestine, small intestines and urinary bladder organs to points on the leg.

Organ	Jing-well wood/yin metal/yang 井穴	Ying-spring fire/yin water/yang 荣穴	Shu-stream earth/yin wood/yang 输穴	Jing-river metal/yin fire/yang 经穴	He-sea water/yin earth/yang 合穴	Lower He-sea 下合穴
LU	11	10	9	8	5	
LI	1	2	3	5	11	ST 37
ST	45	44	43	41	36	
SP	1	2	4	5	9	
HT	9	8	7	4	3	
SI	9	1	2	3	5	ST 39
BL	67	66	65	60	40	
KI	1	2	3	7	10	
PC	9	8	7	5	3	
SJ	1	2	3	6	10	BL 39
GB	44	43	41	38	34	
LV	1	2	3	4	8	

Yuan/source points (yuán xué, 原穴)

The yuan/source points are where the yuan qi gathers. Because the yuan qi is brought from the kidney to the organs through the sanjiao, the yuan/source points can activate the associated organs. Most of the yuan/source points are on the wrists and ankles where pulses can be felt. The yuan/source points can be combined with the luo-connecting divergent collateral of its external-internal channel. For example, if the stomach is the primary issue then ST 42 (chōng yáng, 冲阳) can be needled as the yuan/source (the host) and the luo-connecting divergent collateral SP 4 (gōng sūn, 公孙) can also be used (the guest). If the large intestine were the main problem then the source point of the large intestine, LI 4 (hé gǔ, 合谷) (the host) would be needled and the luo-connecting divergent collateral of the lung, LU 7 (liè quē, 列缺), would be used in conjunction (guest).

Four command points (sì zǒng xué, 四总穴) and eight gathering points (jiāo huì xué, 交会穴)

The command and gathering points (also called "influential" points) have a broad effect on specialized aspects and areas of the body.

Four Command Points	
Head and Neck	LU 7
Face and Mouth	LI 4
Abdomen	ST 36
Back	BL 40

Eight Gathering Points			
Zang-organs	LV 13	Marrow	GB 39
Fu-organs	RN 12	Bone	BL 11
Qi	RN 17	Sinews	GB 34
Blood	BL 17	Vessels	LU 9

Confluence points (*bā mài jiāo huì xué*, 八脉交会穴)

Confluence points have been considered to be useful for accessing the eight extraordinary vessels. Because the eight extraordinary vessels are paired, the two upper and lower points of the pairs may be used either separately or together.

Eight Extraordinary Vessels – Confluence Points			
Ren	LU 7	*Yin Qiao*	K 6
Du	SI 3	*Yang Qiao*	BL 62
Chong	SP 4	*Yin Wei*	PC 6
Dai	GB 41	*Yang Wei*	SJ 5

In further studies and practice, the student and practitioner will have a chance to become familiar with other points such as the entry and exit points, window of the sky and ghost points. Yet acupuncture points are not like buttons on a vending machine that then spits out a product of a cure. Dr. Wang elegantly states, "As a doctor, when one treats a patient, that person's channels should be treated delicately and with respect. One should create effects in the channel system that is like the music of an experienced musician. Don't beat on the strings or play indiscriminately. A successful treatment should be like conducting a piece of beautiful music."[1]

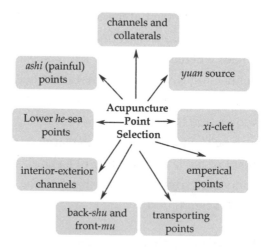

Herbs and the Channels

Chinese herbs are said to have "four properties and five flavors" that are closely related with channel theory. Clinically, different disease patterns of the organs and channels have their specific demands for treatment. Therefore, herbs also have channel affinities (tropism). An herb is commonly chosen because of the channel it is

---

①   Ju-yi Wang, Jason D. Roberston. *Applied Channel Theory in Chinese Medicine*. Seattle: Eastland Press; 2008. p. 548.

said to "enter" or have an effect on. For example, each of the following herbs acts to cool fire but go to different channels. *Huáng lián* (Coptis Rhizoma) drains heart fire, *huáng qín* (Scutellariae Radix) drains lung fire, *chái hú* (Bupleuri Radix) drains liver-gallbladder and *sanjiao* fire, *bái sháo* (Paeoniae Radix Alba) clears spleen fire, *zhī mǔ* (Anemarrhenae Rhizoma) drains kidney fire, *mù tōng* (Akebiae Caulis) cools small intestine fire, and *shí gāo* (Gypsum Fibrosum) clears stomach fire. Obviously using herbs based on the channel affinities can lead to a more accurate treatment of complex illnesses.

The above examples apply to the channels and the organs. Certain herbs however have affinity to the collaterals. This is especially important in treating pain and dermatological cases. *Jī xuè téng* (Spatholobi Caulis) is one such herb that not only moves the blood but has special properties to invigorate the blood in the collaterals.

Section 2   Twelve Channels

NAMES OF THE TWELVE CHANNELS

The twelve channels symmetrically distribute on the two sides of the body, respectively running along the medial or lateral sides of the upper or lower limbs and each of them affiliates itself with a *zang-* or *fu-* organ respectively. The naming of the twelve channels is based on their distribution in the hand or foot, medial or lateral side, the organs they belong to, and their yin or yang attributes.

Hand or Foot

The channels that run in the upper limb, and start or end at the hand are called "hand channels" while the channels in the lower limb that start or end at the foot are called "foot channels".

Yin or Yang

Yin channels are affiliated with the *zang* (yin) -organs, while yang channels are affiliated with the *fu* (yang)-organs. Most of the channels that run on the medial side of the limbs are "yin channels", while all the channels that run on the lateral sides of the limbs are "yang channels". Yin channels all run on the front of the body and the yang channels run on the sides or back of the body. (The exception is the yang *yangming* stomach channel which runs up the front of the body and face.) According to the principles of yin and yang, yin is further divided into *taiyin, jueyin* and *shaoyin* and yang is divided into *yangming, shaoyang* and *taiyang*.

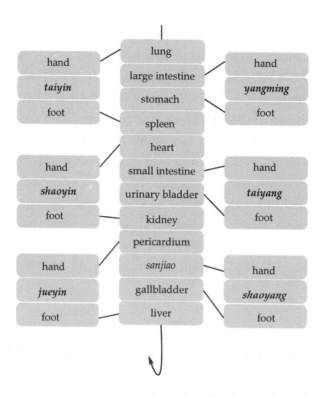

COURSE AND CONNECTION OF THE TWELVE CHANNELS

The directions of continual movement of the twelve channels are as follows: the three hand yin channels run from the internal organs in the abdomen to the ends of fingers. From the fingers, these yin channels connect with the three hand yang channels. The three hand yang channels run from the fingers to the head and face and connect with the three foot yang channels there. Then the three foot yang channels run from the head and face to the ends of toes where they connect the three foot yin channels. The three foot yin channels run from the toes to the abdomen and connect with the first three hand yin channels we mentioned. In this way, the twelve channels form a complete cycle in which yin and yang channels circulate and connect with each other. The order of the entire circuit is the lung, large intestine, stomach, spleen, heart, small intestine, urinary bladder, kidney, pericardium, *sanjiao*, gall bladder and liver. The end of the liver channel connects again with the lung. The following gives a more detailed description of how the external-internally related yin and yang channels connect on the four limbs based on several perspectives.

(1) The external-internally related three hand yin and yang channels connect at the ends of the toes or fingers.

For the hands, the hand *taiyin* lung channel and the hand *yangming* large intestine channel connect at the end of the index finger. The hand *shaoyin* heart channel and the hand *taiyang* small intestine channel connect at the end of the little finger. The hand *jueyin* pericardium channel and the hand *shaoyang sanjiao* channel connect at end of the ring finger.

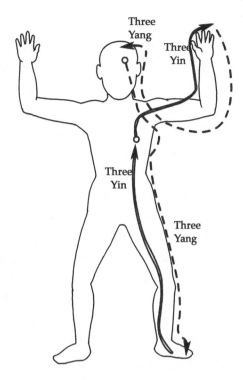

For the feet, the foot *yangming* stomach channel and the foot *taiyin* spleen channel connect at the end of the big toe. The foot *taiyang* bladder channel and the foot *shaoyin* kidney channel connect at the end of the little toe. The foot *shaoyang* gallbladder channel and the foot *jueyin* liver channel connect at the end of posterior side of the big toe.

(2) For the yang channels, the hand and foot yang channels with the same name connect in the head and face. For example, the foot and hand *shaoyang* channels. There are three pairs of hand and foot yang channels with the same name. The three pairs all connect in the head and face. Specifically, the hand *yangming* large intestine channel and the foot *yangming* stomach channel connect at the side of nose. The hand *taiyang* small intestine channel and the foot *taiyang* bladder channel connect at the inner canthus. The hand *shaoyang* sanjiao channel and the foot *shaoyang* gallbladder channel connect at the outer canthus.

(3) For the yin channels, the foot and hand yin channels connect in the thorax. There are also three pairs of foot and hand yin channels. The three pairs all connect to the internal organs of the thorax. Specifically, the foot *taiyin* spleen channel and the hand *shaoyin* heart channel connect in the heart; the foot *shaoyin* kidney channel and the hand *jueyin* pericardium channel connect in the chest; and the foot *jueyin* liver channel and the hand *taiyin* lung channel connect in the lung.

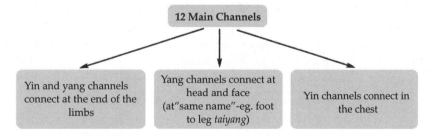

DISTRIBUTION OF THE TWELVE CHANNELS

The distribution of the twelve channels in the body is circuitous and although they sometimes cross each other, they mainly run vertically or up and down. Yin channels run on the medial sides of the limbs and chest-abdominal aspect of the trunk, and yang channels run in the lateral sides of the limbs and dorsal aspect of the trunk (with the exception of the foot *yangming* stomach channel). The hand channels start or end in the hands, while the foot channels start or end in the legs.

The three hand yang channels run from the hand to the head and the three foot yang channels run from the head to the foot. Therefore, all the yang channels pass through the head and face. The two *yangming* (large intestine and stomach) channels travel on the front of the face while the *shaoyang* (gall bladder and *sanjiao*) channels travel on the lateral sides of the head. The hand *taiyang* (small intestine) channel runs mainly to the zygomatic region and the foot *taiyang* (urinary bladder) channel goes to the vertex and the posterior part of the head.

On the trunk, the three hand yin channels all go from the thorax to the axilla (armpit) while the three hand yang channels pass through the shoulder and scapular region. Of the three foot yang channels, the foot *yangming* channel runs on the anterior aspect (pectoral and abdominal areas), urinary bladder *taiyang* channel in the back and the gallbladder *shaoyang* channel on the lateral side of the chest. The three foot yin channels all run on the abdomen and chest.

The twelve channels run symmetrically on the left and right sides of the body in the trunk, head and face, and four limbs. So there are 12 channels on each side. The channels on the left and right sides do not go to the opposite side (except for the hand *yangming* large intestine channel which goes to the opposite side of the face).

Summary
- The three hand yin channels run from the thorax to the hand, the three hand yang channels from the hand to the head, the three foot yang channels from the head to the foot and the three foot yin channel from the foot to the abdomen.
- The exterior-interiorly related yin and yang channels connect with each other at the ends of limbs. The hand and foot yang channels with the same name connect in the head and face and the foot and hand yin channels connect in the internal organs of thorax.
- Therefore, the yang channels start at the head or the hands and the yin channels start at the center of the body or the feet. If the hands are held above the head, then the yang channels go downward and the yin upward.

EXTERIOR-INTERIOR RELATIONSHIPS OF THE TWELVE CHANNELS

The hand or foot three yin channels and the hand or foot three yang channels form six pairs of exterior-interior relationship through communication of their channel divergences and divergent collaterals.

External-internally related channels all connect at the ends of the four limbs, run in the opposite regions of the medial and lateral sides of the limbs and connect with their external-internally related organs. External-internally related channels may also affect each other pathologically. For example, an invasion of the lung channel by pathogens may block the movement of qi of the large intestine and cause constipation. Excess heart fire may spread down along the channels to the small intestine and thus cause burning pain and reddish urine. In treatment, one has the option to use the acupuncture points of either of the external-internally paired channels.

FLOW ORDER OF THE TWELVE CHANNELS

The twelve channels are the main passageways for the circulation of qi and blood. They communicate with each other by connecting the end of one channel to the beginning of another channel. Qi and blood can then flow orderly from one channel to another. The qi and blood of the whole body comes mainly from food and drink transformed and transported by the spleen and stomach. Therefore, one connection of the qi and blood flow of the twelve channels is that it starts at the hand *taiyin* lung channel (that originates from the middle *jiao*), and then it flows orderly into other channels until it finally goes to the foot *jueyin* liver channel. From there, it flows back into the hand *taiyin* lung channel and starts the next cycle without stopping.

The flow order of the main channels starts with the hand *taiyin* lung to go to the hand *yangming* large intestine and then to the foot *yangming* and then to foot *taiyin* spleen and through the rest of the channels. The order then goes hand, hand, foot, foot, hand, hand, foot, foot, hand, hand, foot, foot.

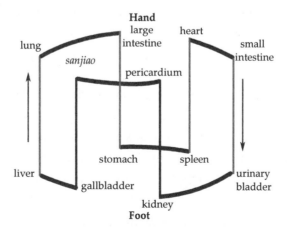

The flow order mentioned above is the major model of the qi and blood circulation of the twelve channels. There are several additional perspectives to look at the way qi and blood circulates. For example, *ying* qi circulates inside the vessels following the course of the twelve channels while *wei* qi circulates outside the vessels. The *wei* qi flows mainly in the yang areas of the body during the daytime and in the yin areas at night. The qi and blood in the channel divergences circulates mainly in the interior of their paired channels. The qi and blood in the collaterals distributes and spreads over the entire body surface. The qi and blood in the eight extraordinary vessels circulates to play a regulatory role for the other channels. Another model of the qi flow is that qi flows from the tips of the fingers and the toes inward to the organs. This allows for the system of the well, spring, stream, river and sea points on the limbs. All these systems are conceptualized differently yet together constitute an integrated circulation system of qi and blood with the twelve channels as the core.

> The two books which make up *The Yellow Emperor's Inner Classic*, the *Basic Questions* and *The Spiritual Pivot*, give different interpretations of how fast qi passes through the channels. The *Basic Questions* is dependent on the size of the person yet says that generally qi will pass through all the channels in about 20 minutes. In the *Spiritual Pivot*, Chapters 15 & 18, it states that in one day, qi and blood will travel through the body 50 times which is equivalent to one pass in 28 minutes and 48 seconds. For that reason, many acupuncture treatments are between 20 to 30 minutes long.

PATHWAYS OF THE TWELVE CHANNELS

The Hand *Taiyin* Lung Channel

Common symptoms

Cough, panting, shortness of breath, hemoptysis (coughing blood), swelling and pain of the throat, distention and fullness sensation of the chest, pain at the supraclavicular fossa, pain in the anterior border of the flexor aspect of the arm, cold pain in the shoulder and back.

Pathway

- The hand *taiyin* lung channel has 11 points on both the left and right sides of the body.[1]
- The hand *taiyin* lung channel starts from the middle *jiao* which allows us to treat many lung diseases by way of the stomach area and vice versa. It then runs downward to connect with the large intestine which is its *fu* or yang connected organ. It then winds back along the openings of the stomach (the lower opening

---

[1]   All of the channels have their points on both sides of the body.

is the pylorus and the upper one is the cardia), passes through the diaphragm, and affiliates itself to the lung. It then ascends along the lung connections (bronchia, trachea and throat), and runs to the first point of the lung. Emerging from under the armpit, it descends superficially along the anterior border of the upper limb, passing through the elbow and to the wrist where it can be felt for

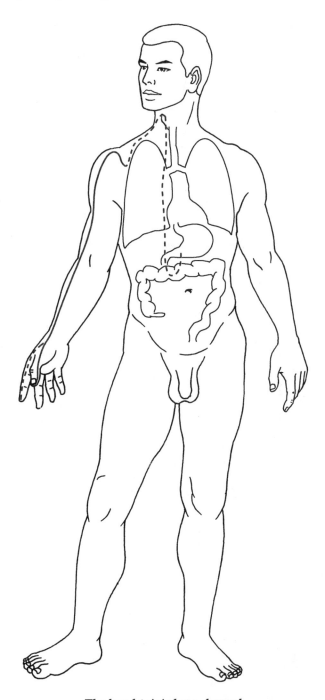

The hand *taiyin* lung channel

the pulse and then to the end of the thumb.

- A branch of the hand *taiyin* emerging from the wrist and then runs to the tip of the index finger, where it links to the hand *yangming* large intestine channel.

The **hand *taiyin* lung divergent collateral** originates from the wrist (LU 7, *liè què*) and goes into the hand *yangming* large intestine channel at the wrist. Its branch

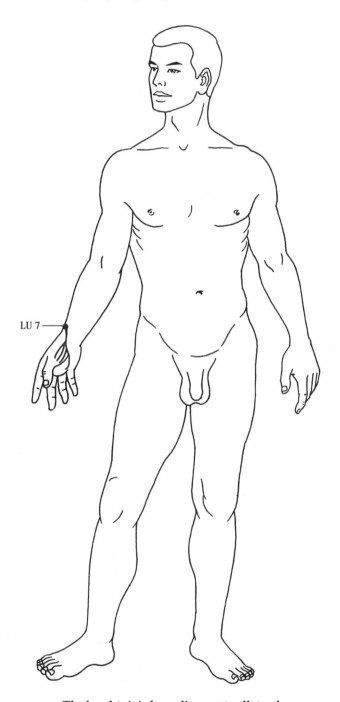

LU 7

The hand *taiyin* lung divergent collateral

joins the hand *taiyin* channel, and then directly enters the palm and spreads over the thumb.

The **hand *taiyin* lung channel divergence** branches out from the axilla and runs to the front of the hand *shaoyin* channel divergence, enters into the thoracic cavity,

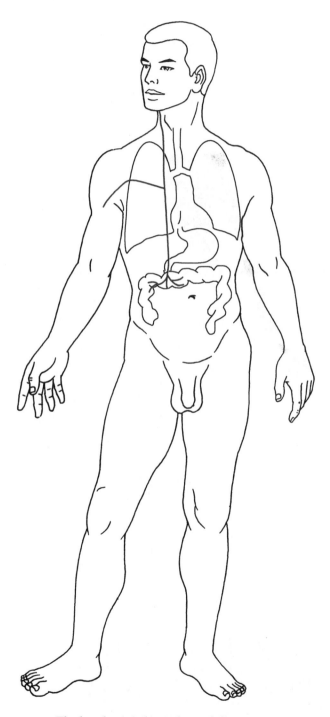

The hand *taiyin* lung channel divergence

goes to the lung, and spreads in the large intestine. From the lung runs up to the supraclavicular fossa and runs superficially, passing by the throat until it finally meets with the hand *yangming* channel.

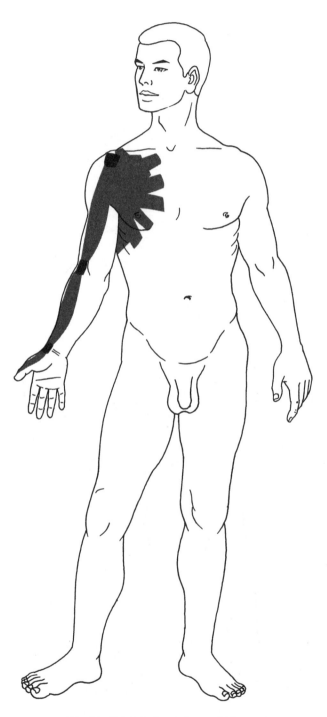

The hand *taiyin* lung channel sinews

Acupoints

Hand *Taiyin* Lung Channel

LU 1	中府	*zhōng fǔ*	Central Treasury
LU 2	云门	*yún mén*	Cloud Gate
LU 3	天府	*tiān fǔ*	Celestial Storehouse
LU 4	侠白	*xiá bái*	Guarding White
LU 5	尺泽	*chǐ zé*	Cubit Marsh
LU 6	孔最	*kǒng zuì*	Collecting Hole
LU 7	列缺	*liè quē*	Broken Sequence
LU 8	经渠	*jīng qú*	Channel Ditch
LU 9	太渊	*tài yuān*	Great Abyss
LU 10	鱼际	*yú jì*	Fish Border
LU 11	少商	*shào shāng*	Lesser Merchant

The Hand *Yangming* Large Intestine Channel

Common symptoms

Toothache, swelling neck, swelling and pain of the throat, dry mouth, hemoptysis, pain in the anterior aspect of the shoulder and anterior border of the extensor aspect of the arm, pain of the thumb and index finger, etc.

Pathway

There are 20 points on the hand *yangming* large intestine channel. Note that the hand *yangming* is the only one of the main channels which crosses from one side of the body to the other.

- The hand *yangming* large intestine channel starts from the radial side of the tip of the index finger, goes to the back of the hand, runs to the upper limb and shoulder joint. Then it runs to the 7th cervical vertebra, to the supraclavicular fossa, to the thoracic cavity to connect with the lung, to the diaphragm, and finally runs down to the large intestine.

- A branch emerges from the supraclavicular fossa, goes to the neck and the cheek, and enters the gums of the lower teeth by the mouth where it crosses to the opposite side above the mouth and to the side of the nose where it links with the foot *yangming* stomach channel. Another branch descends to ST 37 (*shàng jù xū*) which is found on the lower leg (lower *he*-sea point).

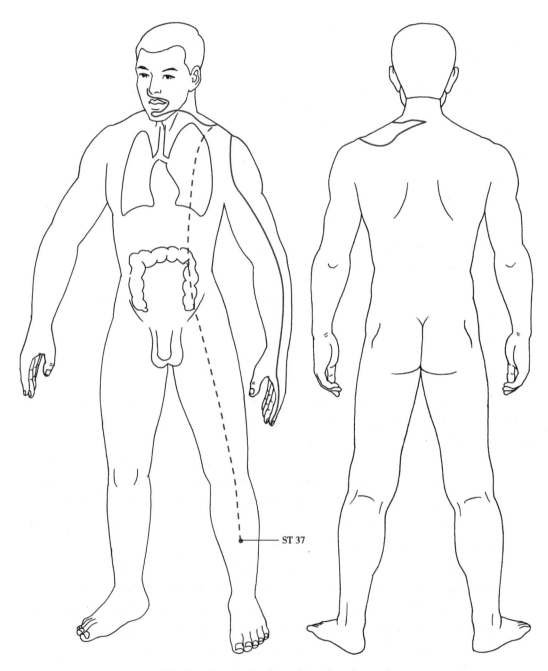

ST 37

The hand *yangming* large intestine channel

The **hand *yangming* divergent collateral** originates from the forearm (LI 6, *piān lì*) and goes upward into the hand *yangming* channel. A branch goes along the arm, arrives at the jaw and spreading over the roots of the teeth. Another branch goes into the ear where it meets several other channels.

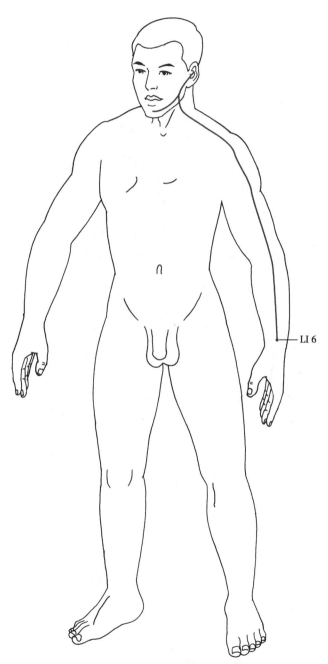

LI 6

The hand *yangming* divergent collateral

The **hand *yangming* channel divergence** branches out at the hand and then ascends to the shoulder at LI 15 (*jiān yú*) and then enters the spinal column from the back of the neck. A branch runs to the large intestine and links with the lung while another branch runs to the throat, to the supraclavicular fossa, and then into the internal branch of the hand *yangming* channel.

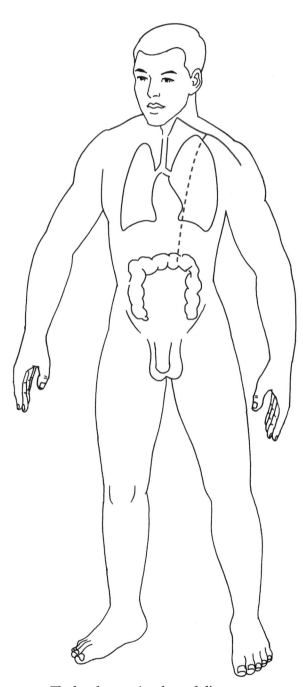

The hand *yangming* channel divergence

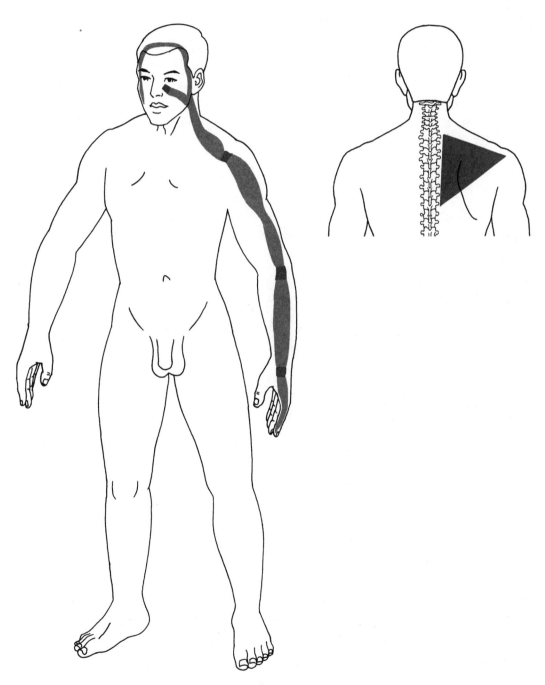

The hand *yangming* channel sinews

Acupoints

Hand *Yangming* Large Intestine Channel

LI 1	商阳	*shāng yáng*	Shang Yang
LI 2	二间	*èr jiān*	Second Space
LI 3	三间	*sān jiān*	Third Space
LI 4	合谷	*hé gǔ*	Union Valley
LI 5	阳溪	*yáng xī*	Yang Ravine
LI 6	偏历	*piān lì*	Veering Passageway
LI 7	温溜	*wēn liū*	Warm Dwelling
LI 8	下廉	*xià lián*	Lower Ridge
LI 9	上廉	*shàng lián*	Upper Ridge
LI 10	手三里	*shǒu sān lǐ*	Three Arm Mile
LI 11	曲池	*qū chí*	Pool Bend
LI 12	肘髎	*zhǒu liáo*	Elbow Bone-Hold
LI 13	手五里	*shǒu wǔ lǐ*	Hand Five Mile
LI 14	臂臑	*bì nào*	Upper Arm
LI 15	肩髃	*jiān yú*	Shoulder Bone
LI 16	巨骨	*jù gǔ*	Great Bone
LI 17	天鼎	*tiān dǐng*	Heaven Tripod
LI 18	扶突	*fú tū*	Protuberance Assistant
LI 19	口禾髎	*kǒu hé liáo*	Grain Bone Hole
LI 20	迎香	*yíng xiāng*	Welcome Fragrance

The Foot *Yangming* Stomach Channel

Common symptoms

Fever, stomachache, vomiting or swift digestion with rapid hunger, thirst, borborygmus, mania and anxiety, abdominal distention, edema, headache, pain of the throat, pain along the channel's pathways in the chest and knee, etc.

Pathway

There are 45 points on the foot *yangming* stomach channel.

- The foot *yangming* stomach channel starts beside the nostril, goes then to the inner canthus of the eye where it meets with the foot *taiyang* channel. Running downward, it enters the upper gums of the teeth, the mouth, and curves around the lips where it meets its opposite channel below the mouth. It then runs along jaw, goes in front of the ear and then to the forehead.

- A branch emerges in the jaw, and runs downward to the neck and throat where it goes to DU 14 (*dà zhuī*). Turning back it runs forward to the supraclavicular fossa, at which it enters the cavity of the body. Descending through the diaphragm, it affiliates itself to the stomach, and connects with the spleen.

- The straight portion: Starting from the neck, it runs downward along the trunk to the inguinal groove.
- The second branch comes out from the lower opening of the stomach (pylorus), where it descends along the inside of the abdomen to ST 30 (*qì chōng*) and joins the vertical portion. Then it runs downward along the thigh to the knee and then to the lateral side of the tip of the 2nd toe.
- The third branch emerges from beside the knee, it descends and enters the

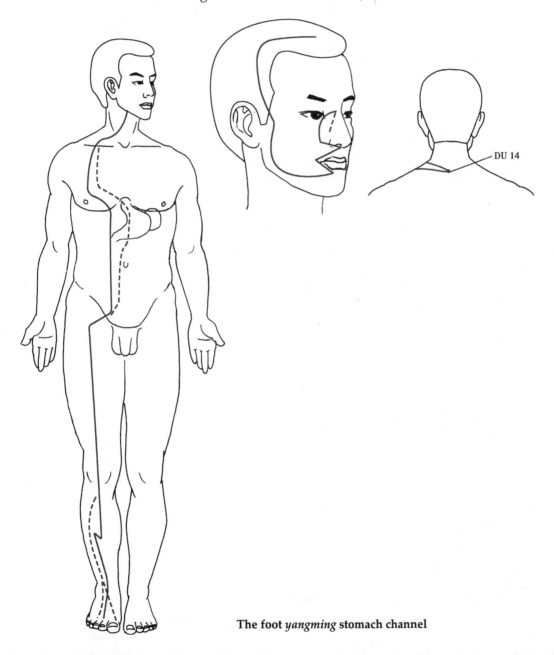

The foot *yangming* stomach channel

lateral side of the tip of the middle toe.

- The last branch arises from the top of the foot, runs forward to the medial side of the tip of the big toe, where it links with the foot *taiyin* spleen channel.

The **foot *yangming* stomach divergent collateral** originates from the middle of the lower leg (ST 40, *fēng lóng*), where it goes to the foot *taiyin* spleen channel. Its branch

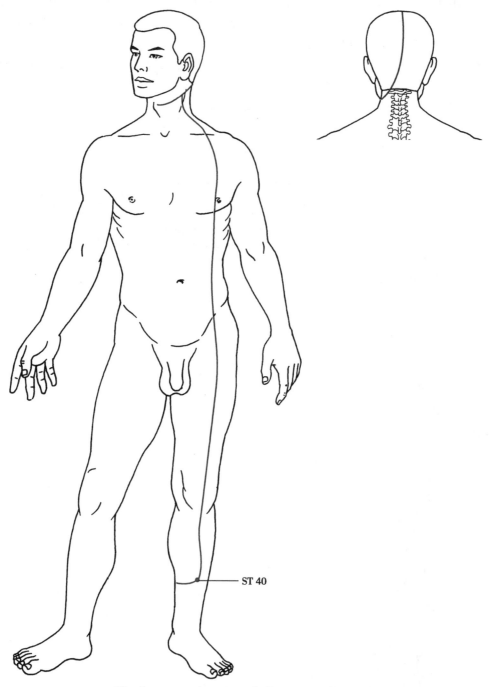

ST 40

The foot *yangming* stomach divergent collateral

runs up along the lateral border of the tibia, and arrives at the just below the back of the skull and meets DU 14 (*dà zhuī*) where it meets several other channels. It then runs downward and ends at the throat.

The **foot *yangming* channel divergence** branches out from the foot *yangming* channel at the anterior aspect of the thigh. It connects and runs to the abdominal

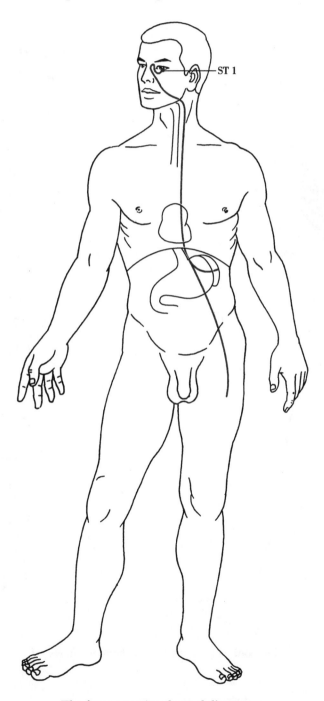

The foot *yangming* channel divergence

cavity, the stomach, spleen, heart, esophagus mouth, root of the nose, infraorbital region, the "eye connector"[1] until it finally goes into the main foot *yangming* channel. The "upper meeting point" of the stomach divergent then is the first point, ST 1 (*chéng qì*), of the stomach's main channel.

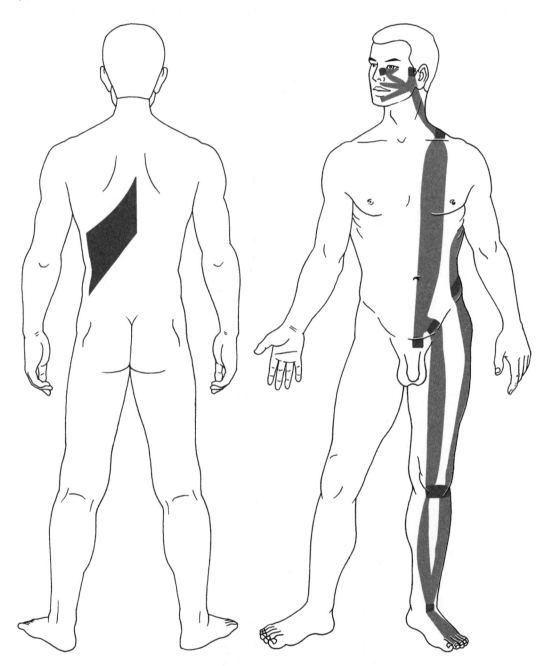

The foot *yangming* stomach channel sinews

---

[1]   The eye connector is considered those tissues which connect the eyes with the brain.

Acupoints

Foot *Yangming* Stomach Channel

ST 1	承泣	*chéng qì*	Tear Container
ST 2	四白	*sì bái*	Four Whites
ST 3	巨髎	*jù liáo*	Great Bone Hole
ST 4	地仓	*dì cāng*	Earth Granary
ST 5	大迎	*dà yíng*	Great Reception
ST 6	颊车	*jiá chē*	Cheek Carriage
ST 7	下关	*xià guān*	Below the Joint
ST 8	头维	*tóu wéi*	Head Corner
ST 9	人迎	*rén yíng*	Man's Prognosis
ST 10	水突	*shuǐ tū*	Water Prominence
ST 11	气舍	*qì shè*	Qi House
ST 12	缺盆	*quē pén*	Empty Basin
ST 13	气户	*qì hù*	Qi Door
ST 14	库房	*kù fáng*	Store Room
ST 15	屋翳	*wū yì*	Roof
ST 16	膺窗	*yīng chuāng*	Breast Window
ST 17	乳中	*rǔ zhōng*	Breast Center
ST 18	乳根	*rǔ gēn*	Breast Root
ST 19	不容	*bù róng*	Not Contained
ST 20	承满	*chéng mǎn*	Assuming Fullness
ST 21	梁门	*liáng mén*	Beam Gate
ST 22	关门	*guān mén*	Pass Gate
ST 23	太乙	*tài yǐ*	Supreme Unity
ST 24	滑肉门	*huá ròu mén*	Slippery Flesh Gate
ST 25	天枢	*tiān shū*	Celestial Pivot
ST 26	外陵	*wài líng*	Outer Mound
ST 27	大巨	*dà jù*	Great Gigantic
ST 28	水道	*shuǐ dào*	Waterway
ST 29	归来	*guī lái*	Return
ST 30	气冲	*qì chōng*	Qi Passageway
ST 31	髀关	*bì guān*	Thigh Joint
ST 32	伏兔	*fú tù*	Crouching Rabbit
ST 33	阴市	*yīn shì*	Yin Market
ST 34	梁丘	*liáng qiū*	Beam Hill

ST 35	犊鼻	dú bí	Calf's Nose
ST 36	足三里	zú sān lǐ	Leg Three Mile
ST 37	上巨虚	shàng jù xū	Upper Great Hollow
ST 38	条口	tiáo kǒu	Ribbon Opening
ST39	下巨虚	xià jù xū	Lower Great Hollow
ST 40	丰隆	fēng lóng	Bountiful Bulge
ST 41	解溪	jiě xī	Ravine Divide
ST 42	冲阳	chōng yáng	Surging Yang
ST 43	陷谷	xiàn gǔ	Sunken Valley
ST 44	内庭	nèi tíng	Inner Court
ST 45	厉兑	lì duì	Severe Mouth

The Foot *Taiyin* Spleen Channel

Common symptoms

Stiff tongue, vomiting, stomachache, abdominal distention, belching, poor appetite, loose stool, lack of strength, jaundice, swelling of the medial side of the knees, cold limbs.

Pathway

There are 21 points on the foot *taiyin* spleen channel.

- The channel starts from the big toe and then passes by the anterior border of the medial malleolus, and then runs upward along the midline of the medial aspect of the leg where it crosses over and further runs in front of the foot *jueyin* liver channel. It ascends along the thigh, enters the abdomen, and then affiliates itself to the spleen and connects with the stomach. Running upward through the diaphragm, reaches the root of the tongue, and scatters its collaterals over the lower surface of the tongue.
- The only branch comes out from the stomach, where it ascends through the diaphragm and enters the heart, linking with the hand *shaoyin* heart channel.

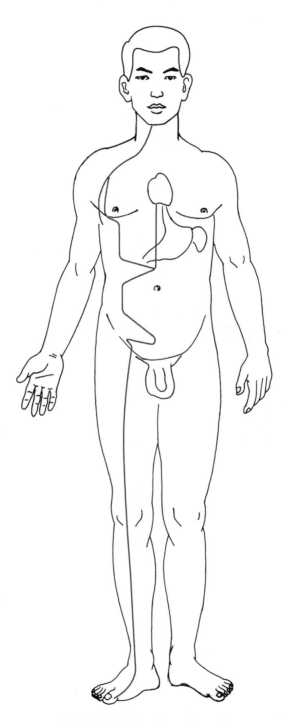

The foot *taiyin* spleen channel

The **foot *taiyin* divergent collateral** begins on the foot (SP 4, *gōng sūn*) where it goes into the foot *yangming* channel. Its branch ascends into the abdomen cavity, linking with the intestines and stomach.

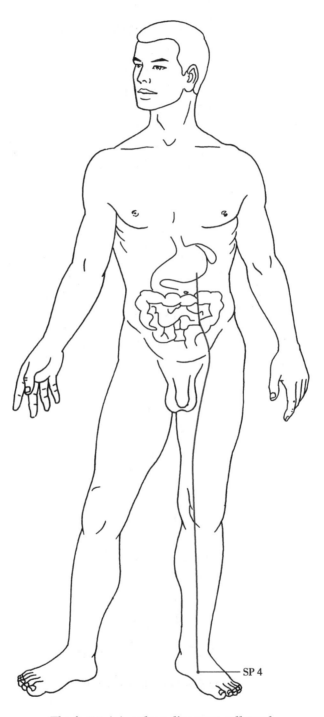

SP 4

The foot *taiyin* spleen divergent collateral

The **foot *taiyin* channel divergence** branches out at the medial side of the thigh. It then joins the foot *yangming* divergence at the thigh. It then goes to the pharynx, and passes through the tongue.

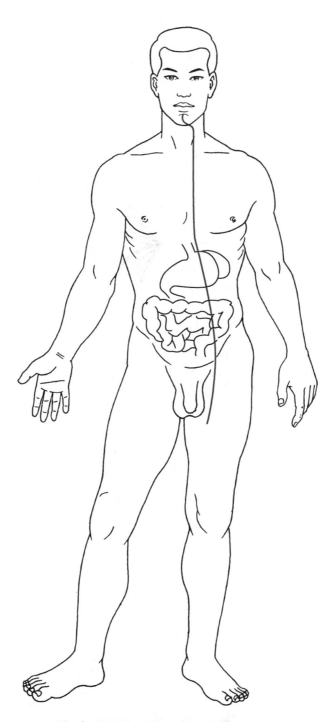

The foot *taiyin* spleen channel divergence

The large collateral of the spleen channel originates from side of the trunk then spreads in the thoracic and hypochondriac regions. This is often referred to as the great *luo* of the spleen.

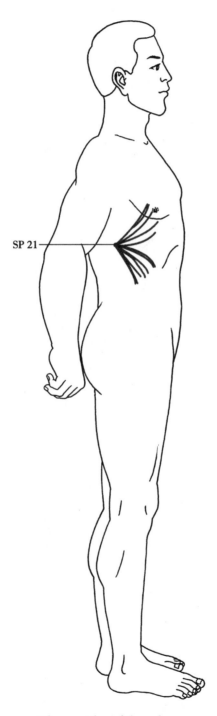

SP 21

The great *luo* of the spleen

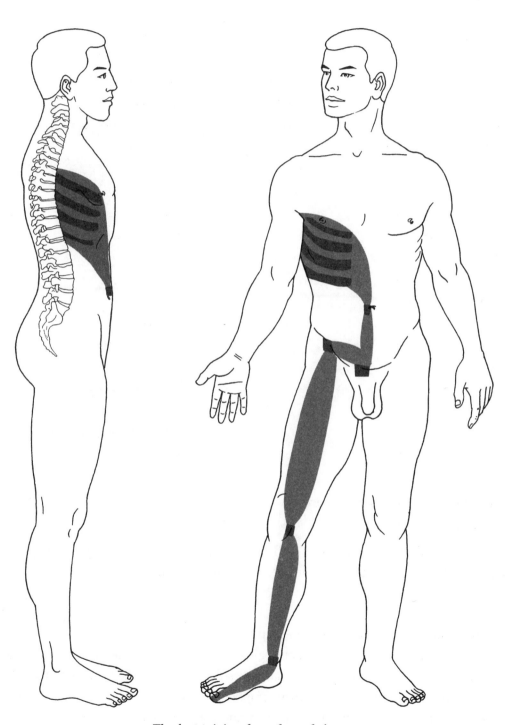

The foot *taiyin* spleen channel sinews

Acupoints

Foot *Taiyin* Spleen Channel

SP 1	隐白	*yǐn bái*	Hidden White
SP 2	大都	*dà dū*	Great Metropolis
SP 3	太白	*tài bái*	Supreme White
SP 4	公孙	*gōng sūn*	Yellow Emperor
SP 5	商丘	*shāng qiū*	Shang Hill
SP 6	三阴交	*sān yīn jiāo*	Three Yin Intersection
SP 7	漏谷	*lòu gǔ*	Leaking Valley
SP 8	地机	*dì jī*	Earth's Link
SP 9	阴陵泉	*yīn líng quán*	Yin Mound Spring
SP 10	血海	*xuè hǎi*	Sea of Blood
SP 11	箕门	*jī mén*	Winnowing Gate
SP 12	冲门	*chōng mén*	Surging Gate
SP 13	府舍	*fǔ shè*	Bowel Abode
SP 14	腹结	*fù jié*	Abdomen Bind
SP 15	大横	*dà héng*	Great Horizontal
SP 16	腹哀	*fù āi*	Abdomen Lament
SP 17	食窦	*shí dòu*	Food Hole
SP 18	天溪	*tiān xī*	Celestial Ravine
SP 19	胸乡	*xiōng xiāng*	Chest Village
SP 20	周荣	*zhōu róng*	All-Round Flourishing
SP 21	大包	*dà bāo*	Great Embracement

The Hand *Shaoyin* Heart Channel

Common symptoms

Heart pain, dry throat, thirst, yellowish sclera, feverish feeling of the palms, hypochondriac pain, anxiety, pain in the flexor side of the arm.

Pathway

The hand *shaoyin* heart channel has 9 points.

- The hand *shaoyin* heart channel begins in the heart, and then enters the "heart connector" (considered to be the large vessels connecting the heart with the other organs), runs downward through the diaphragm and connects with the small intestine.
- A branch comes out from the heart connector, where it runs upward alongside the esophagus to join with the eye connector.

- A branch emerges from the heart connector and runs upward through the lung. Then it descends and runs out from the axilla (armpit) and the first point of the main channel (HT 1, *jí quán*).

- It passes superficially along the posterior border of the medial aspect of the upper limb where it runs and passes through the cubital fossa (interior aspect of the elbow) down to where it enters the palm. Then it runs along the radial side of the little finger to its tip where it connects with the hand *taiyang* small intestine channel.

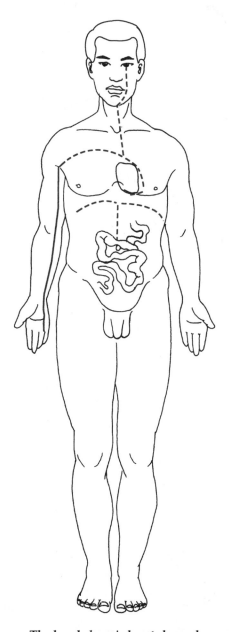

The hand *shaoyin* heart channel

The **hand** *shaoyin* **divergent collateral** originates from the hand (HT 5, *tōng lǐ*), runs up alongside the hand *shaoyin* channel proper, entering the heart. Then it ascends to link the root of the tongue, and joins the connector linking the eye with the brain.

The **hand** *shaoyin* **heart channel divergence** branches out from the hand *shaoyin*

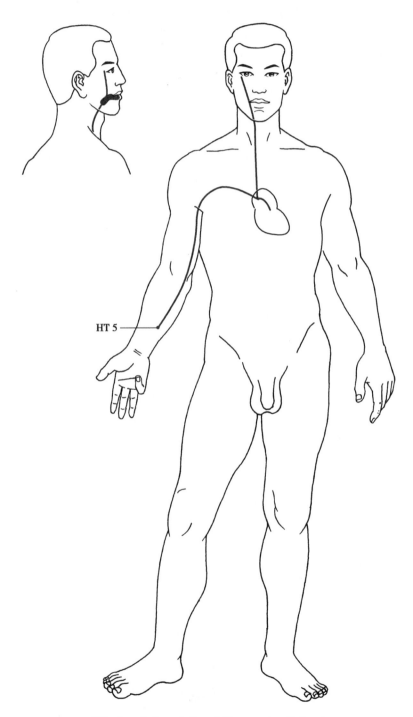

HT 5

The hand *shaoyin* heart divergent collateral

channel in the axilla and then enters the thoracic cavity, and links with heart. The divergence then runs to the throat, then superficially in the face, and finally joins the hand *taiyang* small intestine channel at the inner canthus. This last location of the hand *taiyang* is the first point of the foot *taiyang*, BL 1.

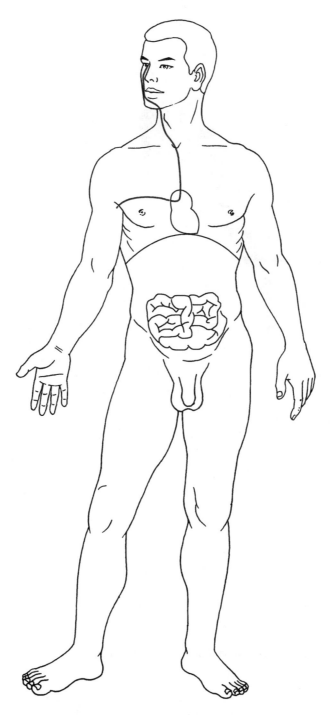

The hand *shaoyin* heart channel divergence

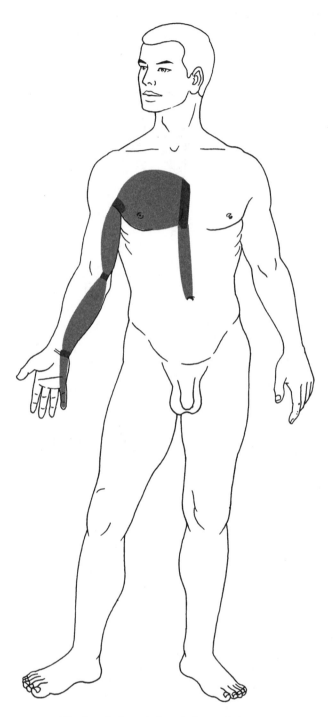

The hand *shaoyin* heart channel sinews

Acupoints

Hand *Shaoyin* Heart Channel

HT 1	极泉	*jí quán*	Highest Spring
HT 2	青灵	*qīng líng*	Blue Green Spirit
HT 3	少海	*shào hǎi*	Lessen Sea
HT 4	灵道	*líng dào*	Spirit Pathway
HT 5	通里	*tōng lǐ*	Connecting Mile
HT 6	阴郄	*yīn xì*	Yin Cleft
HT 7	神门	*shén mén*	Spirit Gate
HT 8	少府	*shào fǔ*	Lesser Mansion
HT 9	少冲	*shào chōng*	Lesser Surge

The Hand *Taiyang* Small Intestine Channel

Common symptoms

Yellowish eyes, tinnitus, swelling and pain in the throat, swelling and pain in the mandibular and cervical region with impairment of the head movement, pain in the posterior border of the extensor side of arm.

Pathway

There are 19 points on the hand *taiyang* small intestine channel.

- The hand *taiyang* small intestine channel starts at the tip of the little finger. It goes up to the cubital (elbow) region, and reaches the region of the shoulder joint. After twisting around in the scapular region it reaches the superior part of the shoulder and to the back and then runs forward to the supraclavicular fossa. From there, it enters the body cavity to connect with the heart. Descending along the esophagus, it passes through the diaphragm, reaches the stomach, and runs down to the small intestine.

- A branch comes out from the supraclavicular fossa and ascends along the neck to the cheek. Arriving at the outer canthus of the eye, it then runs back and enters the ear.

- Another branch arises from the cheek, runs up to the eye region, and then reaches the inner canthus of the eye to link with the foot *taiyang* bladder channel.

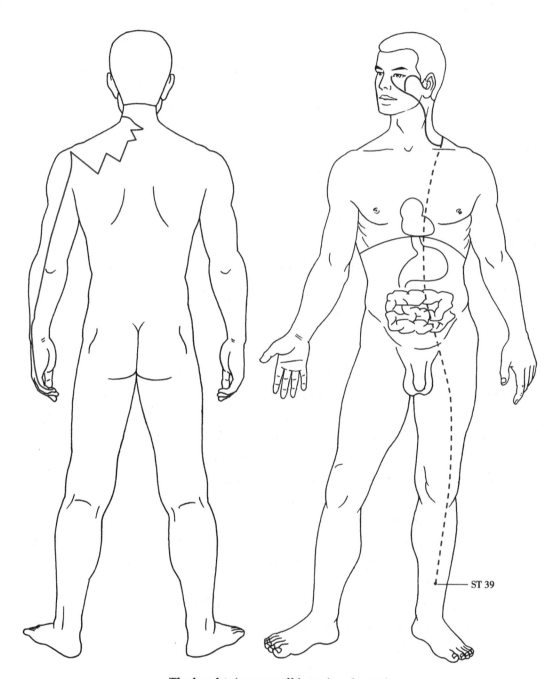

ST 39

The hand *taiyang* **small intestine channel**

The **hand *taiyang* small intestine divergent collateral** originates on the forearm (SI 7, *zhī zhèng*) where it connects into the hand *shaoyin* channel. A branch ascends to the elbow, and then to the shoulder at LI 15 (*jiān yú*).

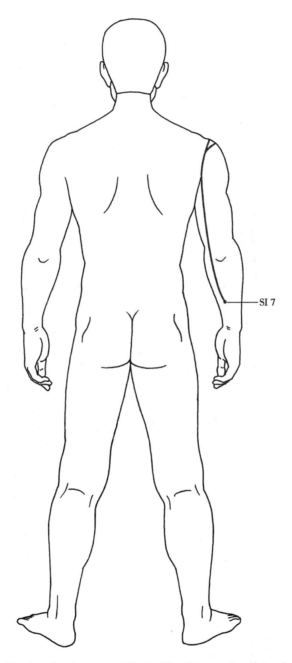

SI 7

The hand *taiyang* small intestine divergent collateral

The **hand *taiyang* channel divergence** branches out from the hand *taiyang* channel in the shoulder joint, runs down to the axilla, then reaches the heart and links with the small intestine.

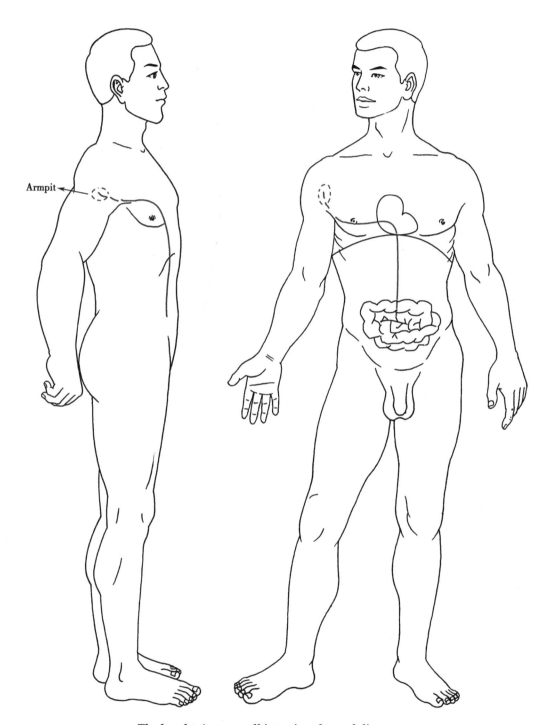

Armpit

The hand *taiyang* small intestine channel divergence

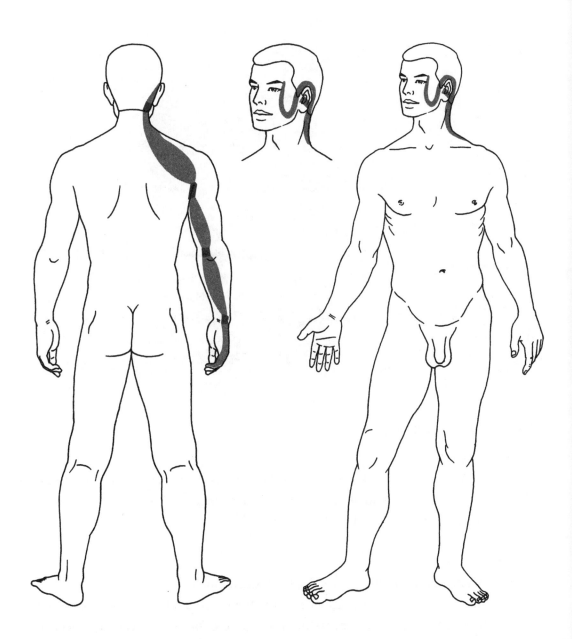

The hand *taiyang* small intestine channel sinews

Acupoints

Hand *Taiyang* Small Intestine Channel

SI 1	少泽	*shào zé*	Lesser Marsh
SI 2	前谷	*qián gǔ*	Front Valley
SI 3	后溪	*hòu xī*	Back Ravine
SI 4	腕骨	*wàn gǔ*	Wrist Bone
SI 5	阳谷	*yáng gǔ*	Yang Valley
SI 6	养老	*yǎng lǎo*	Nourish the Aged
SI 7	支正	*zhī zhèng*	Upright Branch
SI 8	小海	*xiǎo hǎi*	Small Sea
SI 9	肩贞	*jiān zhēn*	True Shoulder
SI 10	臑俞	*nào shù*	Upper Arm Transport
SI 11	天宗	*tiān zōng*	Celestial Gathering
SI 12	秉风	*bǐng fēng*	Grasping the Wind
SI 13	曲垣	*qū yuán*	Crooked Wall
SI 14	肩外俞	*jiān wài shù*	Outer Shoulder Transport
SI 15	肩中俞	*jiān zhōng shù*	Central Shoulder Transport
SI 16	天窗	*tiān chuāng*	Celestial Window
SI 17	天容	*tiān róng*	Celestial Countenance
SI 18	颧髎	*quán liáo*	Cheek Bone Hole
SI 19	听宫	*tīng gōng*	Auditory Palace

The Foot *Taiyang* Bladder Channel

Common symptoms

Headache, painful stiff neck, hemorrhoids, mania, depressive psychosis, lacrimation, yellowish sclera, epistaxis, pain in the waist, back and hip, as well as along the channel's pathways in the posterior side of the lower limb.

Pathway

There are 67 points on the foot *taiyang* bladder channel.

- The foot *taiyang* bladder channel starts at the inner canthus of the eye, ascends to the forehead where it reaches the vertex at the top of the head and meets its channel from the other side of the body.
- A branch comes out from the vertex, and then runs near the top of the ear.
- A branch from the top of the head runs to the back of the head and then enters the cranial cavity to communicate with the brain. It then runs to the back where it

meets its channel from the other side of the body, down to the scapula and parallel with the spine. Arriving at the lower back it connects with the kidney and bladder.

- A branch comes out from the lower back, descends spine, and passes through the gluteal region, following the thigh, it descends to the back of the knee.
- A branch starts at the back of the neck, to the scapula. From the back, it descends alongside the spine to the buttocks and then to the thigh to the back of

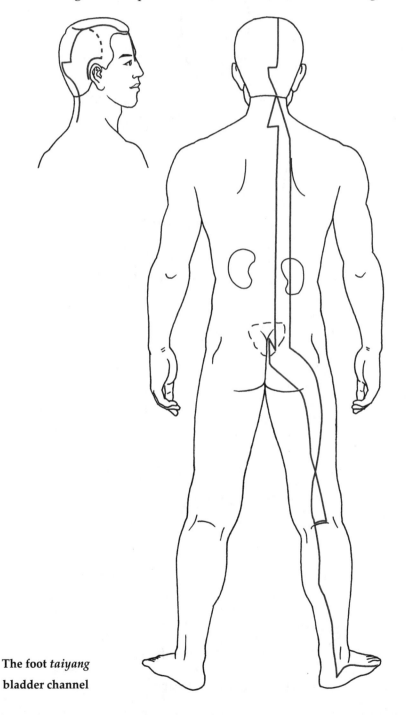

The foot *taiyang*
bladder channel

the knee. It then travels by the ankle to the lateral side of the tip of the little toe, where it links with the foot *shaoyin* kidney channel.

The **foot *taiyang* bladder divergent collateral** originates from the calf of the leg (BL58, *fēi yáng*) and circles it to go into the foot *shaoyin* channel.

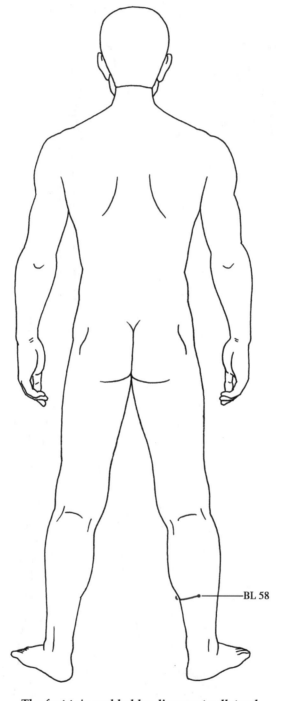

BL 58

The foot *taiyang* bladder divergent collateral

The **foot *taiyang* bladder channel divergence** branches out and runs upward to the sacrum, then the anus, joins the bladder, spreads in the kidney, runs up the back where it spreads in the heart. A vertical branch runs up from the back to the top of the head, and then goes into the main foot *taiyang* channel.

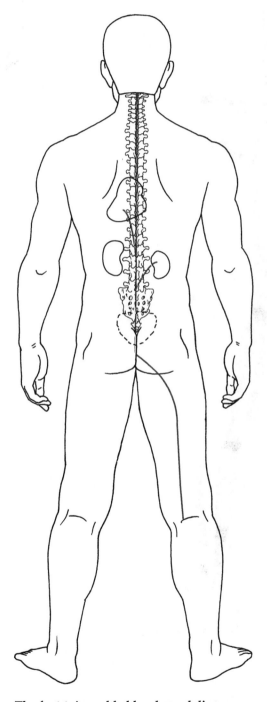

The foot *taiyang* bladder channel divergence

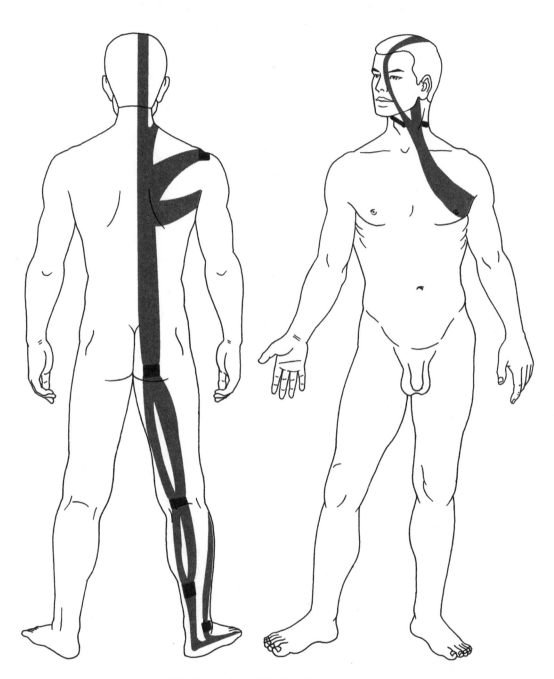

The foot *taiyang* bladder channel sinews

Acupoints

Foot *Taiyang* Bladder Channel

BL 1	睛明	*jīng míng*	Bright Eyes
BL 2	攒竹	*cuán zhú*	Bamboo Gathering
BL 3	眉冲	*méi chōng*	Eyebrow Ascension
BL 4	曲差	*qū chā*	Deviating Turn
BL 5	五处	*wǔ chù*	Fifth Place
BL 6	承光	*chéng guāng*	Light Guard
BL 7	通天	*tōng tiān*	Heaven's Palace
BL 8	络却	*luò què*	Declining Connection
BL 9	玉枕	*yù zhěn*	Jade Pillow
BL 10	天柱	*tiān zhù*	Heaven's Pillar
BL 11	大杼	*dà zhù*	Great Shuttle
BL 12	风门	*fēng mén*	Wind Gate
BL 13	肺俞	*fèi shù*	Lung Shu
BL 14	厥阴俞	*jué yīn shù*	Jue Yin Shu
BL 15	心俞	*xīn shù*	Heart Shu
BL 16	督俞	*dū shù*	Du Shu
BL 17	膈俞	*gé shù*	Diaphragm Shu
BL 18	肝俞	*gān shù*	Liver Shu
BL19	胆俞	*dǎn shù*	Gallbladder Shu
BL 20	脾俞	*pí shù*	Spleen Shu
BL 21	胃俞	*wèi shù*	Stomach Shu
BL 22	三焦俞	*sān jiāo shù*	San Jiao Shu
BL 23	肾俞	*shèn shù*	Kidney Shu
BL 24	气海俞	*qì hǎi shù*	Sea of Qi Shu
BL 25	大肠俞	*dà cháng shù*	Large Intestine Shu
BL 26	关元俞	*guān yuán shù*	Origin Pass Shu
BL 27	小肠俞	*xiǎo cháng shù*	Small Intestine Shu
BL 28	膀胱俞	*páng guāng shù*	Urinary Bladder Shu
BL 29	中膂俞	*zhōng lǚ shù*	Central Background Shu
BL 30	白环俞	*bái huán shù*	White Ring Shu
BL 31	上髎	*shàng liáo*	Upper Bone Hole
BL 32	次髎	*cì liáo*	Second Bone Hole
BL 33	中髎	*zhōng liáo*	Central Bone Hole
BL 34	下髎	*xià liáo*	Lower Bone hole
BL 35	会阳	*huì yáng*	Yang Meeting
BL 36	承扶	*chéng fú*	Support
BL 37	殷门	*yīn mén*	Abundance Gate

BL 38	浮郄	*fú xì*	Superficial Gate
BL 39	委阳	*wěi yáng*	Yang Bend
BL 40	委中	*wěi zhōng*	Center Bend
BL 41	附分	*fù fēn*	Attached Branch
BL 42	魄户	*pò hù*	Po Door
BL 43	膏肓	*gāo huāng (shù)*	Vital Organ Shu
BL 44	神堂	*shén táng*	Spirit Hall
BL 45	譩譆	*yì xī*	Yi Xi
BL 46	膈关	*gé guān*	Diaphragm Pass
BL 47	魂门	*hún mén*	Hun Gate
BL 48	阳纲	*yáng gāng*	Yang Rope
BL 49	意舍	*yì shè*	Yi House
BL 50	胃仓	*wèi cāng*	Stomach Granary
BL 51	肓门	*huāng mén*	Membrane Gate
BL 52	志室	*zhì shì*	Zhi Chamber
BL 53	胞肓	*bāo huāng*	Bladder Membrane
BL 54	秩边	*zhì biān*	Sequence Limit
BL 55	合阳	*hé yáng*	Yang Union
BL 56	承筋	*chéng jīn*	Sinew Support
BL 57	承山	*chéng shān*	Mountain Support
BL 58	飞扬	*fēi yáng*	Taking Flight
BL 59	跗阳	*fū yáng*	Instep Yang
BL 60	昆仑	*kūn lún*	Kun Lun (Mountains)
BL 61	仆参	*pú cān*	Subservient Visitor
BL 62	申脉	*shēn mài*	Extending Vessel
BL 63	金门	*jīn mén*	Metal Gate
BL 64	京骨	*jīng gǔ*	Capital Bone
BL 65	束骨	*shù gǔ*	Bundle Bone
BL 66	足通谷	*zú tōng gǔ*	Valley Passage
BL 67	至阴	*zhì yīn*	Reaching Yin

The Foot *Shaoyin* Kidney Channel

Common symptoms

Dry tongue, swelling and pain in the throat, hemoptysis, panting, edema, waist pain, pain of the medial and posterior aspect of the thigh, feverish feeling of the sole, etc.

Pathway

There are 27 points on the foot *shaoyin* kidney channel.

- The kidney channel starts at the little toe and runs through the center of the sole. It emerges at the heel and ascends along the back of the leg, the thigh, and the vertebral column, enters the kidney and connects with the bladder.

- A branch from the kidney ascends and passes through the liver and diaphragm and then enters the lung, runs along the throat, and finally reaches the two sides of the tongue root.
- A branch arises from the lung, joins with the heart and enters the chest to link with the hand *jueyin* pericardium channel.

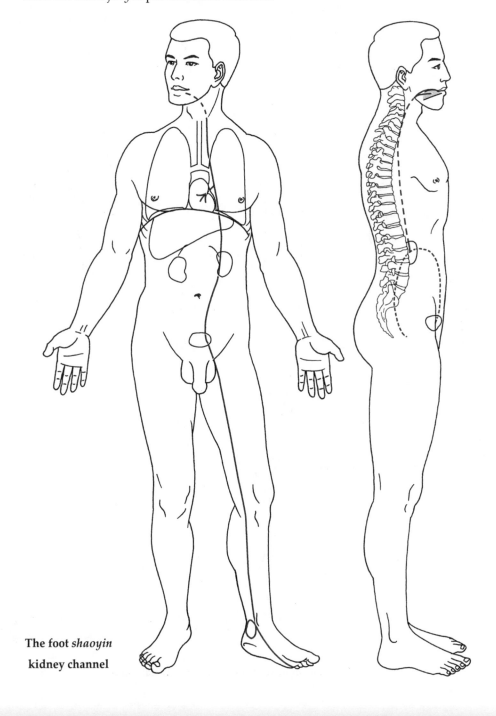

**The foot *shaoyin*
kidney channel**

The **foot *shaoyin* kidney divergent collateral** begins from the inside of the heel at KI4 (*dà zhōng*). Circling about the heel, it goes into the foot *taiyang* channel. It then joins the foot *shaoyin* kidney channel to below the pericardium organ, and then slightly downward to the lower back and the lumbar vertebrae.

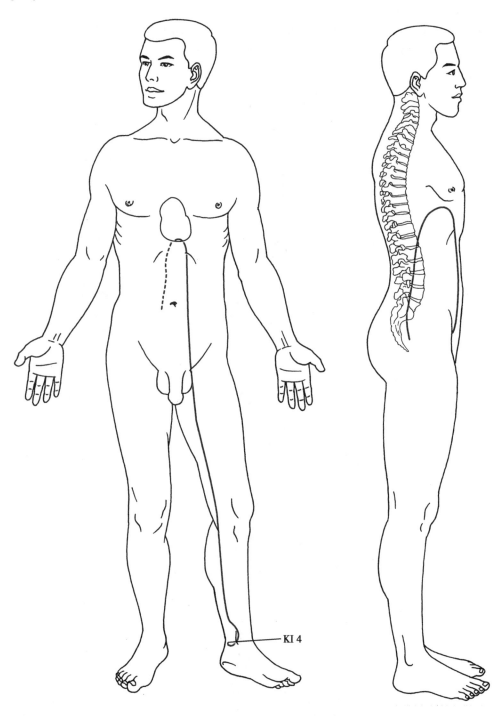

KI 4

The foot *shaoyin* kidney divergent collateral

The **foot** *shaoyin* **kidney channel divergence** branches out from behind the knee, joins the foot *taiyang* channel divergence and runs up to the kidney. At the 2nd lumbar vertebra, it joins the *dai mai*. The vertical branch goes the root of the tongue, then superficially at the nape of the neck, and finally goes into the foot *taiyang* bladder channel.

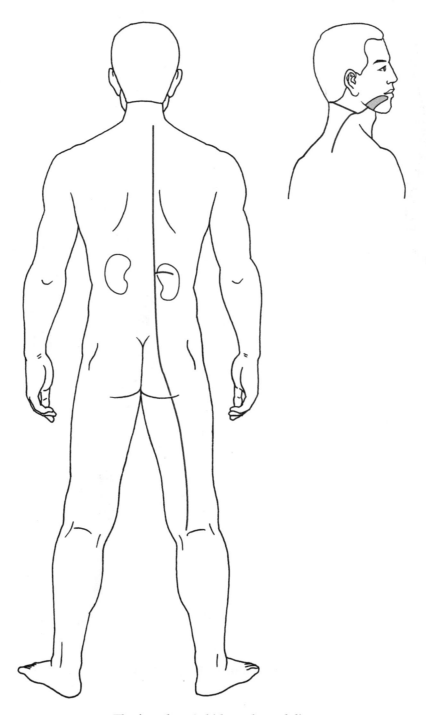

The foot *shaoyin* **kidney channel divergence**

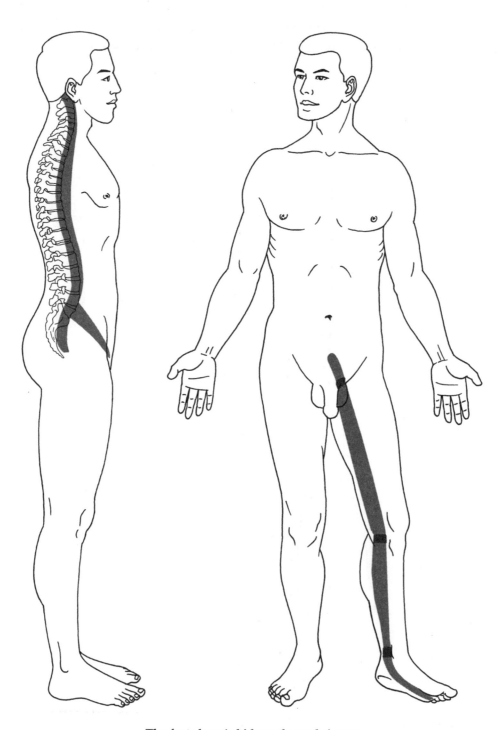

The foot *shaoyin* kidney channel sinews

Acupoints

Foot *Shaoyin* Kidney Channel

KI 1	涌泉	*yǒng quán*	Gushing Spring
KI 2	然谷	*rán gǔ*	Blazing Valley
KI 3	太溪	*tài xī*	Great Stream
KI 4	大钟	*dà zhōng*	Large Goblet
KI 5	水泉	*shuǐ quán*	Water Spring
KI 6	照海	*zhào hǎi*	Shining Sea
KI 7	复溜	*fù liū*	Recover Flow
KI 8	交信	*jiāo xìn*	Reaching Intersection
KI 9	筑宾	*zhù bīn*	Guest House
KI 10	阴谷	*yīn gǔ*	Yin Valley
KI 11	横骨	*héng gǔ*	Pubic Bone
KI 12	大赫	*dà hè*	Great Manifestation
KI 13	气穴	*qì xué*	Qi Point
KI 14	四满	*sì mǎn*	Fourfold Fullness
KI 15	中注	*zhōng zhù*	Central Flow
KI 16	肓俞	*huāng shù*	Membrane Transport
KI 17	商曲	*shāng qū*	Shang Bend
KI 18	石关	*shí guān*	Stone Pass
KI 19	阴都	*yīn dū*	Yin Capital
KI 20	腹通谷	*fù tōng gǔ*	Open Valley
KI 21	幽门	*yōu mén*	Dark Gate
KI 22	步廊	*bù láng*	Corridor Walk
KI 23	神封	*shén fēng*	Spirit Seal
KI 24	灵墟	*líng xū*	Spirit Ruins
KI 25	神藏	*shén cáng*	Spirit Storehouse
KI 26	彧中	*yù zhōng*	Lively Center
KI 27	俞府	*shù fǔ*	Transport Office

The Hand *Jueyin* Pericardium Channel

Common symptoms

Palpitations, heartache, vexation, chest distress, depressive psychosis and mania, arm swelling, spasm of the elbow and arm, feverish feeling of the palm, etc.

Pathway

There are 9 points on the hand *jueyin* pericardium channel.

- The channel starts from the inside of chest where affiliates to the pericardium. Then it descends through the diaphragm to connect with the upper, middle and lower *jiao*.

- An internal branch arises from the inside of chest, then it runs along the inside of the chest and emerges superficially from the costal region near the nipple. Then it ascends to the axilla (armpit) to the upper limb, inside of the elbow, to the wrist, and then to the palm, and the middle finger to its tip.
- Another internal branch out from the palm, then runs to the ring finger to its tip

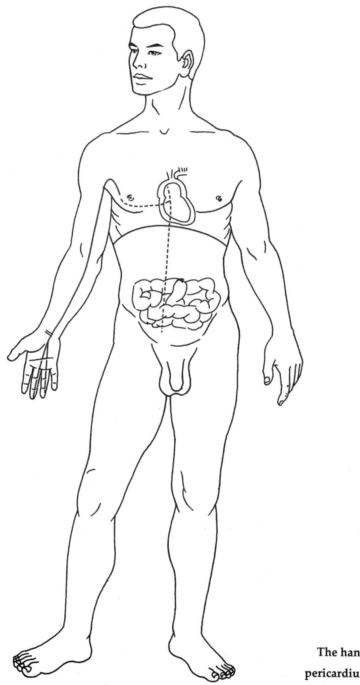

The hand *jueyin*
pericardium channel

and connects with the hand *shaoyang sanjiao* channel.

The **hand *jueyin* pericardium divergent collateral** originates from the inside of the forearm at PC 6 (*nèi guān*). Its branch goes into the hand *shaoyang* channel, runs up along the channel properly and scatters over and connects with the pericardium.

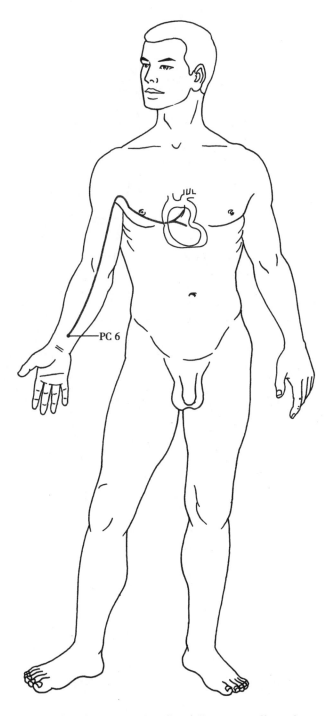

The hand *jueyin* pericardium divergent collateral

The **hand *jueyin* pericardium channel divergence** branches out from the hand *jueyin* channel on the abdomen and then enters the chest and links with the upper, middle and lower *jiao*. It also runs upward along the throat, then behind the ear and joins the hand *shaoyang* channel below the mastoid process.

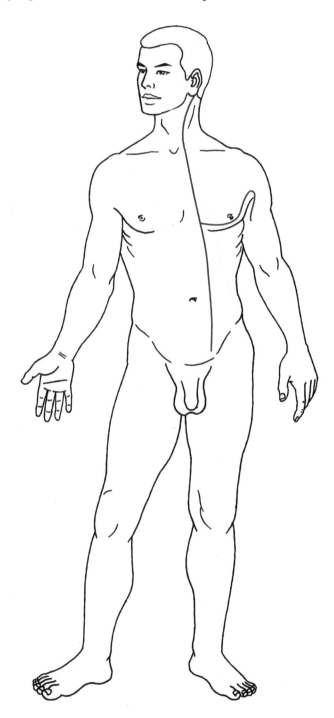

The hand *jueyin* pericardium channel divergence

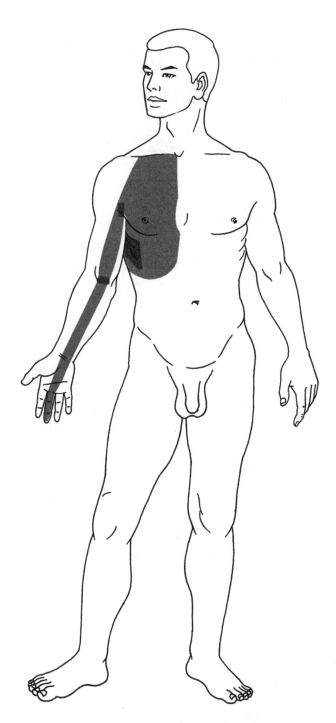

The hand *jueyin* pericardium channel sinews

Acupoints

Hand *Jueyin* Pericardium Channel

PC 1	天池	*tiān chí*	Heaven's Pool
PC 2	天泉	*tiān quán*	Heaven's Spring
PC 3	曲泽	*qū zé*	Marsh Bend
PC 4	郄门	*xì mén*	Cleft Gate
PC 5	间使	*jiān shǐ*	Intermediary courier
PC 6	内关	*nèi guān*	Inner Pass
PC 7	大陵	*dà líng*	Great Mound
PC 8	劳宫	*láo gōng*	Toiling Palace
PC 9	中冲	*zhōng chōng*	Central Hub

The Hand *Shaoyang Sanjiao* Channel

Common symptoms

Abdominal distention, edema, tinnitus, deafness, swelling and pain in the throat, cheek pain, pain of the outer canthus, pain in the retroauricular region and lateral aspect of the shoulder, arm and elbow, etc.

Pathway

There are 23 points on the hand *shaoyang sanjiao* channel.

- The hand *shaoyang sanjiao* channel starts from the ring finger and goes to the wrist, to the upper arm and the shoulder region, to the front of the neck and connects with the pericardium. Passing through the diaphragm, it enters the upper, middle and lower *jiao*.

- An internal branch rises from the pericardium, runs to the neck and to the shoulder region. It goes to the back of the neck, to behind the ear, curves downward to the cheek and arrives at the eye.

- Another branch arises from the ear, enters the ear, comes out in front of the ear and passes the face and cheek. It further runs to the outer canthus of the eye where it links with the foot *shaoyang* gallbladder channel.

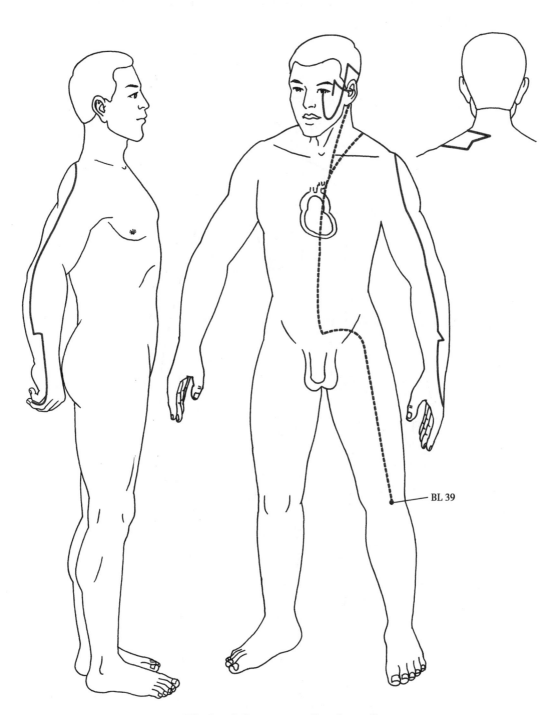

The hand *shaoyang sanjiao* **channel**

The **hand** *shaoyang sanjiao* **divergent collateral** originates from the forearm at SJ 5 (*wài guān*) to the lateral aspect of the arm, and enters the thoracic cavity to join the hand *jueyin* pericardium channel.

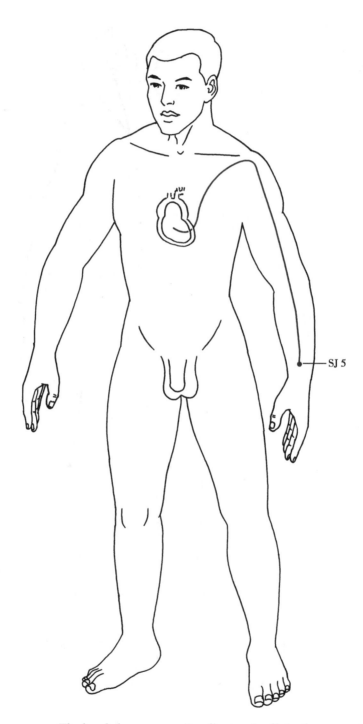

SJ 5

The hand *shaoyang sanjiao* divergent collateral

The **hand *shaoyang sanjiao* channel divergence** branches out from the hand *shaoyang* channel at the vertex to top of the head. It goes down into the supraclavicular fossa, then passes through the upper, middle and lower *jiao* and spreads in the chest.

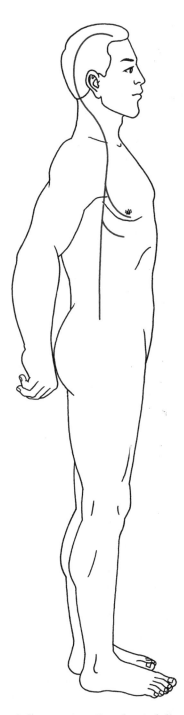

The hand *shaoyang sanjiao* channel divergence

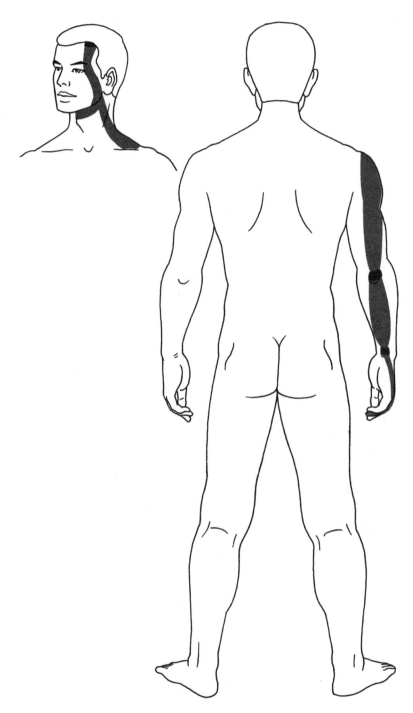

The hand *shaoyang sanjiao* channel sinews

Acupoints

Hand *Shaoyang Sanjiao* Channel

SJ 1	关冲	*guān chōng*	Passage Hub
SJ 2	液门	*yè mén*	Liquid Gate
SJ 3	中渚	*zhōng zhǔ*	Central Islet
SJ 4	阳池	*yáng chí*	Yang Pool
SJ 5	外关	*wài guān*	Outer Pass
SJ 6	支沟	*zhī gōu*	Branch Ditch
SJ 7	会宗	*huì zōng*	Converge and Gather
SJ 8	三阳络	*sān yáng luò*	Three Yang Connection
SJ 9	四渎	*sì dú*	Four Rivers
SJ 10	天井	*tiān jǐng*	Heaven's Well
SJ 11	清冷渊	*qīng lěng yuān*	Clear Cold Abyss
SJ 12	消泺	*xiāo luò*	Dispersing Riverbed
SJ 13	臑会	*nào huì*	Upper Arm Convergence
SJ 14	肩髎	*jiān liáo*	Shoulder Bone Hole
SJ 15	天髎	*tiān liáo*	Heaven's Hone Hole
SJ 16	天牖	*tiān yǒu*	Heaven's Window
SJ 17	翳风	*yì fēng*	Wind Screen
SJ 18	瘈脉	*chì mài*	Tugging Vessel
SJ 19	颅息	*lú xī*	Skull Rest
SJ 20	角孙	*jiǎo sūn*	Angle Vertex
SJ 21	耳门	*ěr mén*	Ear Gate
SJ 22	耳和髎	*ěr hé liáo*	Harmony Bone Hole
SJ 23	丝竹空	*sī zhú kōng*	Silk Bamboo Hole

The Foot *Shaoyang* Gallbladder Channel

Common symptoms

Bitter taste in the mouth, headache, pain of the outer canthus, mandibular pain, malaria, pain at the supraclavicular fossa, swelling, pain in the hypochondrium and lateral side of the lower limb, feverish feeling of the lateral side of the foot, etc.

Pathway

There are 44 points on the foot *shaoyang* gallbladder channel.

- The *shaoyang* gallbladder channel begins from the lateral aspect of the eye area, ascends to the corner of the forehead, to behind the ear and turns back and runs to the forehead and to the eyebrow. It then returns to the neck, to the shoulder, to the center of the back, and then runs forward to the supraclavicular fossa.

- A branch arises by the ear and enters the ear, comes out from in front of the ear and then to the outer canthus of the eye.

- A branch emerges from the outer canthus, goes to the jaw and meets the branch of the hand *shaoyang sanjiao* channel at the cheek. Then it runs up to the infraorbital region; returning it runs down through jaw and neck. From there, it enters the body cavity, passes through the diaphragm to connect with the liver, and enters the gallbladder. It then runs along the inside the hypochondriac region to the inguinal groove where it emerges superficially, circling about the pubic hair, and runs transversely to the hips and buttocks.

- A branch from the supraclavicular fossa runs downward to the axilla, further descends along the lateral aspect of the chest and via the floating rib to hip buttocks, at which it meets the preceding branch. Then it again runs downward along the lateral aspect of the thigh and the lateral side of the knee joint. Going down in front of the fibula, it reaches the lower end of the lower leg. After coming out superficially at the anterior aspect of the external malleolus, it runs along the dorsum of the foot to the lateral aspect of the tip of the 4th toe.

- A branch comes out at the top of the foot and then runs forward to the lateral aspect of the tip of the big toe. Returning, it passes through the nail and arrives at the big toe, where it connects with the foot *jueyin* liver channel.

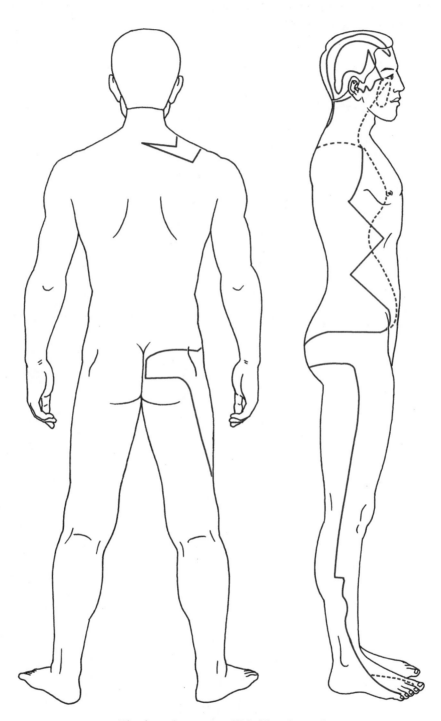

The foot *shaoyang* gallbladder channel

The **foot** *shaoyang* **gallbladder divergent collateral** starts from the lower leg at GB 37 (*guāng míng*), then goes into the foot *jueyin* liver channel, and runs downward to link with the dorsum of the foot.

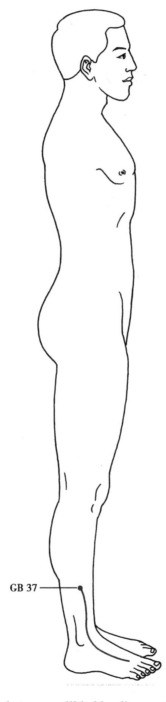

GB 37

The foot *shaoyang* gallbladder divergent collateral

The **foot *shaoyang* gallbladder channel divergence** branches out from the foot *shaoyang* channel at the lateral aspect of the thigh. Circling the anterior part of the thigh it goes into the margin of the pubic hair, where it joins the foot *jueyin* channel divergence. It runs up passing the ribs and along the inside of the thorax. It joins the

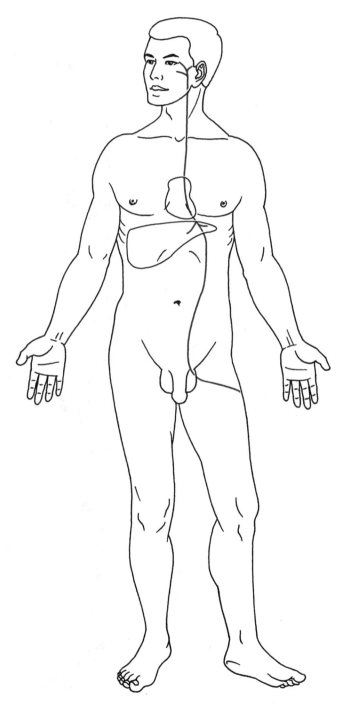

The foot *shaoyang* gallbladder channel divergence

gallbladder and spreads in the liver, then goes through the heart, and further ascends alongside the esophagus. It runs superficially to the jaw, around the mouth, spreads over the face, and connects with the eye connector, where it finally goes into the foot *shaoyang* channel at the outer canthus (GB1, *tóng zǐ liáo*).

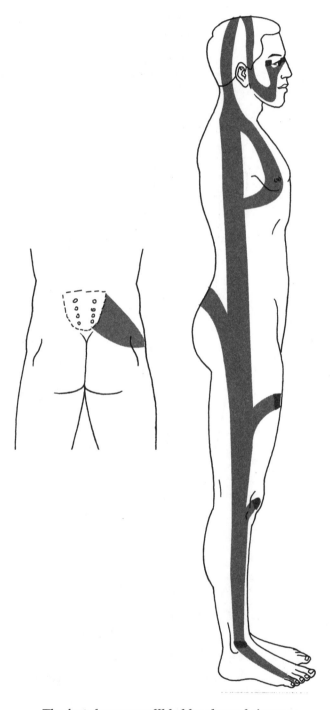

The foot *shaoyang* gallbladder channel sinews

Acupoints

Foot *Shaoyang* Gallbladder Channel

GB 1	瞳子髎	*tóng zǐ liáo*	Pupil Bone Hole
GB 2	听会	*tīng huì*	Hearing Converging
GB 3	上关	*shàng guān*	Upper Gate
GB 4	颔厌	*hán yàn*	Forehead Fullness
GB 5	悬颅	*xuán lú*	Suspended Skull
GB 6	悬厘	*xuán lí*	Suspended Tuft
GB 7	曲鬓	*qū bìn*	Temporal Hairline Curve
GB 8	率谷	*shuài gǔ*	Valley Lead
GB 9	天冲	*tiān chōng*	Heaven's Hub
GB 10	浮白	*fú bái*	Floating White
GB 11	头窍阴	*tóu qiào yīn*	Head Orifice Yin
GB 12	完骨	*wán gǔ*	Completion Bone
GB 13	本神	*běn shén*	Root Spirit
GB 14	阳白	*yáng bái*	Yang White
GB 15	头临泣	*tóu lín qì*	Head Overlooking Tears
GB 16	目窗	*mù chuāng*	Eye Window
GB 17	正营	*zhèng yíng*	Upright Construction
GB 18	承灵	*chéng líng*	Spirit Support
GB 19	脑空	*nǎo kōng*	Brain Hollow
GB 20	风池	*fēng chí*	Wind Pool
GB 21	肩井	*jiān jǐng*	Shoulder Well
GB 22	渊腋	*yuān yè*	Armpit Abyss
GB 23	辄筋	*zhé jīn*	Sinew Seat
GB 24	日月	*rì yuè*	Sun and Moon
GB 25	京门	*jīng mén*	Capital Gate
GB 26	带脉	*dài mài*	Dai Vessel
GB 27	五枢	*wǔ shū*	Fifth Pivot
GB 28	维道	*wéi dào*	Linking Path
GB 29	居髎	*jū liáo*	Squatting Bone Hole
GB 30	环跳	*huán tiào*	Jumping Round
GB 31	风市	*fēng shì*	Wind Market
GB 32	中渎	*zhōng dú*	Central River
GB 33	膝阳关	*xī yáng guān*	Knee Yang Joint
GB 34	阳陵泉	*yáng líng quán*	Yang Mound Spring

GB 35	阳交	*yáng jiāo*	Yang Intersection
GB 36	外丘	*wài qiū*	Outer Hill
GB 37	光明	*guāng míng*	Bright Light
GB 38	阳辅	*yáng fǔ*	Yang Assistance
GB 39	悬钟	*xuán zhōng*	Suspended Bell
GB 40	丘墟	*qiū xū*	Hill Ruins
GB 41	足临泣	*zú lín qì*	Foot Overlooking Tears
GB 42	地五会	*dì wǔ huì*	Earth Five Converging
GB 43	侠溪	*xiá xī*	Pinched Brook
GB 44	足窍阴	*zú qiào yīn*	Foot Orifice Yin

The Foot *Jueyin* Liver Channel

Common symptoms

Chest fullness, vomiting, nausea, waist pain, enuresis, dribbling urinary block, hernia type disorders, distention and pain of the lesser abdomen, etc.

Pathway

There are 14 points on the foot *jueyin* liver channel.

- It starts from the top of the big toe and then runs up the leg to the knee and then the thigh and the pubic region. Curving round the external genitalia, it runs up to the lower abdomen and enters the abdominal cavity, the stomach, the liver, and connects with the gallbladder. After that, it goes through the diaphragm, and to hypochondriac region. Then it runs to the throat and links to the eye connector. From the forehead, it runs up to the top of the head, where it meets the *du* vessel.

- A branch arises from the eye connector, then descends, runs along the inside of the cheek, and curves round the inner surface of the lips.

- A second branch comes out from the liver where it ascends through the diaphragm and enters the lung to link with the hand *taiyin* lung channel.

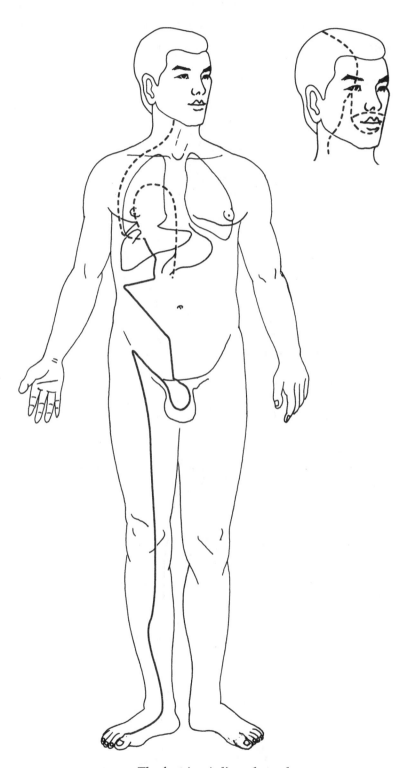

The foot *jueyin* liver channel

The **foot** *jueyin* **liver divergent collateral** originates from LV 5 (*lí gōu*) on the lower leg and then goes into the foot *shaoyang* channel. Its branch moves to the tibial region and ascends to the testicles, and terminates at the penis.

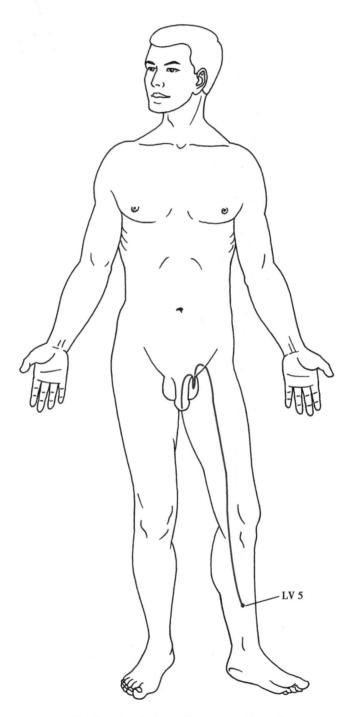

LV 5

The foot *jueyin* **liver divergent collateral**

The **foot *jueyin* liver channel divergence** branches out from the foot *jueyin* channel at the dorsum of the foot. Ascending to the margin of the pubic hair, it joins the *shaoyang* gallbladder channel divergence. Because the GB divergent goes to the eyes, we can understand more fully how the liver channel (foot *jueyin*) can influence the eyes.

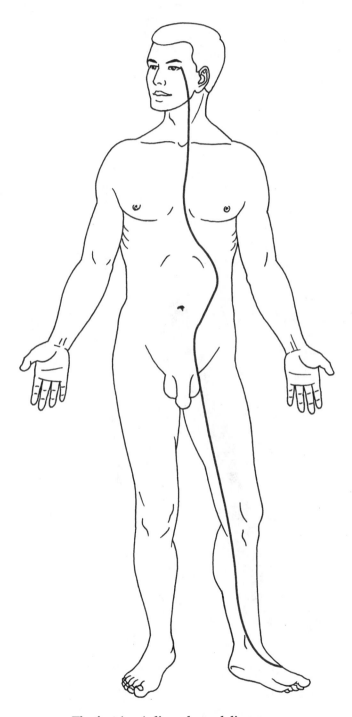

The foot *jueyin* liver channel divergence

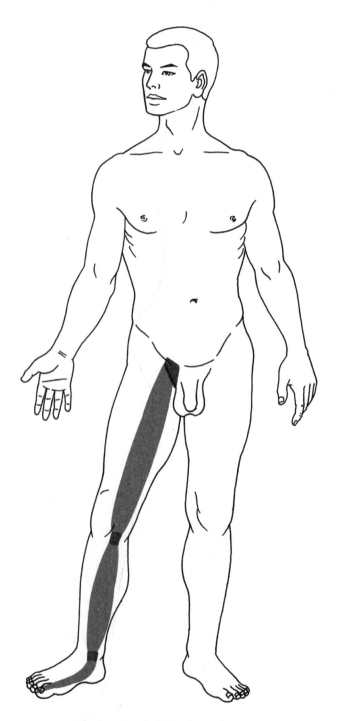

The foot *jueyin* liver channel sinews

Acupoints

Foot *Jueyin* Liver Channel

LV 1	大敦	dà dūn	Large Vessel
LV 2	行间	xíng jiān	Moving Between
LV 3	太冲	tài chōng	Supreme Surging
LV 4	中封	zhōng fēng	Center Mound
LV 5	蠡沟	lí gōu	Woodworm Canal
LV 6	中都	zhōng dū	Central Capital
LV 7	膝关	xī guān	Knee Joint
LV 8	曲泉	qū quán	Spring at the Bend
LV 9	阴包	yīn bāo	Yin Container
LV 10	足五里	zú wǔ lǐ	Foot Five Miles
LV 11	阴廉	yīn lián	Yin Corner
LV 12	急脉	jí mài	Urgent Pulse
LV 13	章门	zhāng mén	Seal Gate
LV 14	期门	qī mén	Cycle Gate

Section 3   Eight Extraordinary Vessels

The eight extraordinary vessels refer to the *du mai, ren mai, chong mai, dai mai, yinqiao mai, yangqiao mai, yinwei mai,* and *yangwei mai*. These eight vessels (*mài*, 脉) differ from the twelve main channels in that they share no direct affiliation with the *zang-fu* organs, have no external-internal relationships among themselves, and their distributions are not as regular; thus they are referred to as "extraordinary vessels".

The eight extraordinary vessels are said to carry the "surplus" qi of the 12 main channels. Li Shi-zhen writes, "The main channels are like irrigation ditches, and the extraordinary channels are like lakes and marshes. When the vessels of the main channels are swollen and abundant, they overflow into the extraordinary channels."

Li also describes a two-way passage between the main channels and the extraordinary vessels. He writes, "The overflow of qi (from the channels and networks) enters the extraordinary vessels to provide reciprocal irrigation and internal warming of the organs."

MAIN PHYSIOLOGICAL FUNCTIONS OF THE EIGHT EXTRAORDINARY VESSELS

The eight extraordinary vessel pathways cross over and connect with the twelve main channels, thus acting to strengthen communication among them. Many of the extraordinary vessels can be classified and grouped according to their characteristic functions.

For example, *du mai* meets the six yang channels of the hands and feet at DU 14 (*dà zhuī*), thus referred to as the "the sea of the yang channels".

The *ren mai* at RN 4 (*guān yuán*) communicates with the three foot yin channels which again link with the three hand yin channels, thus referred to as "the sea of the yin channels".

The *chong mai* runs superiorly, inferiorly, anteriorly and posteriorly, communicating with the three yin and three yang channels, thus referred to as "the sea of the twelve channels".

The *dai mai* binds all the channels which run vertically, communicating especially with the channels running through the waist and abdomen.

The *yangwei mai* regulates all the yang channels and links them with the *du mai*.

The *yinwei mai* regulates all the yin channels and links them with the *ren mai*.

The *yangqiao* and *yinqiao mai* run in pairs on the right and left, thus the saying "the *qiao mai* control the yin and yang channels on both right and left of the body".

The main function of the extraordinary vessels is to store and regulate the qi and blood of the twelve main channels. The eight extraordinary vessels act to supplement the qi and blood of the main channels in the event of insufficiency, while also acting to store qi and blood when there is an overabundance. In this way, the extraordinary vessels help to maintain a relatively constant supply of qi and blood in the main channels.

Although the eight extraordinary vessels have no direct connection with the *zang-fu* organs, they have close relationships with the kidney as well as the brain, marrow, and uterus (three of the extraordinary *fu*-organs). The eight extraordinary vessels also facilitate communication between some of the organs; for example, the *du mai* "enters the cranial cavity to communicate with the brain", "runs along the inside of the spinal column", and "joins the kidney". Regarding the vessels themselves, there is greatest communication between the *ren, du,* and *chong mai* in that they all originate from the lower abdomen.

PATHWAYS AND FUNCTIONS OF THE EIGHT EXTRAORDINARY VESSELS

There are several unique features that should be featured when comparing the extraordinary vessels with the twelve main channels. Because the extraordinary vessels run crosswise over the twelve main channels, their distribution is more irregular. Also, with the exception of the *dai mai*, their pathways run from the lower to the upper areas of the body, while no extraordinary vessel goes to the upper limbs. Furthermore, there is no exterior-interior relationship among the eight extraordinary vessels. Some sources also hold that the eight extraordinary vessels function independently of the five-phase and seasonal correspondences as normally associated with the internal organs and channels.

The eight extraordinary vessels are generally paired into four groups: the *ren* and *du*, the *yinwei* and *yangwei*, the *yinqiao* and *yangqiao*, and the *chong* and *dai mai*.

DU AND *REN MAI*

The *du* and *ren mai* both originate within the lower abdomen, and due to their running course, the pair is often seen as one channel that vertically encircles the body and head. There is a basic qi gong practice called the "microscopic orbit" that promotes the movement of qi through the *du* and *ren mai*; qi in the body is intentionally visualized as moving upward along the back and over the head through the *du mai*, and then downward along the *ren mai* to complete the cycle.

Du Mai

The *du mai* contains 28 points. The pathway begins near the anus and travels upward along the back and over the head, terminating near the upper lip.

Basic functions

The *du mai* is also referred to as the "governing vessel", and because it acts to regulate the qi and blood of the yang channels, it is also known as the "sea of yang channels". In its running course, the *du mai* intersects with the three yang hand and foot channels as well as the *yangwei mai*. For example, it meets with the three yang hand and foot channels at DU 14 (*dà zhuī*) on the upper back, the foot *taiyang* channel at DU 17 (*nǎo hù*) and DU 20 (*bǎi huì*) on the head, and with the *yangwei mai* at points DU 16 (*fēng fǔ*) and DU 15 (*yǎ mén*). Accordingly, as the "sea of yang channels", the *du mai* acts to regulate the qi and blood of all yang channels.

An important *du mai* point on the lower back is DU 4 (*mìng mén*, 命门). The term *ming men* refers to both the name of the point as well as an area in the lower abdomen where kidney qi and essence are especially concentrated and transformed. *Ming men* can be translated literally as "destiny gate", and is associated with the *dan tian* (丹田). The *dan tian* and the *ming men* are emphasized in many martial arts and qi gong exercises as well as in Taoist practices.

The *du mai* runs along the inside of the spinal column and enters the brain, closely related with both the brain and marrow. With the *du mai* pathway passing through the spinal column and brain, typical signs and symptoms of *du mai* disorders include spinal stiffness, and sudden fainting with unconsciousness. The *du mai* also joins the kidney, and because the kidney governs reproduction and is the foundation of the prenatal constitution, infertility, premature aging and senility can all be treated by accessing the *du mai*.

Pathway

- Li Shi-zhen writes, "The *du* is the sea of yang vessels. Its vessel starts from within the gestational membranes below the kidneys, goes to the lower abdomen, the lumbar and then circles the pubic bone, where it links with the end of the urethral opening. In men, it proceeds to the penis and then descends to the perineum. For women, a network goes to the genitals and unites at the perineum." Then it ascends along the inside of the spinal column to the DU 16 (*fēng fǔ*) point at the nape of the neck where it enters the cranial cavity to communicate with the brain. It further runs following the midline of the head, via the vertex, forehead, nose and upper lip, and reaches the upper lip.

- A branch arises from the inside of the spinal column where it joins the kidney. Another branch starts from the interior of the lower abdomen, it vertically runs up, passes through the center of the umbilicus and the heart, and arrives at the throat. It further ascends to the mandibular region, then curves round the lips, and finally terminates at the centers of the inferior regions of the two eyes.

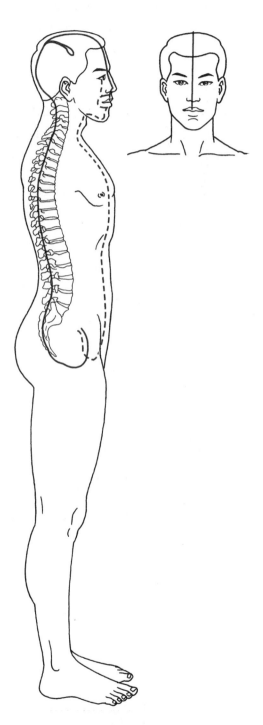

Du mai

The **divergent collateral of** *du mai* originates from DU 1 (*cháng qiáng*). It runs upward alongside the vertebral column and arrives at the nape and spreads over the head. Two downward collaterals start at the scapula regions and go respectively into the foot *taiyang* channels on both left and right, deeply entering the paravertebral muscles.

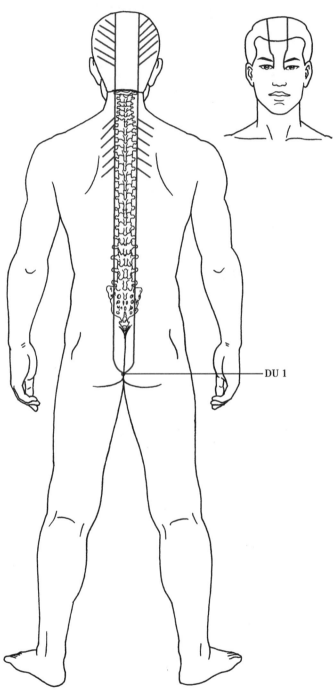

DU 1

The divergent collateral of *du mai*

Acupoints

Du Mai

DU 1	长强	*cháng qiáng*	Long Strong
DU 2	腰俞	*yāo shù*	Lumbar Shu
DU 3	腰阳关	*yāo yáng guān*	Lumbar Yang Pass
DU 4	命门	*mìng mén*	Vitality Gate
DU 5	悬枢	*xuán shū*	Suspended Pivot
DU 6	脊中	*jǐ zhōng*	Spinal Center
DU 7	中枢	*zhōng shū*	Central Pivot
DU 8	筋缩	*jǐn suō*	Sinew Contraction
DU 9	至阳	*zhì yáng*	Extremity of Yang
DU 10	灵台	*líng tái*	Spirit Tower
DU 11	神道	*shén dào*	Spirit Path
DU 12	身柱	*shēn zhù*	Body Pillar
DU 13	陶道	*táo dào*	Kiln Pathway
DU 14	大椎	*dà zhuī*	Great Hammer
DU 15	哑门	*yǎ mén*	Mute's Gate
DU 16	风府	*fēng fǔ*	Wind Office
DU 17	脑户	*nǎo hù*	Brain's Door
DU 18	强间	*qiáng jiān*	Unyielding Space
DU 19	后顶	*hòu dǐng*	Behind the Vertex
DU 20	百会	*bǎi huì*	Hundred Convergences
DU 21	前顶	*qián dǐng*	Before the Vertex
DU 22	囟会	*xìn huì*	Fontanel Meeting
DU 23	上星	*shàng xīng*	Upper Star
DU 24	神庭	*shén tíng*	Spirit Court
DU 25	素髎	*sù liáo*	White Bone Hole
DU 26	水沟	*shuǐ gōu*	Water Trough
DU 27	兑端	*duì duān*	Mouth Extremity
DU 28	龈交	*yín jiāo*	Gum Intersection

Ren Mai

Basic functions

Because of its association with women's physiology and fertility, the *ren mai* is often translated as the "conception vessel". In a commentary on the *Classic of Difficult Issues* (*Nàn Jīng*, 难经), Yang Shang-shan stated that "*Ren* means to be pregnant; this is the root of human life and its nourishment. " Wang Bing's commentary on Chapter 60 of *Basic Questions* states, "The reason for the *ren* vessel being named so is because it is the means by which women become pregnant. Therefore, *The Yellow Emperor's Inner Classic* states that, 'If this vessel is diseased, the woman will be infertile.'"

The main functions of the *ren* vessel are to regulate the qi and blood of the yin channels. The *ren* vessel runs along the front midline where it meets several times with the three foot yang channels and also the *yinwei mai*. Accordingly, the *ren mai* communicates between the yin channels to regulate their qi and blood, thus the *ren mai* is referred to as "the sea of the yin channels".

The *ren* vessel also controls the development of the embryo and fetus. The *ren mai* originates from the deep within the lower abdomen and specifically the womb for a female. The *ren mai* is thus associated with menstruation, conception and fetal development.

Pathway

The *ren mai* runs mainly on the front of the body, but the direction of its flow remains debatable. Some hold that the *ren mai* involves two pathways along the front of the body that run in both upward and downward directions.

- The *ren mai* originates from the interior of the lower abdomen. Descending, it emerges at the perineum between the legs. It then ascends via the mons pubis and along the midline of the abdomen and chest to the throat. It further runs upward to the jaw, curves round the lips, and passes through the cheek where it then divides to reach the eyes.
- A branch starts from deeply in the lower abdomen, and runs upward in front of the spinal column together with a branch of the *chong mai*.

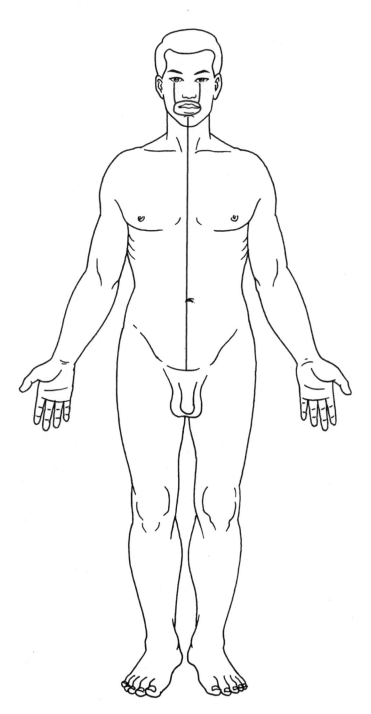

Ren mai

The **divergent collateral of the *ren mai*** originates at RN 15 (*jiū wěi*) and then runs downward from the sternal xiphoid to spread over the abdomen.

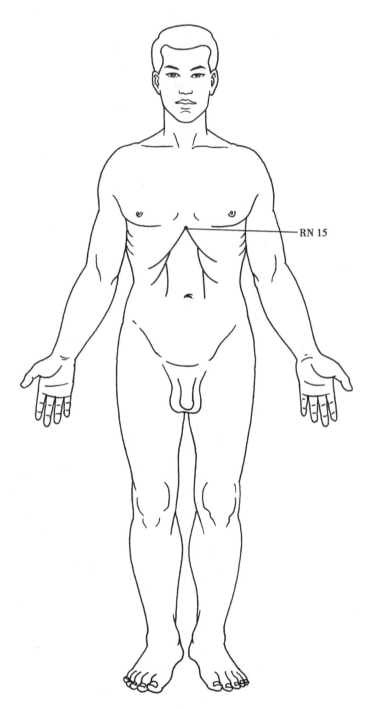

The divergent collateral of the *ren mai*

Acupoints

Ren Mai

RN 1	会阴	*huì yīn*	Yin Meeting
RN 2	曲骨	*qū gǔ*	Curved Bone
RN 3	中极	*zhōng jí*	Central Pole
RN 4	关元	*guān yuán*	Origin Gate
RN 5	石门	*shí mén*	Stone Gate
RN 6	气海	*qì hǎi*	Sea of Qi
RN 7	阴交	*yīn jiāo*	Yin Intersection
RN 8	神阙	*shén què*	Spirit Gate Tower
RN 9	水分	*shuǐ fēn*	Water Divide
RN 10	下脘	*xià wǎn*	Lower Stomach Duct
RN 11	建里	*jiàn lǐ*	Interior Strengthening
RN 12	中脘	*zhōng wǎn*	Central Stomach Duct
RN 13	上脘	*shàng wǎn*	Upper Stomach Duct
RN 14	巨阙	*jù què*	Great Tower Gate
RN 15	鸠尾	*jiū wěi*	Turtle Dove Tail
RN 16	中庭	*zhōng tíng*	Central Palace
RN 17	膻中	*dàn zhōng*	Chest Center
RN 18	玉堂	*yù táng*	Jade Hall
RN 19	紫宫	*zǐ gōng*	Purple Palace
RN 20	华盖	*huá gài*	Florid Canopy
RN 21	璇玑	*xuán jī*	Jade Swivel
RN 22	天突	*tiān tū*	Heaven's Chimney
RN 23	廉泉	*lián quán*	Ridge Spring
RN 24	承浆	*chéng jiāng*	Sauce Receptacle

CHONG AND *DAI MAI*

The *chong mai* is the most interior of all the vessels and channels and acts to unite them from the interior. The *dai mai* circles around the entire body, binding all of the channels together like a string holding together a group of sticks. Together, the *chong* and *dai mai* can then be seen as the most interior and exterior respectively of the eight extraordinary vessels.

Chong Mai

Basic functions

The *chong mai* acts to regulate both qi and blood of the twelve channels. The *chong mai* is therefore called the "sea of blood" and the "sea of the channels". The *chong mai* runs upward to the head, downward to the foot, posterior on the back, and anterior at the abdomen and chest. Because the *chong mai* runs throughout most of the body, its functions are also quite extensive. It serves as the hub of circulation for qi and blood, acting to regulate qi and blood of all twelve main channels. An ascending part runs inside the spinal column, opening into all yang channels, while a descending part runs to the lower limb, opening into all yin channels. Consequently, it receives and regulates the qi and blood of both the main channels and the *zang-fu* organs.

Clinically, the *chong mai* is strongly related with menstruation and pregnancy, which are both said to be based upon blood and *tian gui*. The *chong mai* originates deeply in the lower abdomen, and its attributions are extensive. Only when the *chong* and *ren mai* maintain an abundant supply of qi and blood can blood flow downward into the womb where it is discharged as menses or remains to nourish the fetus during pregnancy. If the qi and blood of the *chong mai* and *ren mai* become deficient or its flow becomes impeded, menstrual irregularities, menopause or infertility may result. For this reason, the *chong mai* and *ren mai* are both extremely important in the clinical treatment of menstrual disorders and infertility.

The *Basic Questions*, Chapter 1 states, "At the age of seven, the kidney qi in women is abundant, they grow their second teeth and their hair grows. At fourteen, menstruation arrives. The *ren mai* is activated, the supreme *chong mai* is strong, the monthly cycles occur regularly, and thus they can have children ... At the age of 49, the *ren mai* becomes insufficient, the supreme *chong mai* weakens and becomes scarce, the monthly flow ceases and the reproductive system is no longer active, so the body deteriorates and loses fertility."[1]

The *Spiritual Pivot* describes one interesting manifestation of a *chong mai* disorder, stating that if there is an "excess of the sea of blood, one has constant sensation of a large body, and one becomes ill at ease (anxious and unhappy) without knowing where the illness is located. If there is an insufficiency of the sea of blood, one has the sensation of a small body, and one becomes cramped without knowing where the illness is located".

Pathway

- The *chong mai* originates from the interior of the lower abdomen. Descending, it

---

① Mei Jiang-han. The Extraordinary Channel Chong Mai and its Clinical Applications. Journal of Chinese Medicine; Sept1993: 27.

emerges at the perineum. From there, it joins the foot *shaoyin* kidney channel to ascend to the navel, and spreading to the chest. Then it runs up through to the throat and curves around the lips, terminating at the eye region.

- One branch starts from the lesser abdomen, it runs to the inferior part of the

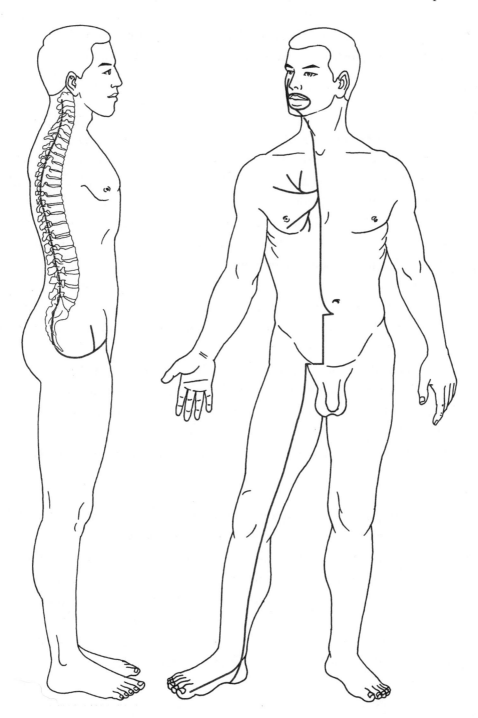

Chong mai

kidney and then to the inguinal region. From there it runs superficially and downward along the medial aspect of the thigh to the popliteal fossa. Then it further descends along the medial side of the tibia to the sole.

- Another branch arises from the area posterior to the medial malleolus, runs forward and obliquely into the dorsum of the foot, and enters the big toe.
- Yet another branch starts from the interior of the lower abdomen, runs backward and joins *du mai*, ascending along the spinal column.

Dai Mai

Basic functions

Dai (带) literally means belt, thus a common translation for *dai mai* is "belt vessel". The *dai mai* pathway runs horizontally (transversely) around the body in order to bind together the twelve main channels and the other seven extraordinary vessels (all of which run vertically) while also acting to regulate their channel-qi. Another image is that of the string or binding used to hold together a bundle of sticks or a bale of hay. The idea of binding together the channels to maintain structure is particularly important for clinical conditions that involve the lower abdominal area.

Another important function of the *dai mai* is to "dominate the white" in women. This means that, in women, if the *dai mai* becomes insufficient and fails to control the channels, there may be leukorrhea with soreness and weakness of the waist and lower back.

Roche de la Vallee writes, "The name for these discharges is *dai xia* (带下). *Xia* means to descend and *dai* is the belt or girdle which gives its name to the extraordinary meridian [vessel]. In some books *dai* is the traditional name for gynaecology or gynaecological pathology. *Dai xia* is a name which can be given to any kind of gynaecological disease but nowadays it is used specifically for vaginal discharges."[1]

Pathway

The *dai mai* originates at the site inferior to the free end of the twelfth rib, runs obliquely downward to the waist, and then curves around waist and abdomen of the body. It then runs forward and downward, then following the superior border of the ilium, and then runs obliquely to the lateral aspect of the lower abdomen. The *dai mai* can be visualized as a wide belt which rides low at the front. It is also thought the *dai mai* not only encircles the channels that pass through the waist, but that its influence also binds all of the channels throughout the body, including the arms and legs. In this way, the *dai mai* is also affiliated with the broader concept of *shaoyang*.

---

[1]   Elizabeth Rochat de la Vallee. *The Essential Woman*. London: Monkey Press; 2007. p. 53.

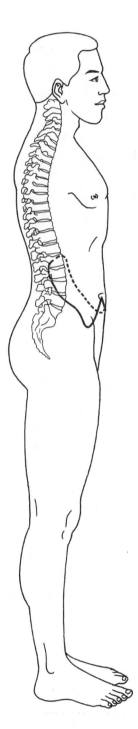

Dai mai

YANGQIAO MAI AND *YINQIAO MAI*

Basic functions

Qiao (蹺) means forceful and nimble as with the heels and ankles, thus common translations for the *qiao mai* include both "heel-vessel" and "motility-vessel". The main functions of *qiao mai* are to dominate the motion of the lower limbs. The *qiao mai* originate from the sites below the ankle and run upward along the medial and lateral sides of the limb, continuing upward to reach the face and head. They communicate with the yin qi and yang qi of the whole body in order to regulate the actions of the limbs and muscles.

Because the *yinqiao mai* and the *yangqiao mai* meet at the inner canthi, the *qiao mai* also control the closing and opening of the eyelids. When a *qiao mai* becomes disordered, the eyelids will fail to close normally so as to cause insomnia or over-sleeping, depending on the condition. The *qiao mai* are also said to be involved with the general balance of yin and yang within the body.

Pathways

- The *yangqiao mai* originates from BL 62 (*shēn mài*) and runs upward along the lateral border of the leg and the thigh. It further runs upward, passing through the abdomen, the lateral aspect of the chest and the shoulder, and then from the lateral side of the neck to the angle of the mouth, then reaching the inner canthus where it meets with both hand and foot *taiyang* channels and the *yinqiao mai*. Then it ascends and enters the anterior hairline, turns downward to the retroauricular region, then meeting the foot *shaoyang* gallbladder channel at the nape of the neck.

- The *yinqiao mai* originates from KI 6 (*zhào hǎi*), a point on the medial malleolus (ankle bone). It then runs directly upward along the medial aspect of the leg and the thigh. Passing the external genitalia, it runs up along the abdomen and chest to the supraclavicular fossa. It then passes by the neck anterior to ST 9 (*rén yíng*), where it then runs by the bridge of the nose to the inner canthus and meets with both hand and foot *taiyang* channels and the *yangqiao mai*.

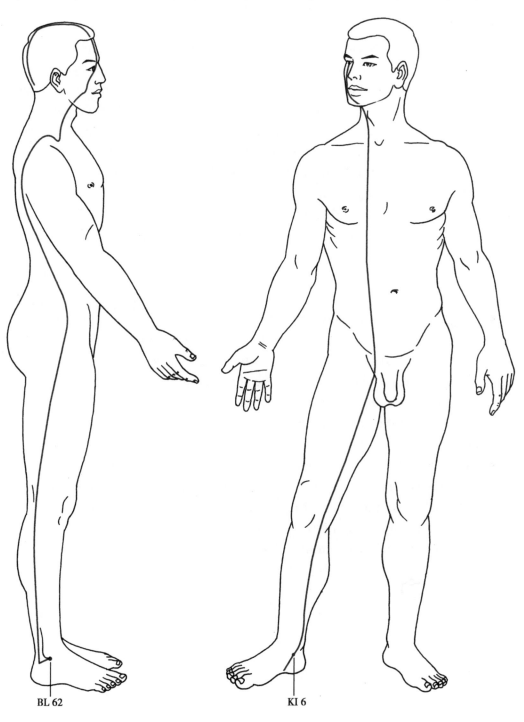

BL 62

Yangqiao mai

KI 6

Yingqiao mai

YANGWEI MAI AND *YINWEI MAI*

Basic functions

Wei (维) refers to regulating and connecting and the *yinwei mai* is commonly translated as the "linking vessel". The *yinwei mai* meets the three foot yin channels and joins with the *ren mai*, while the *yangwei mai* meets the three foot yang channels and joins with the *du mai*. Thusly, the *yinwei mai* regulates and connects the yin channels of the whole body, while the *yangwei mai* regulates and connects the all of yang channels.

Wei mai disorders often manifest with signs and symptoms that suggest psychological issues. Shima and Chase write, "The *yang wei* vessel binds to the yang and the *yin wei* vessel binds to the yin such that when yin and yang are unable to bind with one another, one then experiences such disappointment that one loses one's sense of purpose. One becomes sluggish and unable to support oneself."[1]

Pathways

- The *yangwei mai* originates from the site inferior to the external malleolus. It runs upward together with the foot *shaoyang* gallbladder channel, along the lateral side of the lower limb and postero-lateral aspect of the trunk; via the posterior of the axilla it ascends to the shoulder. It further ascends via the neck and behind the ear, runs forward to the forehead, and then spreads over the lateral side of the head and the back of the nape, and then meets with the *du mai*.

- The *yinwei mai* originates from the site at the medial side of the leg where the three foot yin channels meet. It runs upward along the medial side of the lower limb to the abdomen. From there it runs together with the foot *taiyin* spleen channel; arriving at the rib-side, it meets with the foot *jueyin* liver channel. Then it ascends to the throat to meet with the *ren mai*.

---

① Charles Chase, Miki Shima. *An Exposition on the Eight Extraordinary Vessels.* Seattle: Eastland Press;2010. p. 101.

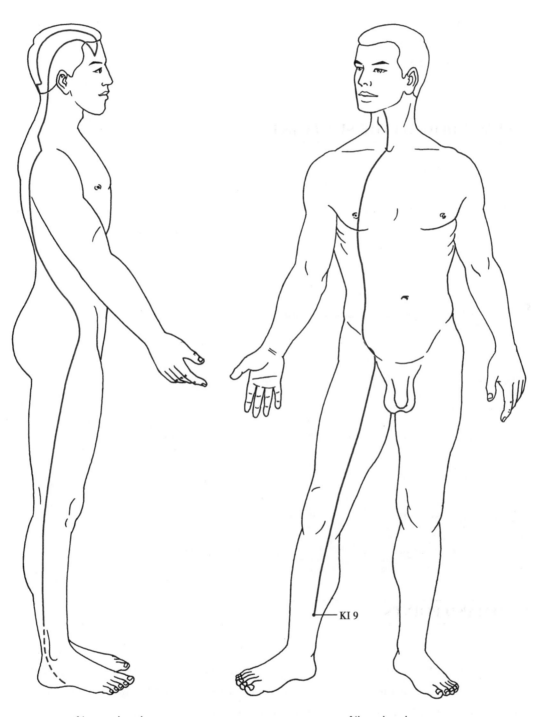

Yangwei mai   *Yinwei mai*

KI 9

Section 4   Miscellaneous Points

Certain points on the channels have special functions as related to their respective channels, while other points are independent of the main channels. Some of these special point categories (such as the *xi*-cleft points and confluence points) have been discussed previously.

FIVE WINDOW TO THE SKY POINTS

The "five window to the sky points" (*tiān yǒu wǔ bù*, 天牖五部) are main channel points located on or near the neck, generally employed for counterflow/rebellious qi flow from the lung and stomach, swellings around the neck, and loss of speech as well as sudden manifestations of internal wind such as twitching, epilepsy and dizziness.[1]

In the *Spiritual Pivot*, chapter *Cold and Febrile Diseases* (*Hán Rè Bìng*, 寒热病) discussed this concept consisting of five points; in the chapter *Fundamental Points* (*Běn Shū*, 本输), there is similar discussion (the concept of seven order channel, *qī cì mài*, 七次脉) involving 10 points, including the 5 points discussed in the chapter *Hán Rè Bìng*.

Five Window to the Sky Points

RN 22	*tiān tū*	天突
ST 9	*rén yíng*	人迎
LI 18	*fú tū*	扶突
SI 16	*tiān chuāng*	天窗
SI 17	*tiān róng*	天容
SJ 16	*tiān yǒu*	天牖
BL 10	*tiān zhù*	天柱
DU 16	*fēng fǔ*	风府
LU 3	*tiān fǔ*	天府
PC 1	*tiān chí*	天池

COMMAND POINTS

As discussed earlier in this chapter, command points have relatively broad effects on large areas of the body, and are often combined with points local to the disorder. For chest pain, a treatment may employ the command point PC 6 (*nèi guān*) on the wrist with RN 17 (*dàn zhōng*), a local point on the chest.

---

[1]   Peter Deadman, Kevin Baker, Mazin Al-Khafaji. *A Manual of Acupuncture*. East Essex:Journal of Chinese Medicine;1998.

Command Points	
LU 7	head and back of neck
LI 4	face
PC 6	chest
ST 36	abdomen
BL 40	lower and upper back

THE FOUR SEAS

The twelve main channels are said to flow into reservoirs and be linked to "seas" of the body. These points are also used to influence large body processes. Listed in the chart below are several of the main points associated with the "four seas".

Four Seas	
Sea of Food	ST 30, ST 36
Sea of Qi	RN 17
Sea of Blood	BL 11, ST 37, ST 39
Sea of Marrow	DU 20, DU 16

EXTRA POINTS

In addition to the main channel points, there are a number of "extra points" with special functions. For example, on the *ren mai* between the eyebrows is extra point *yìn táng* (EX-HN3), a point often employed for its strong calming effect. *Sì shén cōng* (EX-HN1) is a group of four points located on the head which are used to treat the spirit.

ASHI POINTS

Ashi points (lit. ouch points) are reactive or painful points often associated with the channel sinews, often used to treat muscular aches and pains.

OTHER POINTS

Other special (and less used) acupuncture point groupings include those of the Sun Si-miao Thirteen Ghost Points, the Nine Needles for Returning Yang, and the Twelve Heavenly Star Points of Ma Dan-Yan[1].

---

[1]   Andrew Nugent-Head. The Heavenly Star Points of Ma Danyang. Journal of Chinese Medicine. Feb 2012.

Section 6 Additional Systems of Acupuncture

There are several systems of acupuncture that rely upon Western understanding of anatomy and not so much on channels and collaterals. In France, "auricular (ear) acupuncture" was developed by Paul Nogier, soon fully embraced within China and further expanded upon in Europe. National Acupuncture Detoxification Association (NADA) style acupuncture (SMART in England) utilizes simple auricular prescriptions to treat a variety of addictions and stress related disorders.

In China, doctors (Jiao, Tang, Fang, Zhu) began working with representations of the brain to develop "scalp acupuncture" while others (Zhang) created various forms of "wrist and ankle" acupuncture. Electro-acupuncture is also commonly used in many clinics today. Interested students may want to refer to *A Practical Handbook on Scalp Acupuncture* and *A Practical Handbook on Auricular Acupuncture*, both published by the People's Medical Publishing House.

Many other acupuncture systems can be studied in the West, including Tung-style acupuncture, Korean hand acupuncture, Japanese Toyo-hari, and others. Some Western physicians practice a system of "medical acupuncture" which places greater emphasis on modern scientific theories and anatomical studies.

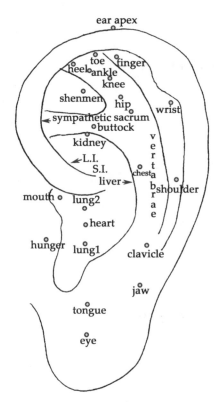

Simple Auricular Chart

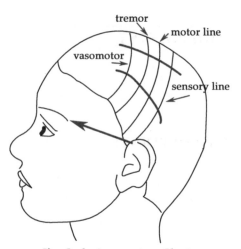

Jiao Scalp Acupuncture Chart

Chapter 11

The History of Chinese Medical Theory

When looking at a history of 5000 years of Chinese medicine, we must consider the range of practices from court doctors, academic writers, herb store owners, practitioners at the highest levels, and traveling (itinerant) doctors treating patients along the way. Many doctors had access to the libraries of the emperor, while others were illiterate, having learned from their families or simply on their own. Some doctors may have set up shop and developed a great following, and others may have lost all due to bad business practices. There were traditions of herbology, acupuncture, moxibustion, tui na/massage, diet and lifestyle counseling as well as Chinese astrology and qi gong energy healing. All of these modalities were taken up by studied practitioners as well as martial artists, parents with ill children, Taoist priests, and lay practitioners. What they knew, what they practiced and how well their patients responded will for the most part remain a mystery, although both art and historical records provide clues. To understand the history of Chinese medicine, we can first look at the extant literature of named and unnamed writers who have left their legacy.

It is said that long ago, the Yellow Emperor (*huáng dì*, 黄帝) ruled the center of the universe, and the Fire Emperor (*yán dì*, 炎帝) ruled the south. The Yellow Emperor had many ministers with whom he invented mathematics, musical instruments, the bow and arrow, boats and many other useful devices. One of his ministers, Wu Peng, invented medicine; and three doctors became prominent, Lei Gong, Yu Fu and Qi Bo. The Fire Emperor, taught humans to plant and sow and thus discovered medicinal herbs which he first tasted, and then observed the results. The Fire Emperor would become called the Divine Farmer (*shén nóng*, 神农). It would be several thousand years before the herbal discoveries of the Divine Farmer would be written down, as well as the conversations between the Yellow Emperor and Qi Bo (*qí bó*, 岐伯).

If the above is a matter of myth, we do know that Neolithic Chinese civilizations existed along the Yellow River and Yangtze River from as early as 7000 BCE. The Neolithic period was hardly primitive as there were clans, noble families, agriculture, and pictograph writing and art. There is evidence that some form of acupuncture with stones was practiced during the time. The later Xia (2100-1600 BCE) and Shang (1700-1046 BCE) Periods saw a furthering of civilization. During this time period, shamans were asked to consult departed ancestors for advice on illness or the meanings of dreams.[1] The *History of Chinese Medicine* states, "In the Li-Yun (*Lǐ Yùn*, 礼运) we read that during the Zhou Dynasty 1056-225 BCE, kings frequently employed sorcerers to protect them from special evils. Special ceremonies against pestilence were performed in spring as well as in autumn."[2]

Following the Shang Period, the concept of ancestors as the cause of disease was beginning to be replaced by a belief that demons that were not tied to blood lineage could cause disease. Herbs could help kill these demons, and needles could puncture spots of swelling or redness wherein the demons were living.

During the process of treating disease with stone needling, people in ancient times had gradually discovered physical lines of transmission that followed from the sensation of needling. Over time, they associated these lines with the internal organs, and from there, in the Han Dynasty the concept of the twelve channels was eventually established. Later came recognition of the eight extraordinary vessels, twelve channel divergences, twelve channel sinews, twelve cutaneous regions and fifteen divergent collaterals.

The development of acupuncture and moxibustion was earlier than that of pharmacotherapy (herbal medicine) in Chinese medicine. They were created in the Neolithic Period and developed rapidly during the Spring-Autumn Warring States Period. At that time, many doctors applied acupuncture and moxibustion in the treatment of disease.

Paleolithic

Neolithic

Xia Dynasty (2100-1600 BCE)

Shang Dynasty (1700-1046 BCE)

Zhou Dynasty (1046-256 BCE)

Spring- Autumn Period (722-476 BCE)

Warring States Period (476-221 BCE)

Qin Dynasty (221-206 BCE)

Han Dynasty (202 BCE-AD 220)

Wei and Jin Periods (AD 265-420)

---

①   Dominique Hoizey, Marie-Joseph Hoizey. *A History of Chinese Medicine*. Edinburgh: Edinburgh University Press; 1993. p. 3.

②   K. Chimin Wong and Wu Lien-teh. *History of Chinese Medicine*. Shanghai: Shanghai Southern Material Center;1936.p. 68.

The Sixteen Barbarian States Period (AD 300-430)

Southern and Northern Dynasties (AD 420-589)

Sui Dynasty (AD 581-618)

Tang Dynasty (AD 618-907)

Five Dynasties and Ten Kingdoms (AD 907-960)

Song, Liao, Jin, and Western Xia Dynasties (AD 960-1234)

Yuan Dynasty (AD 1271-1368)

Ming Dynasty (AD 1368-1644)

Qing Dynasty (AD 1644-1911)

Modern era

Republic of China (AD 1911-1949)

People's Republic of China (AD 1949 to Present)

SPRING-AUTUMN PERIOD (722-476 BCE)

In the Spring-Autumn Period, moxibustion, acupuncture and medicinal herbs were commonly used. The emergence of professional doctors created beneficial conditions for the creation of medical theory. The famous physician Yi He created a theory in which six climatic factors explain the causes of disease. This led to concept of an etiology and a pathomechanism, and the beginning phase of Chinese medical theory.

"The history of Chinese medicine is not so much a succession of ever newer theoretical explanatory models and corresponding practical therapies, but rather a constant enrichment of already existing knowledge. The notion of progress, at least as an ideal, which has determined the history of medicine in the West- whereby previous knowledge is considered to be obsolete and discarded as it "progresses"- is viewed in China as an amplification of knowledge in which old views are never considered to be outdated and continuously updated."[1]

WARRING STATES AND THE HAN DYNASTY (202-195 BCE)

In the period of Warring States Period, various philosophers and scholars rose to prominence, and as a result "a hundred schools of thought contended". This is the development of "modern" concepts such as Taoism, Confucianism, and the Yin-Yang School as well the Legalist School and Warring Strategist School. This cultural

---

[1]　Paul Unschuld. *Medicine in China: Historical Artifacts and Images*. Prestel Verlag GmbH Company; 2000. p. 10.

atmosphere greatly influenced the establishment and development of the theoretical system of Chinese medicine. Taoist investigations into the origin of the world exerted a profound influence and permeated all aspects of Chinese medicine. The enterprising spirit and ethical idea of "self-discipline and social commitment" proposed by Confucians also had a deep impact on medical practitioners' own cultivation and the development of medical ethics.

Chinese society went through great changes during the period of Warring States (476-221 BCE). Consequently, the agriculture-based economic structure set up centuries earlier consolidated and developed along with innovations in astronomy, calendar, agriculture, botany, mineralogy and smelting technologies. Medical knowledge advanced rapidly because of the increasing number of professional doctors.

The major aspects of the theoretical system of Chinese medicine were established during the period of the Warring States and the Han Dynasty. It was during this time that many medical classics were written, including *The Yellow Emperor's Inner Classic* (*Huáng Dì Nèi Jīng*, 黄帝内经), *Classic of Difficult Issues* (*Nàn Jīng*, 难经), *Treatise on Cold Damage* and *Miscellaneous Diseases* (*Shāng Hán Zá Bìng Lùn*, 伤寒杂病论) and *Shen Nong's Classic of the Materia Medica* (*Shén Nóng Běn Cǎo Jīng*, 神农本草经).

During this time, the concept of demons affecting the health of an individual was being replaced by that of "external pathogens". "Wind" (*fēng*, 风) which had been perceived as supernatural, was now simply a force of nature manifesting as qi, heat, cold and dampness. Building on texts such as *The Yellow Emperor's Inner Classic*, the body was seen as having a circulation system of qi and blood that included not only the 12 channels, but also those of "collateral vessels" and "secondary vessels". The body was thought, like nature, to be harmonized when everything was in place. Medicine was incorporating yin-yang theory together with the "five phases" and thus supplanting demonology. Illness and health now had a cause and effect. This has been called the "medicine of systematic correspondence"[1] because health and nature (and social structures) now all moved to the same laws.

Mawangdui

Archeologists in the early 1970's discovered a large tomb complex, called Mawangdui, in Hunan, China dating from 168 BCE. Buried in the tomb were three persons, the Marquis of Dai, his wife and their son. Within the complex are some of the earliest records of medical practices in China. In a silk writing, *Formulas for Fifty-two Diseases* (*Wǔ Shí Èr Bìng Fāng*, 五十二病方) were 103 disease names involving internal medicine, surgery, gynecology and pediatrics, as well as 247 herbs and

---

[1]   Paul Unschuld. *Medicine in China*. Berkeley: University of California Press; 1985. p. 6.

medicinal materials with 283 formulas containing groups of herbs. These writings were a compilation of material that provides a record of almost 1000 years of Chinese medical history.

The Yellow Emperor's Inner Classic (*Huáng Dì Nèi Jīng,* 黄帝内经)

The writing of *The Yellow Emperor's Inner Classic* is the result of medical developments spanning hundreds of years previous. It includes two parts called *Basic Questions* (*Sù Wèn,* 素问) and the *Spiritual Pivot* (*Líng Shū,* 灵枢). In total, there are 18 volumes and 162 chapters covering a wide range of ideas including the relationship between man and nature, human physiology and pathology, diagnosis, and the prevention and treatment of diseases. The therapies recorded in *The Yellow Emperor's Inner Classic* mostly concern acupuncture and moxibustion.

Classic of Difficult Issues (*Nàn Jīng,* 难经)

The *Classic of Difficult Issues* is a book associated with *The Yellow Emperor's Inner Classic,* said to be written by Qin Yue-ren (Bian Que). The contents cover various aspects of physiology, pathology, disease patterns, diagnostics, pulses, and therapeutics. The *Classic of Difficult Issues* goes further in explaining channel and collateral theory, the gate of vitality (*mìng mén*) and the *sanjiao* in the organ theory. *The Yellow Emperor's Inner Classic* and *Classic of Difficult Issues* are seen as the cornerstone of development for the theory and practice of Chinese medicine.

Treatise on Cold Damage and Miscellaneous Diseases (*Shāng Hán Zá Bìng Lùn,* 伤寒杂病论)

Zhang Ji (Zhang Zhong-jing[①]) was the writer of the *Treatise on Cold Damage and Miscellaneous Diseases,* which was later divided into two parts: *Treatise on Cold Damage* (*Shāng Hán Lùn,* 伤寒论) and *Essentials of the Golden Cabinet* (*Jīn Guì Yào Lüè,* 金匮要略). Zhang was encouraged to pursue medicine study by a friend and doctor, Zhang Bo-zu. This was a time when epidemics were devastating vast areas of China, where over a period of ten years about two thirds of Zhang's extended family died from various diseases. As a result, Zhang applied himself to collecting herbal formulas and creating a system that closely followed the theories of *The Yellow Emperor's Inner Classic.* The importance of his work in the development of Chinese medicine cannot be underestimated, even up to the present. For the first time, Chinese medicine had a theory based on patterns, each with a clear and direct treatment. Although the book is primarily concerned with herbal medicine, it created a methodology that would be

---

① Zhang is the family name, and Ji is the given name. Zhong-jing is the courtesy name (*zi,* 字) *Zi* is a name bestowed upon at adulthood in addition to one's given name.

used in every phase of the medicine.

Zhang's main contribution was to codify a system where diseases traveled through the six pairs of channels, starting with the most "superficial", the *taiyang*. Diseases were seen to have a progression, and they could be cured through moving the disease appropriately through the channels, either to the outside of the body through sweating, or downwards through defecation or urination. The book has often been called, "the book of mistakes" because it includes many case studies that show what doctors should not do in many situations. The *Treatise on Cold Damage* begins with an inspirational introduction that discusses the attitudes and ethics of his times, which remains surprisingly relevant to the current day.

Zhang's original manuscripts were thought to be lost, but nearly 400 years later Wang Shu-he would resurrect the book and divide it into the *Treatise on Cold Damage* and the *Essentials of the Golden Cabinet*. The latter applies the theory of the *Treatise on Cold Damage* to clinical case studies. There have been numerous versions of both books over the years, and each publication seems to encourage another round of commentary.

Shen Nong's Classic of the Materia Medica (*Shén Nóng Běn Cǎo Jīng*, 神农本草经)

Shen Nong's Classic of the Materia Medica is the earliest monograph of a materia medica (herb encyclopedia) in China. In this book, 365 kinds of herbs, minerals, animal byproducts and other medicinal substances are recorded. They are divided into the three grades of upper, middle and lower agents. The upper grades are for boosting qi, the middle agents are for treating diseases and supplementing deficiency, and the lower agents are for eliminating pathogens and breaking up accumulations. Also recorded are the properties, actions and indications of each herb[1]. The theory of "four properties and five flavors" is presented, with definite principles for each medication given. Another concept introduced here is "the seven relations of medicinal compatibility" or medicinal herb-combining theory, which to this day provides us with an important theoretical basis for herbal formulation and prescription.

WEI, JIN, SUI, AND TANG DYNASTIES (AD 265-907)

The Wei, Jin, Sui, and Tang Dynasties saw a progression in politics, economics and culture along with improved medical theory and techniques. Trade brought medical and intellectual relations with other cultures from East Asia, and the Arab

---

[1] Although we often refer to "herbs" in this text, it is recognized that Chinese "herbs" include minerals, resins and animal products. Others have translated "herbs" as "medicinals".

world. Buddhism came from India in the Han Dynasty and spread throughout China enriching both culture and medicine. It was during the earlier part of this period when the famous Buddhist cliff-cave monasteries were built in Southern China.

The Pulse Classic (Mài Jīng, 脉经)

The Pulse Classic by Wang Shu-he of the Jin Dynasty is the earliest monograph concerning pulse diagnosis. In the work, the pulse was comprehensively discussed for the first time, from basic theory to clinical practicalities. Pulse-taking at the wrist was promoted over those of the neck and ankle. A total of 24 kinds of pulses, with descriptions such as floating, hollow, surging, slippery, rapid, hasty, wiry, and tight remain as a standard used up to the present time. This emphasis on the pulse was important because it was the same Wang who had also resurrected the *Treatise on Cold Damage*, which itself draws much upon successfully interpreting the pulse.

The Systematic Classic of Acupuncture and Moxibustion (Zhēn Jiǔ Jiǎ Yǐ Jīng, 针灸甲乙经)

The Systematic Classic of Acupuncture and Moxibustion by Huang-Fu Mi (215-282) of the Jin Dynasty is the earliest existing monograph of acupuncture and moxibustion in China. The contents include descriptions of organ manifestations, channels and collaterals, acupuncture points, branch and root, the nine needles, needling, diagnostic methods, disease patterns, and therapeutic methods. *The Systematic Classic of Acupuncture and Moxibustion* was a compilation and distillation of all acupuncture and moxibustion books up to that time; it still plays a major role in modern acupuncture and is the current subject of numerous English translations. Huang-Fu Mi was a poet and writer who contracted a rheumatic condition in his mid-40's which impelled him to study medicine for the rest of his life.

Treatise on the Origins and Manifestations of Various Diseases (Zhū Bìng Yuán Hòu Lùn, 诸病源候论)

Treatise on the Origins and Manifestations of Various Diseases by Chao Yuan-fang is the first monograph on etiology, pathomechanism and symptomology in China. In this book the etiologies, pathomechanisms and signs and symptoms of diseases involving internal, surgery, gynecologic, patriotic, ENT and dermatologic departments were discussed in 1729 sections. Chao discussed many pathogenic factors such as the fact that scabies was caused by mites, tapeworm disease resulted from eating raw beef, "lacquer dermatitis" was associated with constitutional factors, and that some infectious diseases were due to "transmission from one to another". The author acted as physician to the emperor at the time, and Chao's name, through his writings, has become better known than the emperor which he served. The many diseases he saw in practice included what we now recognize as leprosy, kidney stones, and rickets.

Important Formulas Worth a Thousand Gold Pieces (*Qiān Jīn Yào Fāng*, 千金要方) & *Supplement to 'Important Formulas Worth a Thousand Gold Pieces'* (*Qiān Jīn Yì Fāng*, 千金翼方)

Important Formulas Worth a Thousand Gold Pieces and *Supplement to 'Important Formulas Worth a Thousand Gold Pieces'* by Sun Si-miao (581-682) of the Tang Dynasty can be called the first medical encyclopedia in China. Sun was a scholar and student of Buddhism, Taoism and Confucians. While his two books concerned both herbology and acupuncture-moxibustion, he is perhaps equally known for his emphasis on medical ethics. He, undoubtedly echoing Buddhist ideas, noted the levels of suffering in his patients and stated that "of high or low rank, wealthy or poor, adult or child, educated or illiterate, engaging or repellent, Chinese or foreigner, intelligent or foolish, the patient should be treated with the same consideration as a near relative".[1] Sun drew heavily upon the *Treatise on Cold Damage*, and has been called "the king of herbs and prescriptions". Sun emphasized the care of pregnant women, including procedures for non-breathing infants. He proposed that epidemics were not caused by demons, but by tainted water and food. Sun Si-miao is considered as one of the giants of Chinese medicine, and no short description of his work is adequate.[2]

SONG, JIN AND YUAN DYNASTIES (AD 960-1230)

The previous Tang Dynasty ended in chaos, and the Song Dynasty began a period of reform and technological innovation; it was during this time that printing of books was greatly expanded by the use of movable type. With the development of a scientific culture, medicine also progressed greatly. At the turn of the millennium, Confucianism was resurrected into what we now call Neo-Confucianism. In 1057, the Bureau for the Re-editing of Medical Books began to publish existing medical texts by allowing physicians and scholars to examine the classic texts and to analyze herbal prescriptions found in hundreds of books.

Chen Yan of the Southern Song Dynasty, in his book *Treatise on Diseases, Patterns, and Formulas Related to the Unification of the Three Etiologies* (*Sān Yīn Jí Yī Bìng Zhèng Fāng Lùn*, 三因极一病证方论) divided the causes of diseases into three categories that include conditions associated with external contraction by six external pathogenic

---

[1]   Dominique Hoizey, Marie-Joseph Hoizey. *A History of Chinese Medicine*. Edinburgh: Edinburgh University Press; 1993. p. 66.

[2]   Interested readers may refer to *A History of Chinese Medicine* (Hoizey) and http://www.itmonline.org/arts/sunsimiao.htm.

factors, internal damage by seven emotions, injuries from improper diet, violent crying, insects or animals, falls, poisoning, or wounds. This summarization is still referred to in modern fundamentals text books.

During the Jin-Yuan Dynasties, Liu Wan-su, Zhang Cong-zheng, Li Gao, and Zhu Zhen-heng made important contributions to development of medical theory, thus respectfully referred to as the "four great physicians of the Jin-Yuan Dynasties".

Four Great Physicians of the Jin-Yuan Dynasties
- Liu Wan-su—School of Cold Disease
- Zhang Cong-zheng—School of Eliminating Pathogens
- Li Gao—School of Supplementing Earth
- Zhu Dan-xi—School of Enriching Yin

Liu Wan-su (known as Shou-zhen and He-jian) created the "He-jian School", which advocated the "heat-fire doctrine". Liu was pressured many times to become a royal court physician but steadfastly insisted that he continue to treat the common people. Liu studied the *Basic Questions* closely, basing his treatments on the five-phase movements and the six influences of qi. He held that the major causes of disease involved environment and extreme emotions transforming into heat or fire within the body, thus he advocated cold-natured herbs in many prescriptions. His representative works include *Explanation of Mysterious Pathogeneses and Etiologies Based on the 'Basic Questions' (Sù Wèn Xuān Jī Yuán Bìng Shì, 素问玄机原病式)* and *Collected Writings on the Mechanism of Disease, Suitability of Qi, and Safeguarding of Life as Discussed in the 'Basic Questions' (Sù Wèn Bìng Jī Qì Yí Bǎo Mìng Jí, 素问病机气宜保命集)*.

Zhang Cong-zheng (known as Zi-he and Dai-ren) was a former military doctor who studied under Liu Wan-su. He viewed pathogens as foreign to the body and so wrote that "*zheng* qi will set itself as the pathogen is eliminated", and warned against the abuse of supplementation methods. He mainly used the three therapies of sweating, vomiting and purgation to eliminate pathogens, later known as "the school of purging pathogens". His representative work is *Confucians' Duties to Their Parents (Rú Mén Shì Qīn, 儒门事亲)*, and he is perhaps best-known for the controversial statement, "prescriptions of former times cannot completely cure the illnesses of today".

Li Gao (known as Li Dong-yuan and Ming-zhi) came from a privileged background and was fascinated by medicine at an early age, later studying under Zhang Yuan-su (known as Jie-gu). Li Dong-yuan created the Earth or Spleen-Stomach School which emphasized the role of spleen and stomach qi. He wrote, "Hundreds of diseases result from deficiency of the spleen and stomach", and thus advocated treatment of the spleen and stomach (supplementing earth) with an emphasis on lifestyle and diet. His representative works are *Treatise on the Spleen and Stomach (Pí Wèi Lùn,* 脾胃论*)* and *Clarifying Doubts about Damage from Internal and External Causes (Nèi Wài Shāng Biàn Huò Lùn,* 内外伤辨惑论*)*. Many of Li's prescriptions are widely used today as Li's writings have greatly influenced contemporary practice.

Zhu Zhen-heng (known as Yan-xiu and Dan-xi) carried on the writings of He-jian, and held that "yang is often excessive, while yin is often insufficient". Therapeutically, he advocated "enriching yin and subduing fire", later associated with "the school of enriching yin". His representative work is *Further Discourses on the Acquisition of Knowledge through Profound Study (Gé Zhì Yú Lùn,* 格致余论*)*.

Leading up to the Ming Dynasty, schools of Chinese medicine were being re-established and standards were raised. In 1317, physicians were tested once again, and those that failed risked having their licenses revoked. Those that excelled were appointed to the court, while those who did less well were often delegated to teaching or administration. In this time, women were also given official status as full doctors.[1]

MING AND QING DYNASTIES (AD 1368-1911)

The Ming and Qing begin the modern era of China, with the Forbidden City in Beijing under construction in 1406. Great power was given and taken by the eunuchs, who formed a potent autocracy. In 1552, China greeted visitors from through the Jesuits, led by Matteo Ricci. His writings on Chinese medicine would filter back to Europe to form the first impressions of acupuncture in the West. The Chinese would be introduced to Western medicine and anatomy and begin an incorporation of the two that remains both important and controversial to this day. During this time, a great number of medical books, compilations and general encyclopedias continued to be published.

Ming Dynasty physician Zhang Jie-bin first posited the theory of "non-excess of yang" and "insufficiency of genuine yin", and so advocated supplementation of both kidney yin and yang, and Zhao Xian-ke further held that the gate of vitality (*mìng mén*) acts as the governor of the entire body. Zhao's book *Key Link of Medicine (Yī Guàn,* 医贯*)* emphasizes the significance of the "*mìng mén* fire" in disease prevention. The *mìng mén* theory greatly impacted Chinese medicine regarding its role in disease prevention as well as in the treatment of chronic and geriatric diseases.

---

[1]   Dominique Hoizey, Marie-Joseph Hoizey. *A History of Chinese Medicine*. Edinburgh: Edinburgh University Press; 1993. p. 97.

Warm Disease Theory in the Ming and Qing Dynasties

The development of "warm disease" (*rè bìng*, 热病) theory was a significant breakthrough in Chinese medicine. Warm disease is a general term for heat diseases analogous to epidemic infection. This theory originated from *The Yellow Emperor's Inner Classic, Classic of Difficult Issues*, and *Treatise on Cold Damage and Miscellaneous Diseases* and was constantly supplemented and developed by medical experts over time until the theory matured by the Ming and Qing Dynasties. Ming Dynasty physician Wu You-xing and Ye Gui, Xue Xue and Wu Ju-tong of the Qing Dynasty each made outstanding contributions to warm disease theory.

Wu You-xing (known as You-ke) wrote the *Treatise on Warm-Heat Pestilence (Wēn Yì Lùn*, 瘟疫论), created the "epidemic pathogen" theory, and wrote that the cause of warm-epidemic diseases is not the general six pathogenic factors, but rather due to "epidemic pathogens", which often invade the body "via the mouth and nose". These conditions are infectious with pandemic outbreaks and similar signs and symptoms, although epidemics tend to vary depending on the season in which they attack. This was a remarkable point of view in light of the fact that it came two hundred years before the discovery of bacteria and other microorganisms.

Ye Gui (known as Tian-shi and Xiang-yan) compiled *Treatise on Warm-Heat Diseases (Wēn Rè Lùn*, 温热论), which concerns the law of epidemic warm diseases in their onset and development; he created the theory known as four-level pattern identification which built upon and complemented the *Shāng Hán Lùn* system of six-level pattern identification. Ye Gui played a major role in ushering in the future development of the warm disease theory in the Qing Dynasty.

Wu Tang (Wu Ju-tong) compiled the *Systematic Differentiation of Warm Diseases (Wēn Bìng Tiáo Biàn*, 温病条辨), also creating the theory of *sanjiao* pattern differentiation for warm diseases.

Xue Xue (Sheng-bai) wrote *Systematic Differentiation of Damp-Heat Disorders (Shī Rè Tiáo Biàn*, 湿热条辨) which expanded upon the causes, symptoms, laws of transmission and change in heat diseases along with therapeutic principles and treatment methods for damp-heat diseases (a kind of warm disease) based on *sanjiao* pattern identification. This text was also a great contribution to warm disease theory.

In addition, Wang Qing-ren (known as Xun-chen) of the Qing Dynasty wrote *Correction of Errors in Medical Works (Yī Lín Gǎi Cuò*, 医林改错), which concerns mistakes found in the medical classics regarding human anatomy, while also first proposing that "human intelligence and memory do not come from the heart, but from the brain". He also developed theories and several effective formulas for conditions of blood stasis.

MODERN CHINA

In the later stage of Qing Dynasty, Western countries brought their medicine to China. By this time, China was seen as lagging behind both in technology and medicine. In 1911, Qing Dynasty was overthrown by the revolutional party, and a new republic was formed. It was clear that all medical care was inadequate for the great number of people, and with the help of Western organizations, Western medicine was established and encouraged. For the most part, the traditions of Chinese medicine were seen by the ruling government of the time as backward and superstitious. Yet, attempts to ban traditional medicine were resisted by the existing traditional medicine schools and organizations.

The Japan-China war interrupted all reforms, and afterwards, fighting between the two major political forces in China, the Nationalists and the Communists, resumed. The Nationalists were defeated in 1949 and retreated to the island of Taiwan. Some traditional medical practitioners left the mainland of China to Taiwan, and have since helped to spread traditions from there.

MODERN TIMES

In the late 1950's, following the establishment of the People's Republic of China (PRC) in 1949, China made a commitment to revive the traditions of Chinese medicine as well as to integrate with existing Western medical institutions. Re-establishing traditional Chinese medicine served several purposes. First, if not always officially encouraged for several decades, it was well-entrenched among the populace. China has always suffered from a drastic lack of doctors from all disciplines, and it was recognized that a people's revolution would only succeed to the extent that the people were healthy. Secondly, Chinese medicine is very inexpensive in comparison to Western medicine, and thus allowed China to attempt to distance its material needs from Western and Soviet influence. As all of the physical needs of Chinese medicine were available within China there would be no need to import expensive medications and technology. In the end, Chinese medicine remains resolutely "Chinese", and a great source of national pride.

As a result of these factors, Chinese medicine began to be taught on the same scale as other medical and academic disciplines to students who came from diverse backgrounds and outside of family lineages. It was recognized that a uniform, national classroom curriculum was needed, and that theories from a vast canon would need to be organized. For the first time, academic textbooks on Chinese medicine would be written. From 1956 to 1962, nine academies of traditional Chinese medicine were set up around the country.

Qin Bo-wei (1901-1970) was a revered Chinese doctor and writer at the forefront of moving modern Chinese medicine and education forward. Throughout his life, Qin was instrumental in preserving the traditions of Chinese medicine, and actively protested when the medicine was in danger of being "overly integrated" into the Western model. Perhaps his biggest contribution was his work in the 1950's and 60's to develop medical education. During this time, medical textbooks accessible to the beginning student had to written for the first time. Indeed, almost every TCM textbook written in China has a direct lineage from the texts written during this period. This book, therefore, is also a direct descendant of Qin Bo-wei and his colleagues' work.

During this time, several medical and political groups within China had to reach a consensus as how to best approach the establishment regarding a national health policy. The result was a system that largely persists to this day. All medical practitioners in China have some training in both traditional and modern Western medicine, although students may choose to emphasize one modality over another. Graduates of Chinese medicine who work at hospitals are licensed to prescribe Western drugs. The hospitals themselves are designated as being weighted in three ways, traditional Chinese medicine, Western medicine, or a full integration of both. This three-tiered system may be the envy of Western practitioners, yet this arrangement is not without controversy and debate, even within China.

Volker Scheid in *Currents of Tradition in Chinese Medicine* has written how generations of doctors in a town near Shanghai (Menghe) influenced the development of Chinese medicine up to the present time. For several hundred years, Menghe was host to a community of doctors, during a time of immense change in China. By the 1950's, it was natural that the descendants of this tradition would be called upon to help create the components of the Chinese medical national institution. For the last 60 years, these doctors and their students helped mold the medicine people in the West know as Traditional Chinese Medicine (TCM).

CHINESE MEDICINE OUTSIDE OF CHINA

The range of influence of Chinese medicine throughout world culture and history is immense. The intersection between Chinese, Japanese, Korean and Vietnamese medicines is intertwined with economic, cultural and political histories of the same. Perhaps less obvious is the influence between what we now call the Arab States and the Chinese, in that many "Chinese" herbs obviously originated from that region. Although the "silk road" from China through India to Persia would flower in the 8th century, trade routes had been established as early as 100 BCE. By AD 300, merchants in the Persian Gulf and Canton were trading "flax, hemp, walnuts, bamboo and saffron".[1]

Asia

As early as the Zhou Dynasty, cultural exchanges took place between Confucian pre-Buddhist China and Korea, where early artifacts of acupuncture have been found Korea also played an important part in the transmission of Chinese medicine to Japan.[2] Koreans also brought hundreds of core texts of Chinese medicine to Japan in the sixth century through traveling Buddhists priests, and over the centuries, Japanese practitioners created several different schools, including the *Goseiha* and *Kohoha* Schools. Using the principles of Chinese medicine, Japan established an academy with a seven-year acupuncture and moxibustion program where students could begin study at the age of thirteen.[3] For the most part, educated doctors served the royal family and other aristocrats, and the poor were served by Buddhist monks.

In the seventh century, China and Japan made direct contact where exchanges occurred not just in medicine, but in all aspects of the two cultures. Classical Chinese texts became the core of Japanese and Korean medicine, and as medicine in China evolved and changed, both Japanese and Korean medicine roots remained traditionally Chinese. In the early twentieth century, a group of Japanese acupuncturists developed "meridian therapy", a system said to be "distilled from the classics of Chinese medicine".[4] The periodic and relative openness of Japan, Korea and Vietnam (as compared to China) also helped to spread Chinese medicine throughout the rest of Asia as well as to the West.

The above provides only the briefest outline of close to two thousand years of complex history. Needless to say Chinese medicine continues to develop, adapt and thrive throughout all of Asia.

Europe

Chinese medicine had been discussed in European circles for as long as Europeans had knowledge of China. Many Jesuit missionaries were fascinated by both herbs and acupuncture and wrote extensively, if not always accurately, about them. In 1671, the French Jesuit Father Placide Harvieu published *"The Secrets of Chinese Medicine"*. European and North American naturalist-physicians began to incorporate Chinese herbs into their own catalogs and *"materia medicas"* (herb books). Westerners had long

---

[1] Pierre Huard and Min Wong. *Chinese Medicine*. New York: McGraw Hill; 1972.

[2] ibid. p. 72.

[3] Yoshiaki Omura. *Acupuncture Medicine, Its Historical and Clinical Background*. Tokyo: Japan Publications; 1982. p. 16.

[4] Shudo Denmei. *Introduction to Meridian Therapy*. Seattle: Eastland Press; 1990. p. 7.

performed cauterization as a major part of medical practice. For many, and perhaps up to the present, moxibustion was considered a form of cauterization. Linda Barnes quotes an 1804 book from Europe: "Sometimes, after puncturing the part with silver needles, they set fire to the leaves of a species of Artemesia upon it, in the same manner as the Moxa in Japan is made use of to cure and even prevent a number of diseases..."[1]

In 1628, Jacob de Bondt, Danish surgeon general of the Dutch East India Company in his book described acupuncture. In the late 1600's, a German doctor, Dr. Engelbert Kaempfer wrote several texts about acupuncture and moxibustion after spending many years in Japan. Dr. Kaempfer coined the word "moxibustion" from the Japanese usage of "mogusa".It is said that Dutch priest Hermann Buschoff invented the word "moxa" from Japanese "mogusa". The word "acupuncture" was created by the Jesuits from the Latin words for needles and puncture (acu and puntura). Since that time, throughout Europe, acupuncture was periodically rediscovered. France, in particular, had several waves where Chinese medicine was embraced. In the early 1800's, in Paris, Dr. Berlioz was treating stomach pain with acupuncture. In the 1920's, Chinese medicine was again very popular. A French diplomat stationed in Shanghai, Solie de Morant, wrote influential, if now controversial, books in the 1930's. These were eventually translated into English, and are often found on the bookshelves of contemporary practitioners.

"The 20th-century interest in acupuncture is closely linked to Georges Soulie de Morant. The story goes that he was very impressed by the achievements of Chinese medicine during a cholera epidemic in 1908 when he was a young Consul in Yunnan-fu (Kunming), and that from then on, the French diplomat pursued an interest in medicine. Back in France, encouraged by P. Ferreyrolles, he translated Chinese medical classics and began to teach acupuncture. Unfortunately he taught his students in the terminology of Western medicine while his translations were interspersed with his own ideas. "[2]

In the 1950's, a French doctor noticed that one of his patients had a burn on his ear that was given by a folk-healer in order to relieve his back pain. Dr. Paul Nogier interviewed the healer, Madame Barrin, who said the treatment originated from an Asian healer. This created an interest in Dr. Nogier, who eventually mapped the ear as a "microcosm" of the entire body. Variations of this "auricular acupuncture" method were soon developed and embraced first by Chinese practitioners and later throughout the world. In the late 1950's, auricular acupuncture was incorporated into

---

[1]   Linda Barnes. *Needles, Herbs, Gods and Ghosts, China Healing and the West to 1848*. Cambridge: First Harvard University Press; 2007. p. 182.

[2]   Elisabeth Hsu. *Outline of the History of Acupuncture in Europe*. Journal of Chinese Medicine, 29/28, January 1989.

a massive study utilizing the Nanjing division of the Chinese army. In the United States, ear acupuncture treatments were incorporated into treating addictions and then other conditions. Although Dr. Nogier died in 1996, his son has taken on much of the work of publishing his father's original research. In addition, other "microsystems" for "scalp acupuncture" and "wrist and ankle acupuncture" have developed over the years.

English-Speaking Countries

In the United States, there has been a long tradition of "sanging", the colloquial term for picking wild ginseng. American ginseng (*xī yáng shēn*, 西洋参) is most often cultivated today but for a long time it could be found in the deep hills of Appalachia where it was picked by "sangers" or country folk and farmers hoping to earn some extra money. In the magazine *Foxfire* it is written, "Our native ginseng first came to the attention of Europeans when Father Joseph Lafitau, who had been a missionary in China, recognized the similar American plant growing near a Mohawk village in Canada. He set up ovens and the Mohawks gathered and cured ginseng for the Chinese market. By 1717, it was being brought from as far away as Green Bay, Wisconsin, by the Fox Indians and shipped to Hongkong via France."[1]

Yet, outside of the Asian communities, acupuncture and Chinese herbs were largely unknown in the United States until the 1970's. At that time, through the "counterculture", different ways of viewing medicine and the body itself were developing. Asian practices of martial arts, acupuncture, meditation, yoga and macrobiotics were effective counterpoints to the excesses of the time. In 1971, the mainstream culture then read of journalist James Reston's acupuncture experiences in China. A community of existing acupuncturists in the United States formed the National Acupuncture Association the next year after Nixon visiting China. A number of acupuncture journals were started by the existing practitioners and institutions.

Although it would be impossible to name all of those who were instrumental in spreading Chinese medicine to the West, we can at least acknowledge a few. Dr. James Tin Yao So (1911-2000) was a well-respected acupuncturist in Guangdong, China and had started his first school in Hong Kong in 1941. After moving to the United States, Dr. So helped create the UCLA Acupuncture Pain Clinic in Los Angeles, as well as starting the first acupuncture schools in the United States, in Boston and Los Angeles. Students and colleagues of Dr. So are quick to praise him as a visionary in the field. In 2001 he was posthumously awarded the title Acupuncturist of the Year by the American Association of Oriental Medicine.

Dr. John Shen (1914-2001) was a well-established physician in Shanghai where he

---

① Foxfire 3 1975, Foxfire Fund ISBN 0-385-02272-7

had studied at the Shanghai Medical College and apprenticed with Dr. Tsi Man Ting. After living in Taiwan, in 1965 he moved to Malaysia and then finally to New York City. He then mentored many Western acupuncturists who would later be influential in their own right, among them Peter Deadman, Giovanni Maciocia and Leon Hammer.

Dr. Hong-Yen Hsu (1917-1991) established the Sun Ten Herbal Company in Taiwan in the early 1960's, which emphasized the Kampo (Japanese medicine) herbal formulas. After moving to the United States he established the OHAI Press, which published several influential books and the Bulletin of the Oriental Healing Arts Institute.

Another key figure in the acceptance of acupuncture in the West is Miriam Lee (1926-2009), a native of China who eventually settled in San Francisco, California. She had a successful practice but was arrested in 1974 because acupuncture was still illegal in California at the time. Her arrest and trial paved the way for California to be the first state to legalize acupuncture. Along with a busy practice, Miriam Lee also spread her influence through teaching and writing.

In England, J.R. Worsley, influenced by many systems of acupuncture, started the unique "5-Element" school of acupuncture. Although the extent to which it conforms to "authentic" Chinese medicine will remain endlessly controversial, like auricular acupuncture, it marked an embrace and then a transformation of the medicine made to fit the particular needs of many contemporary Western patients.

Many people have been exposed to acupuncture through community and addiction treatment. In the late 1960's in New York City, Black and Hispanic empowerment groups, including the Young Lords, had been training in Asian martial arts. By way of the community of martial arts they were made aware of the work of a Hong Kong neurosurgeon, H.L Wen, who was using acupuncture needles in the ear to treat heroin addiction. Through the tumultuous 1970's, a group began to treat patients at Lincoln Hospital in the South Bronx of New York City. In the 1980's, Dr. Michael Smith solidified the efforts of the Lincoln Hospital community and formed the "NADA protocol" into a national and then international movement. This protocol has been broadly adapted from treating addiction to also treating people in crisis and those with other psychological and physical issues.

By the 1990's, the influence of Chinese medicine was spreading throughout the world, and acupuncture was officially recognized as a treatment for many medical conditions in the United States by the National Institutes of Health (NIH). Schools teaching Chinese medicine now exist in many countries, as either a separate discipline or as incorporated within biomedical or alternative departments of medical schools. The policies of P.R. China allowed many of the best practitioners to emigrate to the West, where these doctors were instrumental in raising the standards of

Chinese medicine in the acupuncture schools. Korean, Vietnamese and Japanese acupuncturists also had a great influence on both schools and communities. As of 2011, there are over fifty acupuncture schools in the United States, and many others throughout the world. As well, hundreds of books have been published in non-Asian languages as well as dozens of Chinese medicine journals.

As the number of practitioners and schools grew in the West, pioneering publishers such as Blue Poppy (Bob Flaws and Honora Wolfe), Paradigm Publications (Bob Felt), Ohai Press (Hong-yen Hsu) and Eastland Press (John O'Connor and Daniel Bensky) began providing translations of core texts and original work. In England, Peter Deadman started the Journal of Chinese Medicine, which has continually provided a valuable resource of original and translated texts for English language practitioners. In France, the Jesuit Father Claude Larre (who had spent many years in Asia) and his student Élisabeth Rochat de la Valle published a number of books based on their extensive lectures on Chinese medicine through Monkey Press. In England, Churchill Livingston also began printing a number of influential books. In 2004, Paradigm Publications published *A Practical Dictionary of Chinese Medicine* by Nigel Wiseman and Feng Ye, which standardized English terminology in Chinese medicine. In 1995, ancient Chinese medicine met the digital age with Acupuncture.com, started by Al Stone.[1] More recently in Australia, Steven Clavey founded *The Lantern* journal.

Chinese medicine seems to have a certain fascination for anthropologists, historians, linguists and writers, many of who have contributed greatly to the general understanding of Chinese medicine. These writers include, but are certainly not limited to Paul Unshculd, Volker Scheid, Nigel Wiseman, Vivanne Lo, Judith B. Farquhar, Yanhua Zhang and Elizabeth Hsu. Electronic media and connectivity are allowing practitioners to share information as never before, and computer technologies may eventually give us English translations of the hundreds of thousands of existing Chinese-language books and articles.

The history of Chinese medicine is continually being written. There is no telling which texts from this age will endure into the future. We hope the readers of this book will love this medicine and their future in it.

---

[1]   Since that time, innumerable digital resources have appeared and Dr. Stone's legacy continues at gancao.net.

Bibliography (English)

Dan Bensky, Andrew Gamble. *Materia Medica*. Seattle: Eastland Press; 1993.

Dan Bensky, Randall Barolet. *Formulas and Strategies*. Seattle: Eastland Press; 1990.

Richard Bertschinger. *The Golden Needle*. London: Churchill Livingston; 1991.

David Bohn. *Wholeness and the Implicate Order*. London: Routeledge and Paul; 1980.

Charles Chace, Miki Shima. *An Exposition on the Eight Extraordinary Vessels*. Seattle: Eastland Press; 2010.

Cheng Xinnong. *Chinese Acupuncture and Moxibustion*. Beijing: Foreign Language Press; 1987.

Peter Deadman, Kevin Baker, Al-Khafaji. *A Manual of Acupuncture*. East Essex: Journal of Chinese Medicine Publications; 1998.

Denmai Shudo. *Introduction to Meridian Therapy*. Seattle: Eastland Press; 1990.

Peter Eckman. *In the Footsteps of the Yellow Emperor*. San Francisco: Cypress Book Company; 1996.

Bob Flaws, Daniel Finney. *A Compendium of TCM Patterns and Treatments*. Boulder: Blue Poppy; 1996.

Charlotte Furth. *A Flourishing Yin*. Berkeley: University of California Press; 1999.

Donald Harper. *Early Chinese Medical Literature*. New York: Columbia University Press; 1998.

Elisabeth Hsu (ed). *Innovation in Chinese Medicine*. Cambridge: Cambridge University Press; 2001.

Pierre Huard, Ming Wong. *Chinese Medicine*. New York: McGraw-Hill; 1968.

Dominique Hoizey, Marie Joseph Hoizey. *A History of Chinese Medicine*. Edinburgh: Edinburgh University Press; 1988.

Jeffery Jacob. *The Acupuncturist's Clinical Handbook*. New York: Integrative Wellness Inc; 2002.

Jiao Shu-de. *Ten Lecture on the Use of Medicinals*. Taos: Paradigm Publications; 2003.

Jiao Shu-de. *Ten Lecture on the Use of Formulas*. Taos: Paradigm Publications; 2005.

Jiao Shu-de. *Case Studies on Pattern Identification*. Taos: Paradigm Publications; 2006.

Larre, Schatz, Rochat de la Vallee. *Survey of Traditional Chinese Medicine*. Paris: Institut Ricci; 1986.

Larre, Schatz, Rochat de la Vallee. *Rooted in Spirit*. Barrytown: Station Hill Press; 1995.

Larre and Rochat de la Vallee. *The Eight Extraordinary Meridians*. London: Monkey Press; 1997.

Larre and Rochat de la Vallee. *The Lung*. London: Monkey Press; 1992.

Li Dong-yuan. *Treatise on the Spleen and Stomach*. Boulder: Blue Poppy; 2004.

Guohui Liu . *Warm Pathogen Diseases*. Seattle: Eastland Press; 2005.

Liu Zhan-wen, Liu Liang (ed). *Essentials of Chinese Medicine*. Volume 1. London: Springer; 2009.

Jane Lyttleton. *Treatment of Infertility with Chinese Medicine*. London: Churchill Livingston; 2004.

Giovanni Maciocia. *Tongue Diagnosis in Chinese Medicine*. Seattle: Eastland Press; 1987.

Giovanni Maciocia. *The Channels of Acupuncture*. Oxford: Elsevier; 2006.

Giovanni Maciocia. *The Foundations of Chinese Medicine*. Oxford: Elsevier; 1989.

Will Maclean, Jane Lyttleton. *Clinical Handbook of Internal Medicine*. Volumes 1-3. Pangolin Press; 2010.

Kiiko Matsumoto, Stephen Birch. *Extraordinary Vessels*. Taos: Paradigm Publications; 1986.

Huang-Fu Mi (Yang and Chace trans.) *The Systematic Classic of Acupuncture and Moxibustion*. Boulder: Blue Poppy; 2004.

Gunter Neeb. *Blood Stasis*. London: Churchill Livingston; 2007.

Yitian Ni. *Navigating the Channels of Traditional Chinese Medicine*. San Diego: Oriental Medicine Center; 1996.

John O'Connor, Dan Bensky (trans). *Acupuncture: A Comprehensive Text*. Seattle: Eastland Press; 1981.

Academy of Traditional Chinese Medicine. *An Outline of Chinese Acupuncture*. Beijing: Foreign Languages Press; 1975.

Qiao Yi, Al Stone. *Diagnosis Study Guide*. Seattle: Eastland Press; 2008.

Isabelle Robinet. *Taoist Meditation: the Mao-shan Tradition of Great Purity*. Albany: State University of New York Press; 1993.

Elizabeth Rochat de la Vallee. *The Essential Woman*. London: Monkey Press; 2007.

Elisa Rossi. *Shen: Psycho-Emotional Aspects of Chinese Medicine*. London: Churchill Livingston; 2007.

Volker Sheid. *Currents in Chinese Medicine 1626-2006*. Seattle: Eastland Press; 2007.

Volker Scheid, Dan Bensky, Andrew Ellis, Randoll Barolet. *Formulas and Strategies*. 2nd ed. Seattle: Eastland Press; 2009.

Paul Unshuld. *Medicine in China: Historical Artifacts and Images*. Munich: Prestel Verlag; 2000.

Paul Unshuld. *Medicine in China: A History of Ideas.* Berkeley: University of California Press; 1985, 2010.

Ju-yi Wang, Jason Robertson. *Applied Channel Theory in Chinese Medicine.* Seattle: Eastland Press; 2003.

Wang Fu-chun. *Scalp Acupuncture Therapy.* Beijing: People's Medical Publishing House; 2007.

Wang Shou-sheng. *Advanced Textbook on Traditional Chinese Medicine and Pharmacology.* Beijing: New World Press; 1996.

Nigel Wiseman, Ye Feng. *The Practical Dictionary of Chinese Medicine.* Taos: Paradigm Publications; 1998.

Yan Shi-Lin. *Pathomechanisms of the Spleen.* Taos: Paradigm Publications; 2009.

Yanhua Zhang. *Transforming Emotions in Chinese Medicine.* Albany: State University of New York Press; 2007.

Greta Young, Robin Marchment. *Shang Han Lun Explained.* London: Churchill Livingston; 2009.

Yellow Emperor's Canon Internal Medicine. Beijing: China Science and Technology Press; 2002.

Yin Huihe. *Fundamentals of Traditional Chinese Medicine.* Beijing: China Science and Technology Press; 1992.

Online:
Journal of Chinese Medicine. jcm.co.uk
The Lantern. thelantern.com.au
Jason Blalack. chinesemedicinedoc.com
Al Stone. gancao.net
Dharmanda, Subhuti. Itmonline.org

Glossary

adequate/sufficient/ample	充足	*chōng zú*
agitation/vexed	心烦	*xīn fán*
area below the left nipple	虚里	*xū lǐ*
blocked sensation	痞	*pǐ*
blood level	血分	*xuè fēn*
can be excessive but not able to be full	实而不能满	*shí ér bù néng mǎn*
channel/ warp/ stage (*Shāng Hán Lùn*)	经	*jīng*
chaos/ confusion/ disorder and/or messy	乱	*luàn*
contrary transmission	逆传	*nì chuán*
dead blood	死血	*sǐ xuè*
deficient/vacuous	虚	*xū*
discharging the exterior	发表	*fā biǎo*
dispel/ move/ drive away	祛	*qū*
dissolve phlegm	化痰	*huà tán*
dredge the water passages and convey water	疏通	*shū tōng*
epidemic qi	疠气	*lì qì*
essence	精	*jīng*
excess/replete	实	*shí*
expel dampness	逐饮	*zhú yǐn*
fair judge	中正	*zhōng zhèng*
firm and impatient	刚强躁急	*gāng qiáng zào jí*
flooding and spotting	崩漏	*bēng lòu*
fluid-retention in stomach and intestines	痰饮	*tán yǐn*
fluid-retention in the hypochodrium	悬饮	*xuán yǐn*
free flowing and descent	通降	*tōng jiàng*
full but cannot be excessive	满而不能实	*mǎn ér bù néng shí*
full/ ample	充	*chōng*
full/substantial/real/replete	实	*shí*
gate of vitality	命门	*mìng mén*
govern qi and control respiration	主气司呼吸	*zhǔ qì sī hū xī*

grease	膏	*gāo*
heart-spirit	心神	*xīn shén*
immediate attack	感邪即发	*gǎn xié jí fā*
impartial and unbiased	不偏不倚	*bù piān bù yǐ*
impotence	阳痿	*yáng wěi*
lower abdominal masses (comparable to uterine fibroids or endometriosis)	癥瘕	*zhēng jiǎ*
mental overwork	劳神过度	*láo shén guò dù*
minor fire	少火	*shào huǒ*
move outward	向外	*xiàng wài*
move upward	向上	*xiàng shàng*
not discharge	不泻	*bù xiè*
obstruction illness	痹病	*bì bìng*
onset of disease	发病	*fā bìng*
original	元	*yuán*
over-ease	过逸	*guò yì*
overwork (overstraining)	过劳	*guò láo*
pathogenic qi	邪气	*xié qì*
phlegm and fluid concentration or retention	痰饮凝聚	*tán yǐn níng jù*
physical overwork	劳力过度	*láo lì guò dù*
progression	从化	*cóng huà*
center qi/chest qi/ ancestral/governing qi	宗气	*zōng qì*
qi constraint or mental depression	郁	*yù*
qi knotted	气结	*qì jié*
qi overbearing/ forceful qi	气盛	*qì shèng*
qi stagnation	气滞	*qì zhì*
qi transformation	气化	*qì huà*
qi movement	气机	*qì jī*
satisfied/full	满	*mǎn*
saliva	涎	*xián*
seep out	渗出	*shèn chū*
separating the clear from the turbid	泌别清浊	*mì bié qīng zhuó*
seven emotional injuries	七情内伤	*qī qíng nèi shāng*
sexual overstraining	房劳过度	*fáng láo guò dù*
skin and pores/grain of the skin	腠理	*còu lǐ*
slippery fetus/habitual abortion	滑胎	*huá tāi*
smooth the qi and rectify the gallbladder	理气利胆	*lǐ qì lì dǎn*

smooth/free the overall qi movement	调畅气机	*tiáo chàng qì jī*
soothe the liver and regulate the qi	疏肝理气	*shū gān lǐ qì*
sovereign	君主	*jūn zhǔ*
sperm/ essence child or essence seed	精子	*jīng zǐ*
stagnation	郁滞	*yù zhì*
store spirit	藏神	*cáng shén*
subcutaneous fluid-retention in the limbs	溢饮	*yì yǐn*
tendon	筋	*jīn*
the sea of water and grains	水谷之海	*shuǐ gǔ zhī hǎi*
thoracic fluid-retention above the diaphragm	支饮	*zhī yǐn*
thought	思	*sī*
turbid fluids blocked	湿浊困阻	*shī zhuó kùn zǔ*
unimpeded	畅通	*chàng tōng*
unsmooth or stagnant	涩滞	*sè zhì*
upright qi not enough	正气不足	*zhèng qì bù zú*
upward and outward	向上向外	*xiàng shàng xiàng wài*
water fluids remain stored or retained	水液贮留	*shuǐ yè zhù liú*

Index

Notes

Notes

图书在版编目（CIP）数据

中医基础理论 =Fundamentals of Chinese Medicine：英文 /
孙广仁，（美）爱新·真道，张庆荣主编 . —北京：人民卫
生出版社，2014
国际标准化英文版中医教材
ISBN 978-7-117-18726-8

Ⅰ.①中…　Ⅱ.①孙…②爱…③张…　Ⅲ.①中医医学基础 - 教
材 - 英文　Ⅳ.①R22

中国版本图书馆 CIP 数据核字（2014）第 069088 号

| 人卫社官网 | www.pmph.com | 出版物查询，在线购书 |
| 人卫医学网 | www.ipmph.com | 医学考试辅导，医学数据库服务，医学教育资源，大众健康资讯 |

中医基础理论——国际标准化英文版中医教材

主　　编：孙广仁，（美）爱新·真道，张庆荣
出版发行：人民卫生出版社（中继线 010-59780011）
地　　址：中国北京市朝阳区潘家园南里 19 号
　　　　　世界医药图书大厦 B 座
邮　　编：100021
网　　址：http://www.pmph.com
E - mail：pmph @ pmph.com
购书热线：010-59787592　010-59787584　010-65264830
开　　本：787 × 1092　1/16
版　　次：2014 年 7 月第 1 版　2014 年 7 月第 1 版第 1 次印刷
标准书号：ISBN 978-7-117-18726-8/R·18727
打击盗版举报电话：**010-59787491**　**E-mail：WQ @ pmph.com**
　　（凡属印装质量问题请与本社市场营销中心联系退换）